# Pharmacy Practice

## Second Edition

# Pharmacy Practice

## Second Edition

Edited by

**Geoffrey Harding**
University of Exeter Medical School, Devon, United Kingdom

and

**Kevin Taylor**
UCL School of Pharmacy, United Kingdom

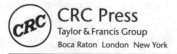

CRC Press
Taylor & Francis Group
Boca Raton London New York

CRC Press is an imprint of the
Taylor & Francis Group, an **informa** business

CRC Press
Taylor & Francis Group
6000 Broken Sound Parkway NW, Suite 300
Boca Raton, FL 33487-2742

© 2016 by Taylor & Francis Group, LLC
CRC Press is an imprint of Taylor & Francis Group, an Informa business

No claim to original U.S. Government works

Printed on acid-free paper
Version Date: 20150805

International Standard Book Number-13: 978-1-4822-5342-9 (Paperback)

**Visit the Taylor & Francis Web site at**
**http://www.taylorandfrancis.com**

**and the CRC Press Web site at**
**http://www.crcpress.com**

# Contents

## SECTION I   The Development and Practice of Pharmacy

# SECTION II    Health, Illness, Well-Being and Medicines Use

# SECTION III    Professional Practice

## SECTION IV   *Measuring and Costing Medicines Use*

## SECTION V   *Undertaking Pharmacy Practice and Health Services Research*

# Preface

As pharmacy evolves from a drug-centred, supply-based activity to one which is increasingly focused on the health and medicines needs of patients, effective pharmacy practitioners increasingly require an understanding of the social, political and economic context within which pharmacy is practised, recognizing the particular needs and circumstances of the users (and funders) of pharmaceutical services and of pharmacy's place within health service provision. With this in mind, we have produced *Pharmacy Practice* to provide a background to the many factors impinging on daily practice and pharmacy's place within health care delivery.

This is the second edition of *Pharmacy Practice*, the first edition having been written in 2001. The content and presentation have been thoroughly revised and new material added to reflect the many changes that have occurred in the intervening years, particularly in pharmacy and health policy and professional regulation and development. The philosophy and aims of this edition remain unchanged from the first. The book is written specifically for those studying or practising pharmacy to provide a background and context for many of the issues impacting on contemporary professional practice and which will directly determine how pharmacy develops in the future. We have drawn on a diverse range of disciplines, including pharmacy, sociology, social policy, psychology, anthropology, history and health economics, with contributors each bringing a unique perspective and insight into the practice of pharmacy. The authors have been purposively chosen for their expertise in a particular subject area, their appreciation of how selected aspects of their speciality inform pharmacy practice and also because of their experience in teaching their subject to students of pharmacy or other health professions.

We hope that by bringing together contributions from this range of disciplines whose knowledge base can, and should, underpin and inform pharmacists' activities, this comprehensive book will equip readers to appreciate the complexities of the social milieu in which pharmacists practice and contribute to their effectiveness as health care practitioners.

**Geoffrey Harding**
*Exeter*

**Kevin Taylor**
*London*

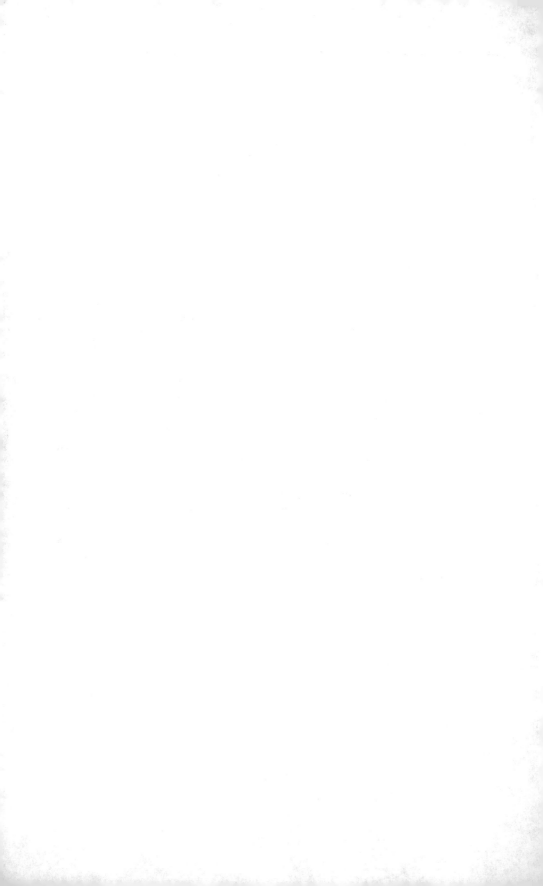

# Acknowledgements

The editors would like to thank the following who have helped with the preparation of this text:

The authors for the time and quality of the effort they have put into their contributions. We know that all are under pressure from many other commitments and that modern life affords little spare time for such activities. The time they have spent in contributing so knowledgeably and professionally to this text is warmly appreciated.

The publishing companies who have given their permissions to reproduce material in this book.

Catherine Baumber (UCL School of Pharmacy) for her excellent secretarial and administrative support during this book's preparation.

Finally, we acknowledge the support of our wives, Sally and Pauline during this and so many other projects we have undertaken together.

# Introduction: Why Pharmacy Practice?

One of the most significant changes in health care delivery in recent years has been the recognition of the importance of patients' biographies as individuals. Pharmaceutical services reflect this, as their focus shifts from being largely drug-product centred to a concern for the patient as an individual, as exemplified by international recognition of the pharmaceutical care concept. This has led to a broadening of pharmacists' activities into areas such as medicines optimization and health promotion. Determining an individual's pharmaceutical and health needs requires a blend of clinical skills, scientific knowledge and social skills if pharmacists are to respond appropriately to symptoms, give medical advice, 'counsel' patients and actively participate in health promotion activities. To be effective requires a sound foundation in the practice of pharmacy. Pharmacy practice is an all-encompassing term which incorporates not only elements of clinical pharmacy and the legal and ethical aspects of professional practice, but also various perspectives which assist in the understanding of the wider social context in which pharmaceutical services are delivered. The academic study of pharmacy practice includes topics such as social pharmacy, behavioural medicine, medicines use, health economics, pharmacoepidemiology and pharmacovigilance.

As with all health professionals, pharmacists' roles and activities are continually changing and developing, and the drivers for this change are multi-factorial, including political, economic and social factors as well as originating from members and leaders of the profession itself. There are also technological drivers for change exemplified by the decline in recent decades of the need for pharmacists to formulate and manufacture medicines extemporaneously. This, together with a trend towards original pack dispensing and the professionalization of pharmacy technicians, has raised the question as to whether the medicines supply function (i.e. routine dispensing supported by IT systems) is the optimal use of pharmacists' extensive and expensively acquired skills.

The impetus for change follows from a number of independent reports and consultations from within the profession suggesting pharmacists (and their skills) have, in the past, been significantly underutilized – an assertion challenged by some commentators in this book. Nevertheless, pharmacy leaders, practitioners, educators and increasingly the funders of health care have embraced what has frequently been termed the pharmacist's extended role (i.e. what pharmacists do above and beyond their traditional medicines supply function). This, allied with the professional development and regulation of pharmacy technicians, has led to a broadening of the services pharmacists offer and has increased their capacity to engage in a range of patient-focused activities. This 'extended role' requires direct interaction with the public, with pharmacists offering a range of services including diagnostic testing, health care advice, therapeutic recommendations and reviewing current medication, as well as ensuring people receive the appropriate medication (prescribed and purchased) and understand how to use it correctly.

Community pharmacists are recognized, and increasingly promoted, as a health care resource within the community, available without appointment and at no direct cost to the public to advise on all matters of health. Arguably, this may represent a return of pharmacists to the role they occupied prior to the industrial production of medicines and the inception in the UK of the National Health Service. Pharmacies have private consultation areas, offer effective proprietary medicines previously available only on prescription (due to extensive medicines reclassification), have acquired prescribing rights within the limits of their professional competence and are remunerated for reviewing the use of medicines by their patients. All this is a far cry from the cliché of 'chemists' chained to their dispensing benches, being little more than counters of tablets and labellers of medicine bottles ('lickers, stickers and pourers').

Hospital pharmacy, meanwhile, has embraced the concepts of clinical and ward pharmacy with the pharmacy workforce being successfully integrated into the health care team as medicines experts. At the same time, hospital pharmacists are able to specialize in, for instance, medicines information, antibiotic management, clinical trials, oncology, paediatrics and technical services, including aseptic services and radiopharmacy.

These developments have led to a wide-ranging evaluation of what pharmacists do, but also an acknowledgement of their potential as health professionals, who, in addition to being experts on medicines (understanding their chemistry, pharmacology and formulation), are capable of taking on greater responsibilities for patients' health status and the outcomes of their drug treatment – a concept frequently referred to as pharmaceutical care.

With these developments in mind, our aim in this book is to provide pharmacy students with a background in some of the issues which are pertinent for effective contemporary pharmacy practice. We have purposely avoided clinical pharmacy and therapeutics *per se*, along with specific aspects of pharmacy law, because these are already comprehensively covered in existing texts. Our focus here is the practice of pharmacy in its social and behavioural context. For instance, how do an individual's beliefs or social circumstances influence their decision to use a pharmacy, and how might pharmaceutical services best be delivered to meet that individual's specific health needs?

In equipping tomorrow's pharmacists for this broader and more demanding spectrum of activities, their education must prepare them to be scholars, scientists, practitioners and professionals. Whether traditional pharmacy courses achieved this has, over the years, been the subject of much heated (and often ill-informed) debate. What is clear is that until recently, the pharmaceutical sciences – chemistry, pharmacology and pharmaceutics – have predominated within the undergraduate pharmacy curriculum. Pharmacy practice as a subject was, at the time of the first edition of this book, ill defined, largely taught by teacher–practitioners and lacked a distinct theoretical and research base (and influence) associated with the pharmaceutical sciences.

Thus, in the Preface to the first edition of *Pharmacy Practice*, published in 2001, we wrote, with some justification:

Undergraduate pharmacy courses remain rooted in the pharmaceutical sciences. Within libraries, social and behavioural science texts are segregated from pharmacy texts, and often found at separate sites. Furthermore, interdisciplinary teaching within pharmacy schools remains the exception rather than the rule.

Fortunately, much has changed in the intervening years. Today, those responsible for regulating, designing and teaching undergraduate pharmacy courses respect and acknowledge the vital importance of both pharmaceutical science and pharmacy practice. Within the curriculum, these should ideally be seamlessly integrated to prepare students for the many professional roles and activities they will undertake on graduation, registration and on into future professional practice. The best contemporary pharmacy programmes achieve this integration (in teaching and assessment) throughout all years of a student's studies, increasingly incorporating opportunities for workplace learning, provide a real-life, practice-based context in which they learn and apply their theoretical knowledge.

In Great Britain, the General Pharmaceutical Council (GPhC) has responsibility for accrediting pharmacy degrees, ensuring that they are fit for purpose. In 2011, the GPhC published *Pharmacists: Standards for the Initial Education and Training of Pharmacists*, outlining the 'standards' and 'outcomes' against which undergraduate pharmacy programmes are accredited and reaccredited. This document states: 'Curricula must be integrated ... the component parts of education and training must be linked in a coherent way', and 'Learning opportunities must be structured to provide an integrated experience of relevant science and pharmacy practice'.

Such statements suggest that pharmacy practice, as an academic discipline, has come of age since publication of the first edition of this book. Pharmacy practice, as a subject, has earned the right to be taught and researched within the formally science-orientated pharmacy schools. In the past 15–20 years, Departments of Pharmacy Practice (or similar) have proliferated, many professors of Pharmacy Practice have been appointed and relevant research journals and conferences have been established or consolidated. Against this background, we believe that this is an opportune time to revisit our book *Pharmacy Practice* to revise and update the content to reflect the seismic changes in the pharmacy profession, the nature of how pharmacy is practised and how pharmacy practice as an academic discipline is taught.

The book is presented in various sections that group chapters into related subject areas. Section I (The Development and Practice of Pharmacy) begins with an outline of the development of pharmacy, from the earliest human records to the present day. Many chapters in this section demonstrate how the changes in what pharmacists do and their occupational status are inextricably linked with wider socio-economic forces and national and international health policy. Past, current and future pharmaceutical service delivery in communities and hospitals is described from several international perspectives. Across the globe, pharmacists have demonstrated their engagement with the concept of pharmaceutical care, such that their activities are no longer centred on the supply of prescribed and over-the-counter medicines, but rather are focused on assuming greater responsibility for patients' health status and optimizing the outcomes of the medicines they (as individuals) are using.

Section II (Health, Illness, Well-Being and Medicines Use) contains chapters which place an individual's experience of health and illness and the ability of health professionals, including pharmacists, to promote better health and the optimal use of medicines in their wider contexts. We learn that there are a number of debunked myths concerning the determinants of individuals' health states and the implications of these for promoting health and the effective use of medicines.

In Section III (Professional Practice), some more pharmacy-specific issues are considered. This section begins with chapters considering the composition of the pharmacy workforce (in particular, focussing on gender and ethnicity), what might be considered professionalism and professional practice (in particular, a consideration of pharmacists' legal duty of care to patients, ethics and professional judgements) and a sociologically informed analysis of the occupational status of pharmacy. The place of pharmacists as members of the multidisciplinary health care team is also considered. Together, these chapters are intended to challenge readers to think deeply about what pharmacists do on a daily basis, the present and future profile of members of the pharmacy workforce, the status of the pharmacy 'profession' and how valued (or otherwise) its activities are from the perspectives of patients, other health professionals and health service funders. This section of the book then continues with a consideration of the health and pharmaceutical needs of a range of particular client groups, including the elderly and their carers, people with mental health problems, ethnic minority groups and drug misusers.

Effective pharmacy practice is based on research evidence and best practice, and original research is referred to, where appropriate, throughout the text. As practice becomes more evidence based, pharmacists increasingly need to evaluate and implement research findings and undertake their own research and professional audits. To this end, we have included sections detailing how medicines use is surveyed and costed in Section IV (Measuring and Costing Medicines Use), together with practical guidance on undertaking pharmacy practice research and evaluating pharmaceutical services in Section V (Undertaking Pharmacy Practice and Health Services Research). We have included introductions to both qualitative and quantitative methods to serve as starting points for the novice researcher.

The contents of this book we hope will provide an introduction to the key discipline of pharmacy practice, highlighting the contexts within which pharmacy is practised and the real potential (which is being increasingly realized) for pharmacists and the wider pharmacy workforce to make significant impacts on the health and well-being of the public they serve.

# Contributors

**Zahraa Mohammed Ali**
Department of Practice and Policy
UCL School of Pharmacy
London, United Kingdom

**Claire Anderson**
The Pharmacy School
University of Nottingham
Nottingham, United Kingdom

**Stuart Anderson**
Centre for History in Public Health
London School of Hygiene and Tropical
    Medicine
London, United Kingdom

**Mohamed Aslam**
Department of Pharmaceutical
    Sciences
School of Pharmacy
University of Nottingham
Nottingham, United Kingdom

**Nick Barber**
The Health Foundation
London, United Kingdom

**Nina Barnett**
North West London Hospitals
    NHS Trust
East and South East England Specialist
    Pharmacy Services
London, United Kingdom

**Lolkje de Jong-van den Berg**
Department of Social Pharmacy,
    Pharmacoepidemiology, and
    Pharmacotherapy
Groningen Institute for Drug Studies
Groningen, the Netherlands

**Alison Blenkinsopp**
Bradford School of Pharmacy
University of Bradford
Bradford, United Kingdom

**Christine Bond**
Department of General Practice and
    Primary Care
University of Aberdeen
Aberdeen, United Kingdom

**Rhiannon Braund**
School of Pharmacy
University of Otago
Dunedin, New Zealand

**Hakan Brodin**
TNO Prevention and Health
Sector HTA
Leiden, the Netherlands

**James Davies**
Department of Practice and Policy
UCL School of Pharmacy
London, United Kingdom

**Corinne de Vries**
Department of Pharmacy and
    Pharmacology
University of Bath
Bath, United Kingdom

**Qian Ding**
Department of Pharmaceutical
    Sciences, College of Pharmacy
Ferris State University
Big Rapids, Michigan

**Mark Exworthy**
School of Social Policy, HSMC
University of Birmingham
Birmingham, United Kingdom

**Sally-Anne Francis**
Department of Practice and Policy
UCL School of Pharmacy
London, United Kingdom

**Madeleine Gantley**
Department of General Practice and
    Primary Care
St Bartholomew's and the Royal London
    School of Medicine and Dentistry
Queen Mary University of London
London, United Kingdom

**Ruth Goldstein**
Medicines Research Unit
School of Health and
    Community Studies
University of Derby
Derby, United Kingdom

**Geoffrey Harding**
Primary Care
University of Exeter Medical School
Exeter, United Kingdom

**Karen Hassell**
College of Pharmacy
California Northstate University
Elk Grove, California

**Robert Horne**
Department of Practice and Policy
UCL School of Pharmacy
London, United Kingdom

**Farheen Jessa**
Department of General Practice
University Hospital
Queens' Medical Centre
Nottingham, United Kingdom

**Jill K. Jesson**
M.E.L. Research Limited
Aston Science Park
Birmingham, United Kingdom

**Dai N. John**
School of Pharmacy and
    Pharmaceutical Science
Cardiff University
Cardiff, United Kingdom

**Joanna Lawrence**
Pharmacy Department
Royal Cornwall Hospitals NHS Trust
Truro, United Kingdom

**Sarah Nettleton**
Department of Sociology
University of York
York, United Kingdom

**Pauline Norris**
School of Pharmacy
University of Otago
Dunedin, New Zealand

**Richard O'Neill**
Department of Pharmacy
University of Hertfordshire
Hertfordshire, United Kingdom

**Rhona Panton**
Worcester NHS Community Trust
Worcester, United Kingdom

**Rob Pocock**
M.E.L. Research Limited
Aston Science Park
Birmingham, United Kingdom

**Jenny Scott**
Department of Pharmacy and
    Pharmacology
University of Bath
Bath, United Kingdom

**Joaquima Serradell**
Pharmasultants Group
Blue Bell
Philadelphia, Pennsylvania

**Janie Sheridan**
School of Pharmacy
University of Auckland
Auckland, New Zealand

**Alesha Smith**
School of Pharmacy
University of Otago
Dunedin, New Zealand

**Felicity Smith**
Department of Practice and Policy
UCL School of Pharmacy
London, United Kingdom

**Sue Symonds**
School of Sociology and Social Policy
University of Nottingham
Nottingham, United Kingdom

**David Taylor**
Department of Practice and Policy
UCL School of Pharmacy
London, United Kingdom

**Kevin Taylor**
UCL School of Pharmacy
London, United Kingdom

**J. W. Foppe van Mil**
Van Mil Consultancy
Zuidlaren, the Netherlands

**Albert I. Wertheimer**
School of Pharmacy
Temple University
Philadelphia, Pennsylvania

**Michael Wilcock**
Prescribing Support Unit
Pharmacy Department
Royal Cornwall Hospitals
    NHS Trust
Truro, United Kingdom

**John Wilson**
Nottingham Health Authority
Nottingham, United Kingdom

# Section I

## The Development and Practice of Pharmacy

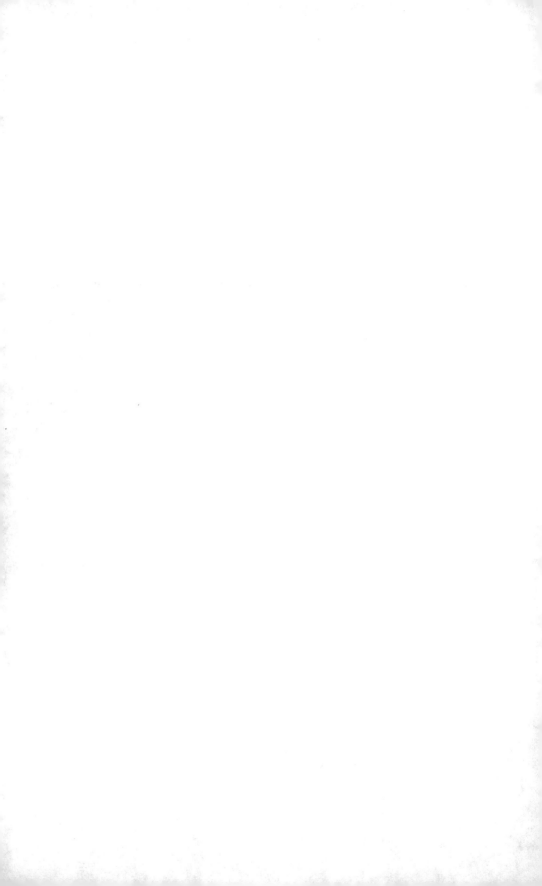

# 1 The Historical Context of Pharmacy and Pharmacy Practice

*Stuart Anderson*

## CONTENTS

## KEY POINTS

- Pharmacy has a history dating back to antiquity.
- Today's pharmacy profession is the product of social, political, economic and technological forces.
- The development of pharmacy in Britain has been influenced by developments in other countries, particularly in Europe, while British pharmacy has influenced the development of pharmacy in other countries.
- The modern history of pharmacy in Britain begins with the founding of the Pharmaceutical Society of Great Britain in 1841.
- During the twentieth century, the nature of pharmaceutical products and their methods of preparation changed dramatically, with products increasingly produced by the pharmaceutical industry.
- The introduction of the National Health Service (NHS) in 1948 had a profound impact on the practice of community pharmacists, with dispensing prescriptions quickly forming the major part of pharmacists' incomes.
- Initiatives since the 1980s have sought to extend pharmacists' activities beyond their dispensing role, promoting them as a 'first port of call' for the public for medicines and health-related activities.
- More recent developments include the creation of the General Pharmaceutical Council, registration for pharmacy technicians and the emergence of consultant pharmacists and pharmacists with prescribing rights.
- Such developments can be viewed as community pharmacists returning to their traditional (pre-NHS) role as a key resource in the community, available without an appointment and at no cost.

## INTRODUCTION

Why is pharmacy practised in the way it is today? Has the dispensing of prescriptions always been the main activity in community pharmacy? How did multiples come to dominate community pharmacy in Britain, but not in other countries? Could pharmacy practice just as easily have developed very differently? The answers to these questions are to be found in pharmacy's history, from its origins in the mists of time to the diversity of practice that is pharmacy today.

This chapter has three objectives: to define the main 'time frames' (periods bounded by key events) within the history of pharmacy; to describe the key 'watersheds' (the defining events) in that history; and to examine the impact which these events have had on the practice of pharmacy. Following a general account of the evolution of pharmacy, the chapter focuses on developments in Britain, illustrating the balance of social, political, economic and technological factors that determine the nature of pharmacy practice in all countries.

## THE ORIGINS OF PHARMACY UP TO 1841

### THE DAWN OF PHARMACY, ANTIQUITY TO 50 BC

The nature of the earliest medicines is lost in the remoteness of history. Cavemen almost certainly rolled the first crude pills in their hands. Pharmacy, as an occupation in which individuals made a living from the sale and supply of medicines, is among the oldest of professions. The earliest known prescriptions date back to at least 2700 BC and were written by the Sumerians, who lived in the land between the Euphrates and Tigris rivers. The practitioners of healing at this time combined the roles of priest, pharmacist and physician.

Chinese pharmacy traces its origins to the emperor Shen Nung in about 2000 BC. He investigated the medicinal value of several hundred herbs and wrote the first *Pen T'sao*, or native herbal, containing 365 drugs. Egyptian medicine dates from around 2900 BC, but the most important Egyptian pharmaceutical record, the *Papyrus Ebers*, was written much later, in about 1500 BC. This is a collection of around 800 prescriptions, in which some 700 different drugs are mentioned. Like the Sumerians, Egyptian pharmacists were also priests, and they learnt and practised their art in the temples.

### THE EMERGENCE OF PHARMACY, 50 BC TO 1231 AD

It was more than another thousand years before the early Greek philosophers began to influence medicine and pharmacy. They not only observed nature, but also sought to explain what they saw, gradually transforming medicine into a science. The traditions of Greek medicine continued with the rise of the Roman Empire. Indeed, the greatest physicians in Rome were nearly all Greek. The transition of pharmacy into a science received a major boost with the work of Dioscorides in the first century AD. In his *Materia Medica*, he describes nearly 500 plants and remedies prepared from animals and metals, and gives precise instructions for preparing them. His texts were considered basic science up to the sixteenth century.

Perhaps the greatest influence on pharmacy was Galen (130–201 AD), who was born in Pergamos and started his career as a physician to the gladiators in his hometown. He moved to Rome in 164 AD, eventually being appointed as physician to the imperial family. Galen practised and taught both pharmacy and medicine. He introduced many previously unknown drugs and was the first to define a drug as anything that acts on the body to bring about a change. His principles for preparing and compounding medicines remained dominant in the Western world for 1,500 years, and he gave his name to pharmaceuticals prepared by mechanical means (galenicals).

The first privately owned drug stores were established by the Arabs in Baghdad in the eighth century. They built on knowledge acquired from both Greece and Rome, developing a wide range of novel preparations, including syrups and alcoholic extracts. One of the greatest of Arab physicians was Rhazes (865–925 AD), who was a Persian born near Teheran. His principal work, *Liber Continens*, was to play an important part in Western medicine. He wrote: 'If you can help with foods, then do not prescribe medicaments; if simples are effective, then do not prescribe compounded remedies'.

These new ideas became assimilated into the practice of pharmacy across Western Europe following the Moslem advance across Africa, Spain and southern France. Perhaps the greatest figure in the science of medicine and pharmacy during this period was the Persian Ali ibn Sina (980–1037 AD), who was known by the Western world as Avicenna. He was the author of books on philosophy, natural history and medicine. His *Canon Medicinae* is a synopsis of Greek and Roman medicine. His teachings were treated as authoritative in the West well into the seventeenth century, and they remain dominant influences in some Eastern countries to this day.

## THE SEPARATION OF PHARMACY FROM MEDICINE: THE EDICT OF PALERMO, 1231

In European countries exposed to Arab influence, pharmacy shops began to appear around the eleventh century. Frederick II of Hohenstaufen, who was Emperor of Germany and King of Sicily, provided a key link between East and West, and it was in Sicily and southern Italy that pharmacy first became legally separated from medicine in 1231 AD. At his palace in Palermo, Frederick presented the first European edict creating a clear distinction between the responsibilities of physicians and those of apothecaries, and he laid down regulations for their professional practice.

Frederick's decree provided the basis of similar legislation elsewhere. The Basle Apothecaries Oath, for example, drawn up in 1271, spelled out the relationship between physicians and apothecaries. It stated that 'no physician who cares for or has cared for the sick shall ever own an apothecary's business in Basle, nor shall he ever become an apothecary'. In other European countries, pharmacy emerged as a separate occupation over the centuries which followed.

The first official pharmacopoeia, to be followed by all apothecaries, originated in Florence. The *Nuovo Receptario*, published in 1498, was the result of a collaboration between the Guild of Apothecaries and the Medical Society, one of the earliest examples of the two professions working constructively together. In Britain, the first official publication was the *London Pharmacopoeia* published in 1617 (Anderson 2013).

## THE MEDICALIZATION OF THE APOTHECARY

In most European countries, the apothecary or pharmacist developed from pepperers or spicers. The evolution of pharmacy in Great Britain from the twelfth to twentieth centuries is illustrated in Figure 1.1. Traders in spices, which included crude drugs and prepared medicines, evolved into either grocers or apothecaries. By the thirteenth century, apothecaries formed a distinct occupational group in many countries, including England and France.

During the Middle Ages, the evolution of French and British pharmacy was almost identical. In due course, the French *apothicaire* developed into the *pharmacien*, while the English apothecary became a general medical practitioner (GP). In Britain, trade in drugs and spices was monopolized by the Guild of Grocers, who had jurisdiction over the apothecaries. However, the apothecaries formed an alliance with court physicians, and they succeeded in persuading James I to grant a Charter in 1617 to form a separate company, the Society of Apothecaries. This was the first organization of pharmacists in the Anglo–Saxon world.

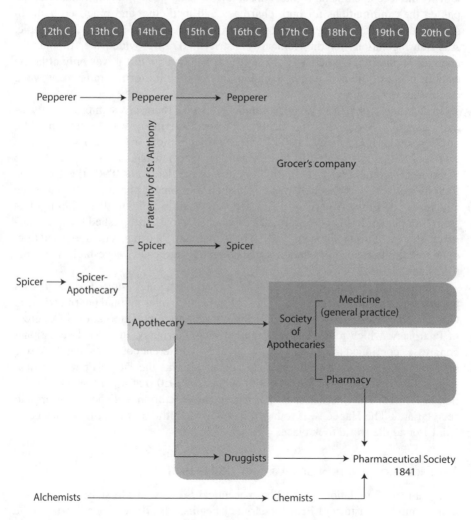

**FIGURE 1.1** Evolution of pharmacy in Great Britain, twelfth to twentieth centuries.

The apothecaries were both physicians (but not surgeons) and pharmacists, diagnosing and dispensing the medicines which they themselves prescribed. There were, however, other groups involved in the sale and supply of medicines: the chemists and druggists. The Apothecaries Act of 1815 confirmed apothecaries as physicians and laid down the training required to practise as such. Most apothecaries subsequently opted to practise exclusively as GPs, and an opportunity was presented to the other groups whose business was the sale and supply of medicines.

## The Organization of Pharmacy

In France, the *pharmacien* received official recognition with the establishment of the College de Pharmacie in 1777, which ushered in modern French pharmacy. During the seventeenth and eighteenth centuries, many people in continental Europe passed the examinations for both pharmacy and medicine, and practised both. In some countries, developments took place on a regional basis. In Italy, for example, Austrian regulations for the Lombardy district in 1778 provided the stimulus for changes in pharmacy practice in the north of the country. But it was only after the establishment of the new Italian Kingdom in 1870 that uniform arrangements were established across Italy.

In Germany, pharmacists in Nuremberg formed themselves into a society as early as 1632. A regional organization for north Germany was formed in 1820, and for southern Germany in 1848. After the federation of German states, these two societies amalgamated to form a national German pharmacists' society, the Deutscher Apothekerverein, in 1872. A few years later, in 1890, the Deutsche Pharamzeutische Gesellschaft was established to promote pharmaceutical science and research. Early American pharmacy was heavily influenced by immigrants from Europe. An Irish apothecary, Christopher Marshall, established the first pharmacy shop in Philadelphia in 1729. The American Pharmaceutical Association, open to 'all pharmaceutists and druggists of good character', was established some time later, in 1852.

International cooperation between pharmacists has a long history. For many years it had been a dream of some pharmacists to establish an international pharmacopoeia. German pharmacists took the initiative to convene the first International Congress of Pharmacy, which took place in Braunschweig, Germany, in 1865. International congresses continued to be held every few years in different countries, but there was no formal mechanism for international contact. It was the Dutch Pharmaceutical Association that proposed at the tenth congress in 1910 that a permanent association be formed. The International Pharmaceutical Federation, with headquarters and secretariat at The Hague, was founded in 1911, when the first meeting of delegates from around the world took place.

## The Professionalization of Pharmacy, 1841–1911

It is with the foundation of the Pharmaceutical Society of Great Britain in 1841 that the modern history of British pharmacy begins. The 70 years leading up to the beginnings of the welfare state in 1911 were a time of rapid social change that saw

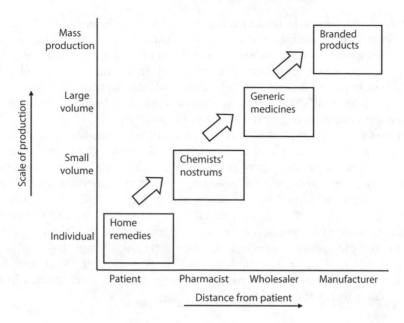

**FIGURE 1.2**  Shift of medicine making from home to factory, 1850–1950.

the increasing professionalization of many occupations, including pharmacy. The period saw the emergence of mass production and the start of a gradual shift in the way medicines were made. The practice in which individual families made up their own home remedies from ingredients they had either gathered themselves or obtained for a few pennies from the chemist slowly declined, with a shift to a greater reliance on remedies made up by the chemist himself, later supplemented by standard preparations made up by wholesalers, and finally to the domination of manufacturers producing and promoting their own branded products (Anderson 2008). The shift is illustrated in Figure 1.2.

Four key developments played defining roles in shaping pharmacy during this period: the foundation of the Pharmaceutical Society of Great Britain; the transformation of the pharmacists' education and qualifications; the emergence of retail pharmacy chains; and changes in the nature of pharmacy practice.

## THE FOUNDATION OF THE PHARMACEUTICAL SOCIETY OF GREAT BRITAIN, 1841

Early in 1841, a Mr Hawes introduced to Parliament a bill that would have made it compulsory for chemists and druggists to pass an examination before being able to carry on their business. If they bandaged a finger or recommended a remedy, they would be deemed to be practising medicine, and hence would need to be medically qualified. The leaders of the chemists and druggists took action, and on 15 April, 1841, a small group met at the Crown and Anchor Tavern in the Strand in London. They included William Allen FRS, John Savory, Thomas Morson and Jacob Bell, the son of a well-known Quaker chemist and druggist, John Bell.

William Allen moved a resolution that 'an Association be now formed under the title of The Pharmaceutical Society of Great Britain'. It was seconded by John Bell and carried by the meeting. The Society was to have three objectives: 'To benefit the public, and elevate the profession of pharmacy, by furnishing the means of proper instruction; to protect the collective and individual interests and privileges of all its members, in the event of any hostile attack in Parliament or otherwise; and to establish a club for the relief of decayed or distressed members'.

At its foundation, the Society was to consist of both members and associates. Full membership was restricted to chemists and druggists who owned their own businesses. Pharmacy managers or assistants, even those who had passed the major examination, could only become associates. Nevertheless, by the end of 1841, the new society had around 800 members, and by May of 1842, membership had increased to nearly 2000. In December 1841, the Society acquired 17 Bloomsbury Square, London, as its headquarters. It was to remain there until September 1976. Jacob Bell began a series of monthly scientific meetings at his own home, and in July 1841, he published *The Transactions of the Pharmaceutical Meetings*, later to be re-titled the *Pharmaceutical Journal*. The Society gained legal recognition with its incorporation by Royal Charter in 1843.

## PHARMACISTS' EDUCATION AND QUALIFICATIONS

From its foundation, one of the main priorities of the Pharmaceutical Society was the setting up of an examination system and a school of pharmacy. The examination system consisted of an entrance requirement, followed by the Minor examination, which was taken at the end of a 4- or 5-year apprenticeship. To become a full member, the associate was required to take the more advanced Major examination. Apprentices and assistants were advised to attend appropriate lectures, but the opportunities to do so were few. The Society set up its own School of Pharmacy within its Bloomsbury Square headquarters in 1842, but this was only available to those with ready access to London.

Branch schools were opened in Manchester, Norwich, Bath and Bristol in 1844, and in Edinburgh soon afterwards. After 1868, privately owned schools of pharmacy began to appear. In 1870, there were seven, only two of which were outside London, but by 1900 the number of schools offering courses in pharmacy had reached 45. The numbers of schools of pharmacy in Britain between 1880 and 2010 are illustrated in Figure 1.3. The last privately owned school, in Liverpool, closed in 1949. In 2003, the first new school of pharmacy since the 1970s opened at the University of East Anglia in Norwich. It was quickly followed by many more: in 2000, the number of schools of pharmacy was 16; by 2013, this figure had increased to 28. But while in 1900 the typical annual student intake was 20, by 2013 it was nearer 200.

The first Register of Pharmaceutical Chemists was established under the Pharmacy Act of 1852. However, there was no requirement at that stage for pharmaceutical chemists (i.e. those whose names appeared on the Register) to become members of the Pharmaceutical Society. The Society was a voluntary association, and those who passed the Major examinations were free to choose whether or not to become members. Only with passage of the Pharmacy and Poisons Act of 1933

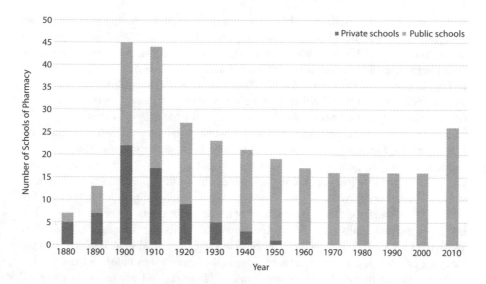

**FIGURE 1.3**   Number of Schools of Pharmacy in Great Britain, 1880 to 2010.

was it made compulsory to be a member of the Pharmaceutical Society in order to practice.

The 1868 Pharmacy Act created a second legal category of pharmacist – the chemists and druggists – whose names appeared on a separate register. The original members of this group came from a wide range of backgrounds. Some had been in business before the Act, some were associate members of the Society, some were assistants who had passed a new modified examination and some had passed the Pharmaceutical Society's Minor examination, which became the sole means of entry. The difference between the pharmaceutical chemist and the chemist and druggist was simply one of educational attainment. This two-tier structure to the pharmaceutical profession in Britain continued until 1954, when pharmaceutical chemists became Fellows of the Society and the two registers merged.

The first woman to register as a pharmaceutical chemist was Isabella Skinner Clarke in 1875. By 1908, the number of registered women pharmacists was 160, representing just 1% of all qualified chemists. By 1937, the figure had risen to 2,227, about 10% of the total. It had reached 26% by 1964, and 36% by 1984. By 2005, more than 65% of new entrants to the register were female; 70% of all pharmacists were employed in community pharmacies, 54% of whom worked for multiple pharmacies.

## THE ORIGINS OF THE MULTIPLES IN COMMUNITY PHARMACY

In securing the 1868 Pharmacy Act, the Pharmaceutical Society was satisfied that it had achieved privileges, including the use of titles, on behalf of proprietor pharmacists. The Society's view was that the professional practice of pharmacy required that qualified pharmacists must retain ownership and control. It maintained that since a corporate body could not sit examinations or be registered as a pharmaceutical chemist, it had no right to operate a chemist's business.

But in the 1870s a number of limited companies, including Cooperative societies and Harrods, began to sell medicines, using the term 'chemist' to describe that part of the shop where this took place. In 1880, the issue of whether companies could own pharmacies was tested in an important legal case, *The Pharmaceutical Society v. The London and Provincial Supply Association*, under the 1868 Pharmacy Act. The Association had been deliberately registered as a company with the intention of enabling an unqualified person to keep open shop for the sale of poisons.

The legal argument was about whether the word 'person' could include a company. If it could not, then companies would not be able to own pharmacies. The Pharmacy Act applied only to persons; a company could not be held guilty of an offence under the Act. The Society lost the case in the County Court, but appealed against the decision to a higher court, where it won. However, the defendants appealed to the Court of Appeal. This court overturned the decision of the previous court, so the Pharmaceutical Society appealed again, this time to the House of Lords. At the hearing on 20 July 1880, the Law Lords confirmed the decision of the Court of Appeal, deciding that the carrying on of a pharmacy business by a limited company was indeed legal.

The decision meant that titles restricted to chemists and druggists by the 1868 Act could now legally be used by companies, provided that a qualified person was employed to carry out the sale of poisons. The decision meant that businesses consisting of large numbers of branches were now possible. The impact was immense; over the next 15 years, more than 200 companies were registered for retail trade in drugs and dispensing. The first limited company that was set up by an unqualified druggist, Jesse Boot, was established in Nottingham (it used an existing shop). Boot called himself a cash chemist, and began opening branches. By 1883 he had 10, and by 1900 he already had by far the largest retail chemist chain, with more than 250 branches.

## THE PRACTICE OF PHARMACY

The emergence of the multiples was not the only threat facing proprietor pharmacists. The nature of retailing was changing, with the emergence of department stores and the growth of the cooperative movement. Sales of proprietary medicines expanded rapidly during this period, but so did the number of outlets from which they were available, and proprietor pharmacists needed to diversify to make a living. Many built up a substantial photographic business, as well as developing their trade in toiletries and cosmetics, wines, spirits and tobacco products (Anderson 2007a).

Figure 1.4 indicates the principal sources of income for independent community pharmacists during the course of the twentieth century. This has been transformed by increasing dependence on income from the National Health Service (NHS) since its introduction in 1948. In 2011, 88% of the revenue of independent pharmacies in Britain came from the NHS.

In late-Victorian Britain, many pharmacists also practised as dentists. Indeed, when the first dental register appeared in 1879, following passage of the first Dentists Act in 1878, two-thirds of those appearing on it combined the practice of dentistry with that of pharmacy. For thousands of pharmacies, the extraction of teeth, making fillings and crowns and supplying false teeth were some of the most profitable parts of the business.

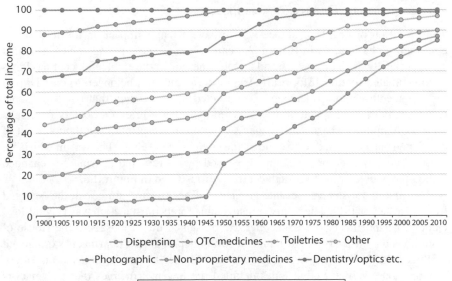

**FIGURE 1.4**   Sources of income of independent community pharmacies, 1900–2010.

Although the Dental Act of 1921 restricted entry to the register to those who had undertaken approved courses of study, it admitted those who had been practising for at least seven years, and for whom dentistry represented a substantial part of their business. As a result, many pharmacists were able to register as dentists and to carry on as before. The Chemists Dental Association, which represented the interests of the chemist–dentists, was finally disbanded in 1949, by which time it had five members.

## NATIONAL INSURANCE TO NATIONAL HEALTH, 1911–1948

The period between 1911 and 1948 is one that was dominated by two world wars. For Britain and for pharmacy, many things had to be put on hold. However, the introduction of the National Insurance Act of 1911 represents a major watershed in the development of pharmacy practice. Post-war plans for the reform of industrial relations were another, leading to another important legal case, which resulted in a change of direction for the Pharmaceutical Society. It is also a period during which the nature of pharmaceutical products changed.

## THE SEPARATION OF DISPENSING FROM PRESCRIBING

The provision of health insurance was to have a major impact on the fortunes of community pharmacists in Britain. An early form of such insurance was provided by the Friendly Societies, which had largely emerged in the eighteenth century. It has been estimated that by 1815, nearly 9% of the population belonged to one. During the nineteenth century, membership continued to grow, such that by 1900, about half the adult male population was covered by either a Friendly Society or a trade union. Community pharmacists began seeing more prescriptions, although most of the dispensing continued to be done by the doctors themselves. The way in which the proportion of written prescriptions dispensed by doctors and pharmacists changed during the course of the twentieth century is illustrated in Figure 1.5.

The first major step in the state provision of health care came with the National Insurance Act of 1912. The minister responsible for its introduction was David Lloyd George, Chancellor of the Exchequer. He presented his proposals to the House of Commons on 4 May 1911. On 1 June, a strong deputation of pharmacists organized by the Society's Council was received by the Chancellor in his rooms at the House of Commons. William Glyn-Jones detailed the Seven Principles that pharmacists wanted incorporated into the National Insurance bill (Box 1.1).

The Seven Principles were quickly agreed upon, and the National Insurance Act became law on 15 July 1912; these principles were to largely shape the practice of community pharmacy in Britain for the rest of the century. The first principle meant that the contract was with the firm or corporate body owning the pharmacy, rather than with the employee pharmacist; the second that the pharmacist had to be present to supervise dispensing; the fourth stated that patients could take their prescription to any pharmacy, rather than being registered with a particular one; and the fifth stated that employees would be paid according to the number of prescriptions dispensed, rather than on the number of patients being treated. A separate salaried service for the dispensing of National Insurance prescriptions

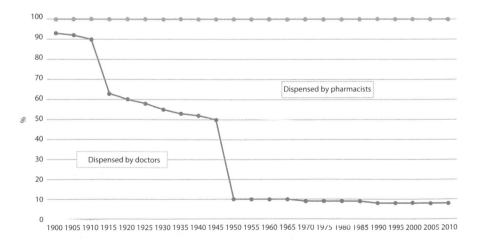

**FIGURE 1.5**   Proportion of prescriptions dispensed by doctors and pharmacists, 1900–2010.

> ### BOX 1.1   SEVEN PRINCIPLES THAT PHARMACISTS WANTED INCORPORATED INTO THE NATIONAL INSURANCE BILL
>
> - No agreement for the supply of medicines for insured persons should be made except with a person, firm or corporate body entitled to carry on the statutory business of a pharmaceutical chemist or chemist and druggist.
> - Dispensing under the Act should be done under the direct supervision of a pharmacist.
> - The control of medical and pharmaceutical services to insured persons: no agreement for the supply of medicines for insured persons should be in the hands of the County Health (later Insurance) Committees, nor under the control of Friendly Societies.
> - A panel of all qualified pharmacists in a particular district willing to supply medicines under the scheme should be set up, so that insured persons could choose their own suppliers.
> - Remuneration for pharmacists should be on a scale system and not on a per capita basis.
> - Pharmacy should be represented on the County Health Committees, the Advisory Committees and the Insurance Commission.
> - Medical benefit should not be extended to persons earning more than £160 per annum.

had been rejected; and special arrangements were agreed to allow doctors to dispense in rural areas where no chemist was available. The immediate impact of the scheme was a threefold increase in the number of prescriptions presented at pharmacies.

The Act itself created a national scheme of insurance against sickness and disability, and applied to all workers over the age of 16 earning no more than £160 per year, amounting to some 14 million men and women. It did not apply to their dependants, although payments were made for the support of the family while the breadwinner was ill. The insurance covered the cost of visiting the doctor and the supply of medicines. It was in the National Health Insurance Act that the first legal distinction was made in Britain between the prescribing and dispensing of medicines. Lloyd George was keen to 'separate the drugs from the doctors'. He was of the opinion that paying doctors to supply medicines encouraged excessive prescribing.

When the National Insurance Scheme was introduced, doctors were given financial incentives to prescribe economically. The total sum for medical care was to be nine shillings per person, of which one shilling and sixpence was available for the supply of drugs. However, a further sixpence (the so-called 'floating sixpence') was to be available for paying chemists if the drug bill exceeded this limit. If it wasn't needed, it was credited to the doctor, thus giving the doctor an incentive to deny patients the use of expensive drugs. This arrangement was to have clear parallels 80 years later with the advent of GP fund-holding practices.

## THE LIMITATION OF THE PHARMACEUTICAL SOCIETY'S FUNCTIONS

One of the major factors in determining the nature of pharmacy practice in Britain has been the powers of the Pharmaceutical Society and the way in which these have been exercised. These powers have regularly been tested in the courts, and many of the cases represent watersheds in the evolution of pharmacy practice. One such was the Jenkin case of 1920.

In the aftermath of the First World War, the government was keen to reform industrial relations in Britain by setting up a number of schemes for negotiating wage rates and other working conditions. The Pharmaceutical Society promoted the instigation of a Joint Industrial Council for this purpose for the whole of the pharmaceutical industry, including manufacturing, wholesaling and retailing. The Society's membership included both employers and employees, and it was well placed to preside over negotiations between them.

The Society's plans came up against some powerful opponents, notably Jesse Boot and pharmacists in Scotland. The latter obtained legal opinion on whether the Society had the powers under its Charter to become involved in negotiations about pay and conditions. The Society decided to test its powers in the courts. Arthur Henry Jenkin was a hospital pharmacist and the only member of the Society's Council who was not a retail chemist. He took out an injunction to restrain the Council of the Society from undertaking a range of activities, including the regulation of pay and conditions of service, to function as an employers' association and to provide legal and insurance services to members.

The injunction was granted. At a hearing on 19 October 1920, the Court decided that the Society did not have powers to regulate wages, hours of business and the prices at which goods were sold, or to provide insurance or legal services. As a result of this decision, and just two months later, a separate body, the Retail Pharmacists Union, was set up as a 'union of retail employer chemists for the protection of trade interests'. It was renamed the National Pharmaceutical Union in 1932, the National Pharmaceutical Association in 1977 and the National Pharmacy Association (NPA) in 2004. At the same time, Jesse Boot established a Managers' Representative Council to represent pharmacist–managers in his branches.

## THE TRIUMPH OF PROFESSIONAL REGULATION

After the Jenkin case, the Society set about redefining its purpose, and changed direction. Indeed, it has been argued that the NPA is the true successor to the aims of the founding fathers of the Pharmaceutical Society. A new Pharmacy and Poisons Act in 1933 clarified the relationship between the Society's Council, the Privy Council and its members. For the first time, every person registered as a pharmacist automatically became a member of the Pharmaceutical Society: the distinction between registration under the Pharmacy Acts and membership of the Society, which until that time had been voluntary, was ended. Membership jumped from 13,800 in 1932 to 20,900 in 1933.

The 1933 Act added substantially to the Pharmaceutical Society's statutory duties. The Society was required to enforce the Act, and had to appoint inspectors, who must be pharmacists themselves, for the purpose. The inspectors had to inspect the conditions under which poisons were stored, the registers of sales and the premises of registered 'authorized sellers of poisons', which included individual proprietor pharmacists and corporate bodies having a superintendent pharmacist. Two thirds of pharmacists had been voluntary members of the Society.

A disciplinary committee, the Statutory Committee, was established. The Committee was given the duty of inquiring into any case where a pharmacist (or other authorized seller of poisons) had been convicted of a criminal offence. The first Statutory Committee met in July 1934, and the first name was removed from the Register shortly after. A code of ethics for the profession followed within a few years. The first *Statement upon Matters of Professional Conduct* was eventually published in the *Pharmaceutical Journal* of 17 June 1944. It was revised and extended in 1953, a process that has continued ever since.

It has been said that with the 1933 Act, 'professional regulation triumphed over protection and trade unionism'. The Jenkin case had removed any prospect of the Society being involved in negotiating terms of service for its members. The 1933 Act ended any hope of the Society amalgamating with the Retail Pharmacists' Union and the Chemists' Defence Association into a 'British Medical Association for Pharmacy'. The objectives of the Society were formally changed through a Supplemental Charter in 1953. The words 'the protection of those who carry on the business of chemists and druggists' were replaced by 'to maintain the honour and safeguard and promote the interests of the members in the exercise of the profession of pharmacy'. The Charter was amended again in 2009.

## PREPARING PHARMACEUTICAL PRODUCTS: FROM BESPOKE TO OFF-THE-PEG

During the course of the twentieth century, the nature of pharmaceutical products, and their modes of preparation, changed beyond all recognition. At the turn of the century, many poor people still bought small quantities of ingredients to make their own home remedies. An important role of pharmacists was to counter prescribe, to suggest a remedy for a cold or a pain. They would usually make their own nostrums, such as cough and indigestion medicines, to their own formulae and using their own labels. There were relatively few proprietary medicines available, and the vast majority of drugs in use were galenicals (liquid medicines extracted mainly from plants) and minerals such as potassium citrate and sodium bicarbonate.

However, the 'therapeutic revolution' of the 1950s and 1960s led to the marketing by pharmaceutical companies of increasing numbers of new chemical entities under brand names, and branded products came to dominate the prescribing habits of many doctors. Prescriptions for branded products exceeded those for generic items for the first time in 1957. This trend continued, reaching a peak of over 80% branded prescription items in 1957. It was only reversed in 1994, with the proportion of generic prescriptions continuing to increase; in 2012, the figure was nearly 84%. Changes in the proportion of branded and generic drugs supplied on prescription during this period are illustrated in Figure 1.6.

Figure 1.7 shows the changes in the nature of the principal dosage forms in use during the twentieth century. This is based on an analysis of the proportion of all

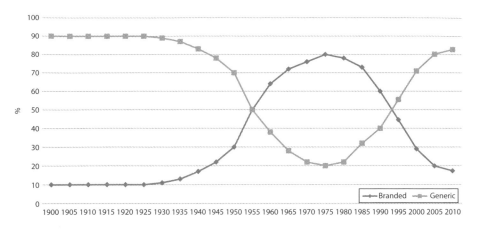

**FIGURE 1.6**    Proportion of prescriptions prescribed by brand or generic name, 1900–2010.

prescriptions dispensed at a south London pharmacy for a particular dosage form. At the beginning of the century, more than 60% of all medicines supplied were oral liquids, mainly mixtures and draughts (single-dose liquid medicines). Only a very small proportion were solid-dosage forms, and these were mainly pills and cachets; less than 2% were tablets. By 1980, more than 70% of all medicines were supplied in oral solid-dosage forms, mainly tablets and capsules; less than 8% were supplied as liquids. The period between 1930 and 1970 was one of great change in the practice of community pharmacy, as the need for extemporaneous dispensing diminished and preparation shifted from the dispensary to the factory.

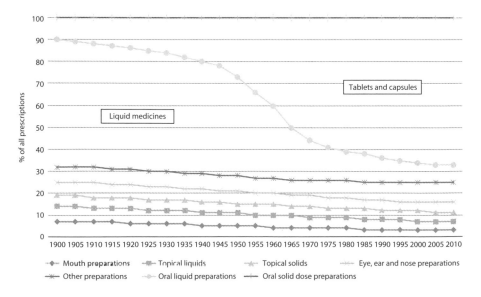

**FIGURE 1.7**    Principal dosage forms prescribed, 1900–2010.

## PHARMACY IN THE NHS, 1948–1986

With the end of the Second World War, the new Labour government set about implementing a programme of reform, including a comprehensive NHS. For pharmacy, its consequences were to be far-reaching. The NHS was to be a major factor in determining the nature of community pharmacy practice for the rest of the century, but it was not the only one. The basic tensions between trade and profession within pharmacy were to surface as the powers of the Society were tested yet again.

### THE IMPACT OF THE NHS

By 1946 around 24 million workers, representing about half the total population, were covered by the National Insurance Scheme, as the income limit was gradually increased. The NHS, introduced on 5 July 1948, made the service available to everyone. It extended provision beyond workers to women, children and the elderly, and included maternity and antenatal services. Before 1948, dispensing prescriptions still accounted for less than 10% of the income of most chemists. After 1948, 94% of the population obtained their medicines from registered pharmacies, and dispensing prescriptions quickly came to form the major part of pharmacists' incomes.

Figure 1.8 illustrates the increase in prescription numbers dispensed during the twentieth century. Within a year of the introduction of the NHS, the number of prescriptions presented at pharmacies almost quadrupled, from 70 million in 1947 to nearly 250 million in 1949. Prescription numbers doubled (from 250 to 500 million) over the 48-year period between 1949 and 1997; they doubled again (from 500 to 1,000 million) over the 15-year period between 1997 and 2012. The average number of prescription items per person increased from 13 in 2003 to 19 in 2013; around 60% of prescriptions are now for people aged 60 or over.

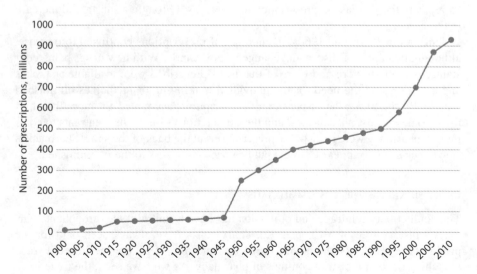

**FIGURE 1.8** Number of prescriptions written in England by doctors and dispensed in pharmacies, 1900–2010.

At the same time as prescription numbers increased, other parts of pharmacists' traditional businesses began to decline. The number of private prescriptions presented dropped markedly, as did both requests for counter prescribing and the sale of proprietary medicines, since all medicines prescribed by the doctor were now available free of charge. Not surprisingly, most people preferred to go to the doctor for a prescription, even for the most minor of complaints, rather than pay for something from the chemist. The drop in the sale of proprietary medicines (Figure 1.4) was to be short lived, however, as manufacturers increased their advertising on television and in magazines from the early 1950s.

The sale of traditional chemists' items, such as toiletries and cosmetics and photographic requisites, was threatened as other retailers entered these markets and specialist shops opened. Dependence on income from secondary occupations, particularly dentistry and optics, which had been common earlier in the century, had virtually ended, and many proprietor pharmacists were persuaded to sell their businesses to the multiples.

## THE 'DISAPPEARING' PHARMACIST

The consequences of the increase in prescription numbers were far-reaching. Almost overnight, many pharmacists effectively migrated from the front of the shop to the back, as they spent much of the working day dispensing prescriptions in the dispensary. At the inception of the NHS, a majority of prescriptions still required the medicines to be compounded. Only a small proportion was available commercially as tablets or capsules.

Many pharmacists took the opportunity to enlarge their dispensaries to meet the demand. Most felt that dispensing was what they had been trained to do, and only a few took the opportunity to train assistants to help with the dispensing. Most were happy with the increase in prescription numbers, as it brought a substantial increase in their income.

During the 1950s and 1960s, the number of prescriptions continued to increase, although the nature of dispensing changed significantly. With new drugs being constantly marketed, more and more of the drugs prescribed were available as tablets and capsules, and the need for the individual making-up of medicines diminished greatly. By this time, the dispensing of prescriptions accounted for more than half the income of most pharmacists, and the expectations of most new entrants to community pharmacy were to dispense prescriptions at the back of the shop. Pharmacists slowly began to disappear from the public's view as access to them diminished.

## PROFESSIONALISM VERSUS COMMERCIALISM

The conflict between trade and profession has been a central issue throughout pharmacy's history (see also Chapter 12). Pharmacists have always been paid for the products they sell, not the advice they give, and almost all engage in retail trade stretching beyond the strict confines of pharmacy. As we have seen, the trade issue became accentuated after 1880, when it was established that companies had the right to establish pharmacy businesses. Throughout its history, the Pharmaceutical

Society has resisted commercial developments, which it perceived as having an adverse effect on the professional standing of pharmacy.

By 1955, there was sufficient concern about the state of community pharmacy for the Council of the Society to appoint a committee to report on the general practice of pharmacy, with particular reference to the maintenance of professional standards. The Committee submitted its report in 1961, and it was eventually published in the *Pharmaceutical Journal* on 20 April 1963. The report suggested that it was undesirable for non-professional business to predominate in a pharmacy, and that the extension of this kind of business in pharmacies should be controlled.

An attempt to incorporate this principle into the Statement upon Matters of Professional Conduct was challenged and led to the Dickson case. A motion was put to the Annual General Meeting of the Society in 1965, but owing to the large attendance no vote could be taken, and a special meeting to consider the recommendation was held at the Royal Albert Hall on 25 July 1965. Mr R.C.M. Dickson, who was a director of the Boots Pure Drug Company, sought an injunction to prevent the holding of the meeting, claiming that the motion was outside the scope of the Society's powers, and that if implemented, would be a restraint on trade.

The Society was unable to satisfy the courts that the professional side of a pharmacy business was adversely affected by other activities. The Society appealed to the House of Lords, who upheld the decision of the lower court. The Society was judged to have no powers to restrict the sale of certain goods from pharmacies. It could make rules affecting the non-professional activities of pharmacists, but only if the rules could be shown to be in the interest of the public and the profession. The Society had attempted to control the commercial aspects of pharmacy. The Dickson case demonstrated that it did not have the power to do so.

## THE EMERGENCE OF 'THE NEW PHARMACY', 1986–2010

By the early 1980s there was widespread uncertainty about the future of pharmacy, particularly community pharmacy. The Minister for Health, Dr Gerard Vaughan, announced at the British Pharmaceutical Conference that 'one knew there was a future for hospital pharmacists, one knew there was a future for industrial pharmacists, but one was not sure that one knew the future for the general practice pharmacist'. Pharmacy needed to re-invent itself. Some important initiatives were taken. In 1982, for example, the National Pharmaceutical Association began its 'Ask Your Pharmacist' campaign, which encouraged the public to make full use of their local pharmacy. But what was really needed was an independent and far-ranging inquiry into the profession. The result was the 'Nuffield Report'.

### THE NUFFIELD REPORT 1986

In October 1983 the trustees of the Nuffield Foundation commissioned an inquiry into pharmacy (Nuffield Committee of Inquiry into Pharmacy 1986). Its terms of reference were 'to consider the present and future structure of the practice of pharmacy in its several branches and its potential contribution to health care and to review the education and training of pharmacists accordingly'. The Committee of Inquiry was chaired by Sir Kenneth Clucas, a former Permanent Secretary at the Department of

Trade, and had 12 members, only half of whom were pharmacists. It made a total of 96 recommendations, 26 of which related to community pharmacy.

The tone of the Nuffield report was very positive: 'We believe that the pharmacy profession has a distinctive and indispensable contribution to make to health care that is capable of still further development'. The years that followed its publication were dominated by the action necessary to implement the recommendations. Two aspects came to dominate the discussion: whether a pharmacist needed to be on the premises in order to supervise activities, and the extended role of pharmacists.

In order to have time to carry out the extended role, the pharmacist would need to be able to leave the pharmacy at times, so that supervision could be exercised in other ways. Eventually, the pharmacy profession rejected this radical suggestion, and in 1989, the Council of the Royal Pharmaceutical Society of Great Britain (it had become 'Royal' in 1988) issued a statement to the effect that 'every prescription for a medicine must be seen by a pharmacist, and a judgement made by him as to what action is necessary'. Pharmacists had not only disappeared from view, but were now shackled to the dispensary bench.

## THE EXTENDED ROLE

The task of considering in what ways the role of community pharmacists might be extended was delegated to a Joint Working Party of the Department of Health and the pharmaceutical profession. This was set up in November 1990 with the following terms of reference: 'to consider ways in which the National Health Service community pharmaceutical services might be developed to increase their contribution to health care; and to make recommendations'.

Its report, *Pharmaceutical Care: the Future for Community Pharmacy* (Department of Health and Royal Pharmaceutical Society of Great Britain 1992), was published in March 1992, and it made a total of 30 recommendations. These included increasing the range of medicines available for sale by pharmacists, the maintenance of patient medication records by pharmacists, the extension of needle and syringe exchange schemes, participation in health promotion campaigns and having separate areas for providing advice and counselling. The recommendations formed the basis for negotiations about the scope of community pharmacy over the years that followed.

By the mid-1990s it was clear that most of the recommendations of the Nuffield report which could be implemented had been. Nuffield was a catalyst for change, but in order to maintain the momentum it was considered necessary to involve the membership as a whole. Over the years that followed, a series of policy documents were developed. The Society launched its 'Pharmacy in a New Age' (PIANA) initiative in October 1995. This aimed to establish a strategy for pharmacy for the next 10–15 years (up to 2010), after involving as many members of the profession as possible in the process. Six papers on factors affecting the future of pharmacy were published in February 1996 as *The Shape of Things to Come*.

In response to feedback from its members, the Society published a further document in September 1996, entitled *The New Horizon* (Royal Pharmaceutical Society of Great Britain 1996). Four key areas for pharmacy involvement were identified: the management of prescribed medicines; the management of chronic conditions; the management of common ailments; and the promotion and support of healthy lifestyles. This was followed in September 1997 by a strategy for a twenty-first century pharmaceutical service, published under the title *Building the Future* (Royal Pharmaceutical Society of Great Britain 1997). This set specific aims and targets for each of the four areas.

## THE NEW SOCIETY

To help it deliver its strategy, the Society agreed a new internal structure based on seven directorates in March 2003. A new Royal Charter, which re-focused the Society's objectives within the context of public benefit, came into force on 7 December 2004. This established a reformed Council of 30 members, 17 of whom were elected pharmacists, 10 were lay members and two were pharmacy technicians.

In the light of the devolution of political power to Scotland and Wales, the Council in 2004 established a review group under Lord Fraser to examine the Society's structure, functions and ways of working. Following the review, the Society established three elected regional boards – the English Pharmacy Board, the Scottish Pharmacy Board and the Welsh Pharmacy Board – during 2006. Policy then became the remit of the three national boards, with the Society only considering issues at the Great Britain and European levels, as well as responding to government consultations and issues raised in the media.

In April 2007, the Society launched its 'Pharmacy 2020' project, aimed at developing a vision of what pharmacy could look like in 2020, and at consolidating pharmacy's position as a clinical profession. Pharmacy 2020 had similar goals to those of the PIANA project launched 12 years earlier.

## REGULATION

From around 2000, a train of events was set in motion which was to lead ultimately to the separation of the Society's regulatory and representative functions and to the creation of a General Pharmaceutical Council. The Kennedy Report of the inquiry into children's heart surgery at Bristol Royal Infirmary published in July 2001 redefined health professional regulation and set an entirely new framework for it.

In February 2007, the government published a White Paper: *Trust, Assurance and Safety: The Regulation of Health Professionals in the 21st Century* (Department of Health 2007). The government announced its intention to establish a General Pharmaceutical Council to regulate the pharmacy profession and proposed the creation of a professional leadership body for the profession. It had concluded that the Society's professional leadership role was potentially in conflict with its role as the profession's regulator. Initially, the Society became subject to oversight by the Council for Healthcare Regulatory Excellence. The Society's response was to commission an independent inquiry into possible options for a new professional leadership body for pharmacy. The Clarke Inquiry (chaired by Nigel Clarke) consulted widely, and reported in 2008.

On 27 September 2010, the General Pharmaceutical Council was established, and the Royal Pharmaceutical Society of Great Britain ceased to be the regulatory body for pharmacy. Instead, it re-emerged as the professional leadership body for pharmacists and pharmacies in Great Britain. Its title became the Royal Pharmaceutical Society, and it extended its membership to include non-pharmacists.

A voluntary register for pharmacy technicians began in January 2005. When statutory regulation of pharmacy technicians came into force on 1 July 2009, there were already more than 7,500 individuals on the voluntary register. Registration of technicians became mandatory on 1 July 2011. A category of non-practising pharmacist membership was established in 2005. In its final year, the Society reported a total membership of 50,374 pharmacists, of whom 41,958 were practising, 5,492 were non-practising and 2,924 were overseas. It also had 8,353 registered pharmacy technicians, 8,320 of whom were practising. The new General Pharmaceutical Council registered only practising pharmacists and pharmacy technicians.

## PHARMACY PRACTICE

Since 2000, the practice of pharmacy has also been subject to a string of policy initiatives. In 2004, the government published *A Vision for Pharmacy in the New NHS*, which outlined 10 key roles for pharmacy (Department of Health 2004). It was largely an update of an earlier policy document, *Pharmacy in the Future – Implementing the NHS Plan*, published in Department of Health (2000). Another important development was seen in 2005 with the publication of a new Community Pharmacy Contractual Framework for England and Wales. The new contract identified three tiers of services (essential, advanced and enhanced) which could be delivered under the NHS. The new contractual framework was designed to provide primary care trusts (PCTs) and pharmacies with the opportunity to work effectively together to meet the needs of their local population. All community pharmacies had to provide essential services, which included dispensing and repeat dispensing, health promotion and healthy lifestyle advice, signposting to other services, support for self-care and disposal of medicines.

Providing the pharmacist and premises were suitably accredited, a pharmacy could also provide advanced services. Originally, there was just one: medicines use review and prescription intervention, where pharmacists review a patient's current medication, but a new medicines service has since been added. A pharmacy can also provide local enhanced services, commissioned by PCTs and following the abolition of PCTs in 2013 by NHS England and Clinical Commissioning Groups (CCGs). The most common of these are stop smoking schemes, supervised administration of medicines, minor ailment schemes and the supply of medicines under patient group directions. Other enhanced services have included out-of-hours services, supplementary prescribing, prescriber support and anti-coagulation monitoring.

The profession has identified public health as an area in which it can potentially make an important contribution (Anderson 2007b). Public health has been defined as 'the science and art of preventing disease, prolonging life and promoting health through the organized efforts and informed choices of society, organizations, communities and individuals'. In 2005, a government paper entitled *Choosing Health through Pharmacy* set out a framework for pharmacy to become more fully engaged in delivering public health services (Department of Health 2005).

In 2011, a Pharmacy and Public Health Forum was established to bring together pharmacy and public health interests. It consolidated pharmacy's growing engagement with public health; for pharmacists, this represented a shift towards a greater focus on population and health issues rather than on individuals and illness. One initiative arising from the shift of focus was the development of Healthy Living Pharmacies. These offer a range of services including smoking cessation services, blood pressure testing and dietary advice. The intention is that all pharmacy staff focus on the health needs of individuals.

In order to lawfully conduct a retail pharmacy business, a registered pharmacist must now be in charge of the registered pharmacy as the responsible pharmacist. The activities that may take place in the pharmacy depend on the level of supervision provided and whether or not the pharmacist is present in the pharmacy. A pharmacist can only be the responsible pharmacist in charge at one pharmacy. In 2006, the UK became the first country in the world to achieve independent prescriber status for pharmacists. By the end of 2007, there were 1,360 supplementary prescribers (those permitted to prescribe medicines in accordance with a clinical management plan) and 310 independent prescribers.

## BEYOND 2010

Following the change of government in 2010, major restructuring of the NHS has taken place. New legislation relating to the practice of pharmacy in Britain has since been enacted or completely revised. The National Health Service (Pharmaceutical Services) Regulations 2012 incorporated market entry provisions, rural dispensing regulations, the terms of service under the community pharmacy contractual framework and fitness to practise provisions for pharmacy contractors. The National Health Service (Pharmaceutical and Local Pharmaceutical Services) Regulations 2013, which came into effect on 1 April 2013, reflected the new NHS architecture, in which NHS England (the NHS commissioning board) became responsible for maintaining pharmaceutical lists, and health and well-being boards were made responsible for developing and publishing pharmaceutical needs assessments, used in the determination of routine applications for new pharmacies.

The Royal Pharmaceutical Society itself has undergone rapid development since 2010. An important focus of the new society has been professional development. It introduced its faculty programme of professional recognition in 2013. At the same time, it replaced its long-standing local branch structure with local practice forums, designed to bring pharmacists from all sectors together for educational activities, networking and mentoring.

In 2013, the English Pharmacy Board commissioned an independent review into future models of care through pharmacy. This resulted in a report, *Now or Never*, which indicated how better integration of pharmacists into the NHS could improve patient care. Achieving this represents one of the greatest challenges for the future.

## A BRIEF HISTORY OF HOSPITAL PHARMACY

The history of pharmacy prior to the start of the twentieth century is largely the history of shop-based pharmacy. Yet pharmacy practice in hospitals can be traced back over many centuries, and the history of hospital pharmacy is closely allied to the history of hospitals. The history of hospital pharmacy can be considered in a number of time frames: an emergent period up to 1897; periods of growing professional identity and standardization up to 1948; and periods of expansion, consolidation and specialization since then.

## THE ORIGINS OF HOSPITAL PHARMACY TO 1897

The first hospitals in Britain in which it is known pharmacy was practised were the Roman military hospitals known as *valetudinaria*. As Britain converted to Christianity, so the Church began to care for the sick and needy. Between 794 and 1547 nearly 800 hospitals were established, of which around 200 were for the care of lepers. However, in medieval times hospitals were ecclesiastical rather than medical institutions, being essentially for the refreshment of the soul rather than the relief of the body. In addition to these hospitals, there were infirmaries attached to many monasteries throughout Europe.

Further hospitals were established by religious and craft guilds in the fourteenth and fifteenth centuries, and a number of pest houses opened in the sixteenth and seventeenth centuries to care for the victims of the plague. Many employed an apothecary and contained a dispensary. The apothecary usually combined the roles of resident medical officer and dispenser of medicines. Larger hospitals, such as St. Bartholomew's and St. Thomas' in London, often also employed an apothecary's assistant or apprentice, and would undertake the preparation of most of their own medicines. Smaller hospitals often employed the services of a visiting apothecary.

Passage of the Apothecaries Act in 1815 put a stop to the early development of hospital pharmacy in Britain, since most hospital apothecaries devoted most of their time to medical matters, and neglected the dispensing side. As the Linstead Report on the hospital pharmaceutical service in 1955 put it: 'The original development of the pharmaceutical service in hospitals was checked when the apothecary obtained recognition as a general practitioner of medicine, and explains why hospital pharmacy had to make a fresh start in the middle of the last century'. During the second half of the nineteenth century, at least in the larger hospitals, the remaining apothecaries were slowly replaced by qualified pharmacists, and some hospitals then began to insist that those appointed be members of the Pharmaceutical Society.

## THE EMERGENCE OF PROFESSIONAL IDENTITY, 1897–1923

There was, however, no legal requirement that only registered pharmacists must be employed in hospitals, and many institutions continued to employ unqualified people with a wide range of backgrounds. Changes in the practice of pharmacy in hospitals in the late-nineteenth century led to the creation of a number of separate professional associations. The Poor Law Dispensers Association was formed in 1897, and in the following year the Public Dispensers Association came into being. The latter Association consisted of London County Council asylum dispensers, prison and charity dispensers and a few hospital dispensers.

These two associations amalgamated in 1900, becoming the Public and Poor Law Dispensers Association. By 1909, the title had become the Public Pharmacists and

Dispensers Association. At this time, many of the pharmacists employed in the public service were women. By 1908 more than 60% of practising women pharmacists were working in hospitals and institutions. In 1916 the organization decided that in future only individuals whose names appeared on the register of chemists and druggists should be elected as members. In 1917, it became the Public Pharmacists Association.

## UNIFICATION AND STANDARDIZATION, 1923–1948

Pharmacists in voluntary hospitals regarded themselves as rather different from their colleagues in other institutions. They formed a separate organization, as a pharmacy section of the Hospital Officers Association. However, in due course the two organizations agreed to merge. The inaugural meeting of the Guild of Public Pharmacists was held on 23 January 1923. There was then a single body to represent pharmacists working in voluntary hospitals, poor law institutions, prisons and other branches of the public service. With the creation of the Guild, public service pharmacy had come of age. The first quarter of the twentieth century represented a period during which the salaries, status and prospects of such pharmacists improved substantially.

The period from 1923 to 1948 represented a period of standardization for the service but differences still remained between pharmacy in voluntary rather than municipal hospitals, since there was no legal requirement to employ a pharmacist in hospitals, and in many the supply of medicines was undertaken by medical staff, nurses or under-qualified dispensers. In 1939, the Pharmaceutical Society carried out the first survey of hospital pharmacy. It found that over two-thirds of the 397 hospitals having 100 or more beds employed a full-time pharmacist, and a further 13 hospitals used the services of a local community pharmacist. Although only 15% of the 543 hospital with less than 100 beds employed a pharmacist, nearly half used a pharmacist outside to supervise the dispensing.

## CONSOLIDATION AND SURVIVAL, 1948–1970

The introduction of the NHS in 1948 provided the opportunity for further development and enhancement of professional aspirations. The Pharmaceutical Whitley Council, at which salaries and conditions of service were negotiated, was the first to be convened. However, initial optimism was soon dashed. Although national pay scales were agreed, poor pay and prospects were to overshadow the practice of hospital pharmacy in Britain throughout the 1950s and 1960s.

Despite these difficulties a number of important innovations were possible at several centres, mainly in teaching hospitals where recruitment difficulties were less severe, where locums could usually be recruited and which tended to have larger establishments. From 1965 onwards, at the Westminster and London Hospitals in London and at Aberdeen Royal Infirmary, developments were implemented that required hospital pharmacists to inspect prescription sheets on the ward rather than in the pharmacy (Anderson 2012).

Quality control for manufacturing was becoming more vigorous, and drug information services were beginning to be developed, initially to support ward pharmacists. However, for most hospitals the capacity to introduce such innovations was severely limited by small establishments, poor recruitment and no obligation on hospital managers to do much to improve matters.

## EXPANSION AND DEVELOPMENT, 1970–1991

Concern about the state of the hospital pharmaceutical service eventually persuaded the government to set up a Committee of Enquiry. The Noel Hall Report was published in 1970 (Report of the Working Party on the Hospital Pharmaceutical Service 1970). At the core of the recommendations was the belief that hospital pharmacy needed to be organized on a larger scale, with several pooling their resources in Noel Hall areas, and that these should be coordinated on a regional basis.

Other reports and health circulars promoted and legitimized many of the innovations that had been developed in a small number of centres. Substantial pay increases were awarded, a proper career structure was established and the early 1970s saw a period of rapid expansion and some specialization. By the end of the 1970s, ward pharmacy was practised in most hospitals, a drug information network had been established and other specialities such as purchasing and radiopharmacy had emerged.

By the 1980s, financial restraint was being applied to the health service. Hospital pharmacy was not immune. It was nevertheless able to establish new activities that contributed to cost control, such as formulary development, and many pharmacists began to specialize in a particular area of clinical pharmacy, such as paediatrics or cardiology.

## RECOGNITION AND SPECIALIZATION, 1991 TO THE PRESENT

The 1990s were to see some contraction of the service, as the more senior posts at district and region levels disappeared following health service changes. A banding system replaced the earlier flexible grading system, and since then, the service has had to contend with further rounds of health service reform, including hospital closures, and found itself with a chronic recruitment crisis, mirroring the experience in the 1950s and 1960s. Opportunities were nevertheless taken to restructure both pharmacy services and staffing.

An important milestone in the history of hospital pharmacy occurred in 2003 with the creation of the first consultant pharmacist posts. This new role was identified in the government White Paper *A Vision for Pharmacy in the New NHS*. It offered an opportunity for pharmacists to make a greater difference to patient care and to build on the success of pharmacists in developing clinical and other specialist roles. The title 'consultant pharmacist' was to apply only to those appointed to approved posts and who met the appropriate level of competence; it was not to be conferred solely in recognition of excellence or innovative practice.

Consultant pharmacists were to be appointed to new and innovative posts. They were to be equally applicable to both PCTs and hospital based services, with posts being based on local need. In practice, most consultant pharmacists work in hospitals; the first consultants were clinical specialist pharmacists. The posts are structured around four functions: expert practice; research, evaluation and service development; education, mentoring and overview of practice; and professional leadership.

Today, consultant pharmacist posts exist in many hospitals, but inevitably progress has proceeded at different rates in different parts of the country. Partly to address this issue, the Royal Pharmaceutical Society published professional standards for hospital pharmacy services in 2012, and in 2014 an updated version placed greater emphasis on patient involvement, organizational transparency and leadership development. Some specialist hospital pharmaceutical services such as aseptic medicines preparation and the provision of medicines information are currently commissioned at the national level.

The greater professional recognition of the pharmacist in the hospital setting was accompanied by an expansion of the role of the pharmacy technician. Increasingly, roles such as dispensary manager – one previously usually held by a pharmacist – are taken by senior and experienced technicians, who also increasingly take on roles not requiring the full range of clinical skills of the modern hospital pharmacist.

## CONCLUSION

This chapter has provided a brief overview of the long and tortuous journey by which pharmacy has become the separate and distinct profession that it is today. It has evolved in different ways at different rates in different countries, but developments in one country have often been strongly influenced by those in another. Through its close ties to Europe, through its colonial past and through its pioneering spirit, pharmacy in Britain has not only adopted ideas from elsewhere but also strongly influenced developments in many countries. Above all, the pharmacy profession today is a product of the social, political, economic and technological forces existing in the country where it is practiced.

Since the formation of the Pharmaceutical Society in 1841, pharmaceutical politicians and commentators have referred to pharmacy being 'at the crossroads' at regular intervals. The metaphor of the crossroads emphasizes the need to make often difficult choices at regular intervals, and it is one of the strengths of pharmacy that it has had many choices to make. The metaphor is less helpful, however, in suggesting that progress is made by choosing the 'right' route and rejecting the others. In fact, successful professions tend to be those that proceed along several routes from the crossroads simultaneously.

With hindsight, it can be seen that pharmacy in Britain suffered during the 1950s and 1960s by proceeding down one route at the expense of others. It was assumed that status, respect and prosperity would follow from increased educational achievement by making the profession degree-only entry. At the same time, there was a lack of attention paid to what pharmacists – particularly those in the community – were actually doing, and the extent to which this contributed to the well-being of the public. The lessons of recent history for pharmacy are that prosperity and survival depend on its capacity to respond quickly to the social, political, economic and technological factors that shape the world in which it operates, and to keep a close eye on the added value it provides, rather than on internal matters of little public interest.

## Is Pharmacy Returning to Its Roots?

Pharmacists in Britain can trace their origins to the apothecaries of the eighteenth and nineteenth centuries. The apothecary was a readily accessible health practitioner, located in shop premises, who diagnosed minor complaints and prescribed something for them and who sold made-up medicines or ingredients for domestic remedies, usually for a few pennies. Some even undertook house visits, although they were not permitted to charge for services rendered, only for any medicines supplied. They were established in the community and known by most of the local inhabitants.

These defining elements of community pharmacy continued well into the twentieth century, but the advent of the NHS increasingly tied the pharmacist to the dispensary, dispensing prescriptions. The 'Ask Your Pharmacist' campaign in the 1980s, the extended role in the 1990s and the 'Pharmacy In A New Age' initiative in the 2000s can be seen as attempts to draw pharmacists out of the dispensary (which was usually at the back of the shop) to the front of the shop, where they would be more accessible to the public and where they could engage in a wide range of pharmacy and health-related activities. Here they would again be the 'first port of call' for the public seeking medical attention, they would be a source of advice and information about medicines to the public and they would prescribe from an increasingly long list of recently deregulated medicines.

At the same time as pharmacists were becoming more accessible, doctors were becoming less accessible, as group practice became the norm, appointment schemes were introduced and prescription charges continued to increase. The changes in pharmacy practice in the last quarter of the twentieth century were also an attempt to move away from a product-orientated approach to medicines towards a more patient-focused one. Despite the fact that the first decades of the twenty-first century have seen further attempts to transform pharmacy and pharmacists, change in public perceptions of the community pharmacist may be hindered by the ever-increasing number of prescriptions being presented and the public's continuing association of the pharmacist with their dispensing.

The creation of the General Pharmaceutical Council in 2010 heralded the start of the most significant period of change in the Pharmaceutical Society's 169-year history. The emergence of consultant and prescribing pharmacists mirrors the role of the apothecary in the eighteenth and nineteenth centuries. The creation of dual registers for pharmacists and pharmacy technicians reflects the dual registers for chemists and druggists and pharmaceutical chemists that existed between 1868 and 1954. The developing role of the pharmacy technician mirrors the additional responsibilities taken on by many dispensers in the first half of the twentieth century. Consultant pharmacists with prescribing rights now often have more in common with some of their medical colleagues than other pharmacists.

In many important ways, developments in the practice of community pharmacy in Britain since the 1986 Nuffield Report can be seen as a return to the traditional role of the community pharmacist as a key health resource in the community, available without appointment and at no cost to the patient – someone with a continuing and knowledgeable relationship with the local community, a relationship that had been heavily eroded following the introduction of the NHS in 1948. History has important lessons to teach those who have the responsibility of shaping the practice of pharmacy in the future.

## FURTHER READING

Anderson, S.C. 2000. Community pharmacy in Great Britain: Mediation at the boundary between professional and lay care 1920 to 1995. In T. Tansey and M. Gijswijt-Hofstra (Eds.), *Remedies and Healing Cultures in Britain and the Netherlands in the Twentieth Century*. Amsterdam: Rodopi, 75–97.

Anderson, S.C. 2005. *Making Medicines: A Brief History of Pharmacy and Pharmaceuticals*. London: Pharmaceutical Press.

Anderson, S.C. and Berridge, V.S. 2000. The role of the community pharmacist in health and welfare 1911 to 1986. In J. Bornat, R.B. Perks, P. Thompson and J. Walmsley (Eds.), *Oral History, Health and Welfare*. London: Routledge, 48–74.

Church, R. and Tansey, E.M. 2007. *Burroughs Wellcome & Co.: Knowledge, Trust, Profit and the Transformation of the British Pharmaceutical Industry 1880–1940*. Lancaster: Crucible Books.

Crellin, J.K. 2004. *A Social History of Medicines in the Twentieth Century: To Be Taken Three Times a Day*. Binghampton, New York: The Howarth Press, Inc.

Greene, J.A. and Watkins, E.S. 2012. *Prescribed: Writing, Filling, Using and Abusing the Prescription in Modern America*. Baltimore, Maryland: The Johns Hopkins University Press.

Hardy, A. 2000. *Health and Medicine in Britain since 1860*. London: Palgrave Macmillan.

Holloway, S.W.F. 1991. *Royal Pharmaceutical Society of Great Britain 1841 to 1991: A Political and Social History*. London: Pharmaceutical Press.

Homan, P.G., Hudson, B. and Rowe, R.C. 2007. *Popular Medicines: An Illustrated History*. London: Pharmaceutical Press.

Hudson, B., with Boylan, M. 2013. *The School of Pharmacy, University of London: Medicines, Science and Society, 1842–2012*. London: Academic Press.

Porter, R. 1999. *The Greatest Benefit to Mankind: A Medical History of Humanity from Antiquity to the Present*. New York: W. W. Norton & Company.

Porter, R. (ed.). 2006. *The Cambridge History of Medicine*. Cambridge: Cambridge University Press.

Risse, G.B. 1990. *Mending Bodies, Saving Souls: A History of Hospitals*. Oxford: Oxford University Press.

Rivett, G. 1998. *From Cradle to Grave: 50 Years of the NHS*. London: The Kings Fund.

## REFERENCES

Anderson, S.C. 2007a. Community pharmacists and tobacco in Great Britain: From selling cigarettes to smoking cessation services. *Addiction*, **102**, 704–712.

Anderson, S.C. 2007b. Community pharmacy and public health in Great Britain 1936 to 2006: How a phoenix rose from the Ashes. *Journal of Epidemiology and Community Health*, **61**, 844–848. Available at http://www.ncbi.nlm.nih.gov/pmc/articles/PMC2652958/pdf/844.pdf.

Anderson, S.C. 2008. From 'bespoke' to 'off-the-peg': Community pharmacists and the retailing of medicines in Great Britain 1900 to 1970. *Pharmacy in History*, **50**(2), 43–69.

Anderson, S.C. 2012. Expert committees, welfare and education: The transformation of the hospital pharmacist in Great Britain 1920 to 1995. *Twentieth Century Studies*, **12**, 289–310.

Anderson, S.C. 2013. Pharmacopoeias of Great Britain. In *A History of the Pharmacopoeias of the World*. Berlin, Germany: International Society for the History of Pharmacy, 1–8. Available at http://www.histpharm.org/ISHPWG%20UK.pdf.

Department of Health. 2000. *Pharmacy in the Future: Implementing the NHS Plan*. London: The Stationery Office.

Department of Health. 2004. *A Vision for Pharmacy in the New NHS*. London: The Stationery Office.

Department of Health. 2005. *Choosing Health Through Pharmacy: A Programme for Pharmaceutical Public Health 2005–2015*. London: The Stationery Office.

Department of Health. 2007. *Trust, Assurance and Safety: The Regulation of Health Professionals in the 21st Century*. London: The Stationery Office.

Department of Health and Royal Pharmaceutical Society of Great Britain. 1992. *Pharmaceutical Care: The Future for Community Pharmacy*. London: Royal Pharmaceutical Society of Great Britain.

Hall, N. (chairman). 1970. *Report of the Working Party on the Hospital Pharmaceutical Service*. London: HMSO.

Nuffield Committee of Inquiry into Pharmacy. 1986. *Pharmacy: A Report to the Nuffield Foundation*. London: Nuffield Foundation.

Royal Pharmaceutical Society of Great Britain. 1996. *Pharmacy in a New Age: The New Horizon*. London: The Royal Pharmaceutical Society of Great Britain.

Royal Pharmaceutical Society of Great Britain. 1997. *Pharmacy in a New Age: Building the Future*. London: The Royal Pharmaceutical Society of Great Britain.

# 2 Pharmacy and Public Health Policy

*David Taylor, Zahraa Mohammed Ali and James Davies*

## CONTENTS

---

### KEY POINTS

- Pharmacists have long acted as both suppliers of medicines and health care providers.
- The roles of the three main health professions – medicine, pharmacy and nursing – are, in the UK, still largely defined by the events surrounding the formation of the National Health Service in 1948.
- New models of pharmacy may be considered as aiming to provide more cost-effective and consumer need-responsive systems of self-care support and primary care provision.

- In addition to supporting optimal use of medicines, pharmacists may contribute to the achievement of health policy goals, such as reducing smoking and obesity.
- Public health roles for community pharmacists may be limited by the timidity of the profession's leaders and a lack of evidence of interventional effectiveness.
- Public health has undergone – and is undergoing – a global transition associated with increasing life expectancies.
- There are many examples of policy and practice initiatives linking public health and community pharmacy development.
- Despite numerous initiatives over recent years, community pharmacy has remained fundamentally a dispensing volume-driven activity.
- A number of issues are critically linked to the future of pharmacy and its capacity to enhance public health, namely: IT developments and robotic dispensing; working relationships with other health care professionals; and payment structures for health care.

## INTRODUCTION

This chapter explores issues relating to the future of community pharmacy and its role not only in supplying medicines, but also in seeking proactively to contribute to improvements in the public's health status. Traditional pharmacy practice has deep roots throughout Europe. The existence of pharmacy predates the industrial production of drugs and their original pack distribution. The profession was fostered by the mediaeval need for a group of practitioners who could earn an adequate income from and (in return for the grant of monopoly rights) be held accountable for the safe compounding, storage and supply of medicines. Medicines traditionally included not only concentrated 'pills' and tablets (which were introduced relatively recently) but also the various tinctures, ointments and dry and fluid mixtures popular in the pre-modern era as 'chemist'-made remedies (see Chapter 1 for a full account of the historical development of pharmacy).

Pharmacists and their predecessors have also long acted as health care providers, offering 'product plus service' combinations involving diagnostic activities as well as treatment and wider health advice. Payment for the latter has typically been incorporated in the price of any medicines supplied, rather than being charged separately.

Fundamental differences between medical and community pharmacy remuneration mechanisms persist today. They are often, if perhaps wrongly, assumed to mark basic differences in the nature of pharmacists as professionals, compared with doctors and nurses.

Members of the medical profession are frequently in 'ideal-type' terms seen as the providers of financially disinterested guidance. They are (specialisms aside) regarded as receiving fees in return for protecting and improving the public's health, rather than marketing particular therapies. Pharmacists, practising in both independent and corporately owned pharmacies, are, by contrast, more likely to be perceived as 'commercially' motivated. That is, their primary motivation is taken to be trade and product-sale related, as opposed to enhancing health outcomes (see Chapter 12 for further discussion of the occupational status of pharmacists). Similar considerations surround the social position of pharmaceutical companies, which today produce innovative medicines in return for the transient financial protections offered by patents and other forms of intellectual property protection.

## PUBLICLY FUNDED HEALTH SERVICES

In the UK, the presently accepted roles of the three main health professions have been defined by events surrounding the establishment of the National Health Service (NHS) in 1948, and the subsequent evolution of health care as a largely state-funded, central command-orientated, economy sector. In the aftermath of World War II, when the UK's political leaders were urgently seeking to redefine the nation's post-imperial domestic identity and its new international role, the UK temporarily led the world in taking forward Soviet-pioneered thinking on publicly resourced (yet not necessarily publicly owned or provided) universal health care provision. However, 'care transition'-associated processes (see Box 2.1) have affected all economically developed nations in the last half century, including the UK.

---

### BOX 2.1   CARE TRANSITION

The terms 'demographic' and 'epidemiological' transition are in common use and refer to the changing patterns of population structure and disease occurrence characteristic of human development in Europe and elsewhere in the last 200 years. By contrast, 'care transition' is used here to refer to the socio-economic changes that societies go through as they move from conditions of poverty, high mortality and short life expectancy to relative affluence and greater longevity.

For the purposes of this chapter, key points to highlight include increasing gender-related equality/equity as birth rates fall and child care requirements change, through to the emergence of universal health care funding systems as individuals and families become more certain of survival into later life. The social status of professionals such as pharmacists tends to rise as transition processes commence, and is to a degree re-normalized as populations become older and more educated. The value of medicines as actual and potential determinates of population health typically increases as communities move through the stages of macro- and micro-environmental improvement and the extrinsic challenges of living with relative plenty towards facing the intrinsic biological challenges associated with average life expectancy at birth rising to more than 80 years.

The creation of the NHS had radical implications in many areas, ranging from assuring individual access to high-cost specialist care, to the formation of public health strategies aimed at optimizing population health within the finite quantum of public funding available. With regard to community pharmacy, the establishment of the NHS in the late 1940s coincided with the start of the first great therapeutic drug revolution and the mass prescribing of antibiotics. As described in Chapter 1, this more or less instantly quadrupled the volume of items dispensed via independently owned community pharmacies in the UK.

Similar developments occurred in the nationalized hospitals. However, the simultaneous provision of free access to general practitioner (GP) care served to narrow the role of community pharmacy around the physical provision of medicines in a way that differed from the hospital pharmacy experience. In the latter context, opportunities emerged (especially after the lessons of thalidomide at the start of the 1960s and with the legal freedoms and finances required to employ pharmacy assistants in hospital dispensaries) for pharmacists to have significant inputs in safely introducing new medicines and in developing the appropriate clinical use of established and innovative therapies in areas such as cardiology, gastroenterology, oncology and psychiatry.

However, because the public – in the main – turned to 'family doctors' for diagnosis and treatment once their services became free at the point of demand (although GPs remained independently contracted professionals), this reduced the use of community pharmacies as intermediate-level health and self-care support centres. While becoming increasingly busy with high-volume NHS dispensing – it is in this sense misleading to describe community pharmacists as 'underutilized' – the positioning of pharmacies as private 'shops' that, as a large part of their trade, supply products that 'NHS doctors' prescribe put them in a marginalized position as far as health care provision was concerned.

The fact that GPs and, following the 'Doctors' Charter of the mid-1960s, their expanding practice teams typically worked in premises apart from those owned by pharmacists and pharmacy companies amplified the consequences of this trend. Combined with the cumulative loss of medicine-making activities that occurred as modern pharmaceutical manufacturing asserted its dominance, this unintended consequence of the NHS's establishment led to progressively more overt questioning of the value of community pharmacy.

The more recent developments of the Internet and computerized dispensing and medicines information technologies has further challenged the 'early NHS' pharmacy and wider primary care model. It has created similar tensions in regions such as North America and other parts of Europe, as well as in countries as far distant as Japan and Australia. Measures aimed at extending the 'public health' roles of pharmacists and establishing 'healthy living' and other revised models of pharmacy can be seen as attempts to counter fears that community pharmacy is becoming – or has become – redundant in its current format.

## Public Health or Clinical Care?

More positively from a public interest perspective, changes to pharmacy models can also be taken as being aimed at providing more cost-effective and consumer need-responsive systems of self-care support and primary care provision. Against this background, this chapter explores, with particular regard to public health activities, the future of pharmacy in the community setting, where in the order of 90% of all Organization for Economic Co-operation and Development (OECD) country pharmacists work. (The 20%–25% figures for hospital pharmacy employment reported in the US and the UK are international outliers.)

Over and above supporting the optimally effective use of medicines and vaccines for the purposes of primary, secondary and tertiary prevention, pharmacists seek to contribute to policy goals such as cutting smoking rates and hazardous alcohol consumption, reducing the harm associated with illicit drug use and lowering obesity levels. They can in addition contribute to sexual health – at least in terms of sexually transmitted infection prevention, detection and treatment – and to emergency and routine birth control, as well as to appropriately informed self-care at all life stages. The latter is important because chronic diseases may take several decades to develop.

The analysis in this chapter centres mainly on English and wider UK policy and practice experience. However, it also draws from studies of the challenges being faced and opportunities available for pharmaceutical care development in other EU member states and in countries such as Australia, New Zealand, Canada, the United States and Japan.

Two further linked sets of introductory points deserve special emphasis. The first is that some observers, well-grounded in established public health practices such as developing fiscal policies and retail sector regulations aimed at facilitating population-level changes in health behaviours, question the extent to which community pharmacists should be seen as providing 'public health' services. Pharmacists can undoubtedly contribute to public health goals, such as reducing the incidence of vascular system diseases and events. However, the degree to which community pharmacists can do this by means other than clinical interventions that closely parallel those already employed by GPs and other conventional health professionals is questionable.

At one level, concerns of this nature can be seen as merely semantic. Yet the view taken here is that approaches which centre on strengthening the 'public health' role of pharmacy are on occasion intended to disguise or at least downplay the extent to which their end is in fact to increase the part independently played by pharmacists in the diagnosis and day-to-day medical treatment of common conditions. Progress of this type could, in theory at least, facilitate changes in the workloads of GPs and in turn those of hospitals, even if not all doctors welcome the prospect of increases in the severity and complexity of the care needs of those they see on a daily basis.

Presentational tactics which lack transparency may be understandable in as much as they are intended to reduce resistance to changes in professional roles. However, they should not obscure policy objectives in ways that undermine social purpose. Although there is a great deal of evidence that pharmacists can usefully provide services that contribute to the achievement of public health goals, there is at the same time little reason to believe that community pharmacists are any better equipped to cost-effectively facilitate health behaviour changes than any other group of primary health care professionals. Indeed, to the extent that many members of the public do not as yet expect to receive authoritative health as opposed to drug use-related advice from pharmacists, they may be at a relative (albeit potentially correctable) disadvantage.

Pharmacists are arguably relatively well positioned to extend their existing diagnostic roles in relation to 'minor'/common illnesses and to take direct responsibility for prescribing treatments as well as supporting medicines use in areas such as cardiovascular and respiratory disease prevention and management. It will not serve UK or other public interests well if a desire to avoid overt competition and/or conflict with the medical profession, and by implication disruption to existing business models and income streams, were to lead pharmacists and their representatives to pursue 'public health' roles of only marginal value to the community, when alternative reforms could deliver more substantive improvements in health and well-being.

Following on from the above, health policy analysts such as Mossialos et al. (2013) have concluded that there is as yet inadequate evidence to support expanding the health care role of community pharmacists. He and allied authors have observed that implementing such developments on a universal basis would (were they to alter system dynamics sufficiently to make significant impacts on care quality and cost effectiveness) require potentially disruptive changes elsewhere in the health economy. Such analysts argue that considerable additional research will be needed to justify major reforms. To date, extending the public health role of community pharmacy in England, America and elsewhere has in the main been confined to making limited and in overall terms largely income- and cost-neutral alterations in medicines management and pharmaceutical care support arrangements, rather more radical interventions.

There is some truth in such assessments. However, fundamental system developments cannot normally be fully justified on the basis of prospectively available evidence. By definition, they need to have taken place before full evaluations are possible. 'Normal' markets function via trial and error, incremental changes and variable rate shifts in public preferences and provider side income streams when new products and services are offered to consumers. In heavily regulated, bureaucratically funded health care settings, user choice-driven 'organic' evolution of this type is very difficult, if not impossible, to achieve. Sometimes, the more that detailed, centrally negotiated, contracts attempt to simulate market conditions, the more they paradoxically serve to preserve the structural status quo.

Having said this, the research undertaken for this chapter indicates that the NHS's record of positive change in relation to both community pharmacy and public health service protection is at least as strong as that of most other health care systems, including those of the United States, Germany, France, Japan and Australia. It has been fundamentally more robust than that of services in countries like, for instance, the Soviet Union/Russian Federation and India in the last half century. Nevertheless, in the eyes of many individual pharmacists and British patient representatives, change has been slow and in some respects disappointing. If the implementation of health policy innovations were to become more dependent on prospective evidence of effectiveness, as distinct from logical and intellectually honest analysis of the limited information available, future progress would, even with increased political will, be likely to remain relatively slow.

The architects of the NHS were not required to present detailed 'proof' of the effectiveness of their proposals before implementation. If this had been the case the UK's new health service would in all probability have been stillborn. The fact that it survived was in large part because in the period during and shortly after the Second World War, Britain was unusually united with regard to its sense of social purpose and common interest. Hence the power of sectional interests to overtly or covertly stand in the way of changes that most people believed desirable was, for a time, muted.

## GLOBAL PUBLIC HEALTH TRANSITION: A TWENTIETH CENTURY SUCCESS

France's unique history involved significant population growth well before the eighteenth century. Nevertheless, the worldwide process of demographic and epidemiological transition that will move towards its close in the coming 50–100 years is conventionally said to have commenced in the Netherlands and Great Britain at the start of the 1800s. The initial steps in the momentous public health shift from short average life expectancies and high age-specific death rates (and dramatically high infant mortality rates) balanced by high birth rates through to long average life expectancies and low birth and age-specific death rates were in large part centred on improved food supply. This enhanced the immune status of young adults, which helped reduce mortality and morbidity rates and increased their working capacity (Figure 2.1).

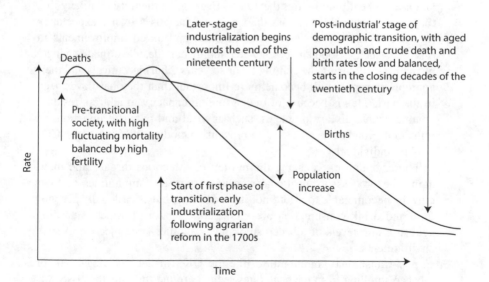

**FIGURE 2.1** In pre-transitional communities, crude birth and death rates may exceed 40 per 1,000 of the population, while in post-transitional settings, they can be under 10. This figure describes Western European experience. Other world regions' transitions have differed in their timing but are following broadly similar paths.

Improved health was driven by better sanitation, access to clean water and enhanced literacy. This subsequently led to better standards of family and self-care. In European and related settings, such developments occurred alongside reduced child death rates and opened the way to the major infant mortality declines seen in the first decades of the twentieth century.

The next main 'stage' of public health development (from approximately the 1970s) was marked by the beginnings of better survival rates for people aged 60 and over. Post-transitional populations are 'older' than pre-transitional communities, in the sense that they have lower birth rates and hence greater proportions of individuals who are older regardless of mortality shifts. Epidemiologically, this is reflected in decreased infectious disease burdens and increased prevalence rates for non-communicable diseases (NCDs), including rheumatic diseases, atherosclerosis, other hypertension-linked disorders, type 2 diabetes, cancers and neurological and allied conditions such as the dementias. However, at the same time, most aspects of age-standardized population health are much better in post-transitional settings than in less-developed environments.

Average global life expectancy at birth has increased by more than 30 years since the start of the twentieth century. Even in less-advantaged countries, life expectancy at birth today is comparable to or better than it was in England at the peak of its imperial power. Such data raise many vital questions, though for the purposes of this chapter, the most important points to note about demographic transition and the changes in public health and the associated health care needs associated with it are:

1. Medicines and vaccines had relatively little capacity to impact upon population-level health until after the 1940s. Even since then, it is unlikely that they have accounted for more than half the increases in life expectancy recorded. However, provided environmental and allied improvements in essentials such as food and clean water supply can (despite climate change) be maintained during the coming 50 or so years, pharmaceuticals and their appropriate supply will become more important than they have ever been in the past. This is because of their growing capacity to address residual communicable disease problems, such as viral and parasitic infections in vulnerable younger people, and to prevent or modify the course of NCDs in older individuals.

2. In poorer countries, reducing the burden of infectious disease and managing the process of nutritional transition seen in communities as their citizens become able to afford not just adequate, but occasionally surplus, food and drink consumption are vital public health priorities. Guarding against rising levels of tobacco smoking is another key objective in such environments.

3. In post-transitional communities, like the UK, further reducing levels of tobacco smoking from the peak rates seen at around the time the NHS was first established remains an important public health priority. Others include meeting the challenges of mental health protection and care and minimizing the harm associated with the patterns of obesity typically found in populations that have experienced more than one or two generations of

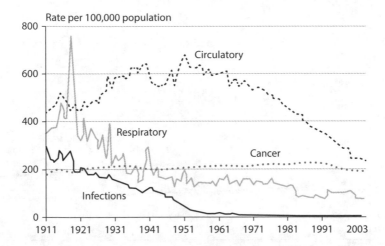

**FIGURE 2.2**  Age-standardized mortality rates for England and Wales from 1911 to 2003 by broad disease group. (From Office of National Statistics.)

plentiful food supply and good health care. In this context, it is important to observe that although rates of diagnosed type 2 diabetes are now higher than at any time in the past, circulatory disease mortality has, in age-adjusted terms, fallen by about two-thirds since the establishment of the NHS (Figures 2.2, 2.3a,b). However, avoidable vascular disease-related disability rates remain high.

4. During the twentieth century, nations spent more of their rising incomes on health care as they became wealthier and attached increasing importance to health and social care provision, even as age-specific levels of risk fell. Such trends can, as has already been noted, be described as part of a process of 'care transition'. Along with increased public and obligatory private insurance-based health service funding, this is also associated with factors such as enhanced gender equality and (initially) the professionalization of many caregiving roles. Later in the human development sequence, this latter trend is likely to be followed by a recovered emphasis on patient-led decision making and informed self-care, as educational standards and personal control-linked expectations rise and new economic pressures emerge.

## UK PUBLIC HEALTH POLICIES

Historically, the development of 'public health' as a multidisciplinary area of health protection and promotion activity, linked to population-wide efforts to initially prevent infections and ensure water and food purity and subsequently to 'improve' lifestyles, has run more or less in parallel with the demographic and epidemiological transitions described above. In Britain, the work of early nineteenth-century pioneers such as Edwin Chadwick (who began his career as Jeremy Bentham's secretary) led on from the initial creation of better sanitation systems, via legislation introduced in the 1830s and 1840s, to changes in the Poor Law and the establishment

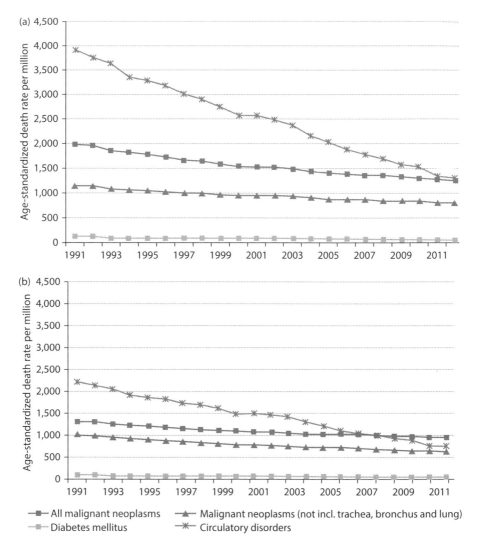

**FIGURE 2.3**  (a) Age-standardized mortality rates for men in England and Wales for selected conditions from 1991 to 2012. (b) Age-standardized mortality rates for women in England and Wales for selected conditions from 1991 to 2012. (From Office of National Statistics.)

of local authority-based Medical Officers of Health. These and other reforms in time facilitated better mother and child care, and in the early to mid-twentieth century promoted enhanced 'home hygiene', followed by a gradually increasing focus on meeting the challenges of living with relative plenty (see also Box 2.2).

There is evidence that people's willingness to collectively fund universal services increases as they become more confident that they, and their children, will survive into later life and tribal and other internal societal divisions grow less important. However, rising tax burdens may in time conflict not only with personal ambitions, but also national abilities to prosper in a competitive global environment.

## BOX 2.2   DEFINING PUBLIC HEALTH AND THE
## PUBLIC HEALTH USE OF MEDICINES

With the effective control of most infectious disease threats having been achieved in Europe through environmental protections, vaccination programmes and medicine use, public health in the richer nations is no longer as medically dominated as it was a century ago. At the start of the 1920s, Charles-Edward Winslow (a Boston-based bacteriologist who played a pioneering role in the establishment of modern public health approaches) first defined public health as 'the science and art of preventing disease, prolonging life and promoting health through the organized efforts and informed choices of society, organizations, public and private, communities and individuals'.

This definition has subsequently been modified, but remains robust. Public health programmes are now typically focused on objectives such as stopping smoking and curbing socially-defined behavioural problems (e.g. physical inactivity and other factors linked to obesity). However, this is not to discount the importance of tasks such as maintaining food safety and controlling outbreaks of food poisoning, or the importance of public health intervention in relation to issues such as atmospheric pollution and the minimization of health inequalities within affluent societies.

From a pharmaceutical perspective, modern public health practice may also be taken to encompass areas such as the mass use of statins and anti-hypertensive medicines for the community-wide reduction of vascular disease risks. This remains a controversial approach among some observers, as indeed is, on occasion, the use of vaccines for the purposes of primary prevention. However, the view taken here is that as biomedicine and the pharmaceutical and allied sciences continue to develop, there will be increasing efforts to use medicines proactively to modify very early disease-linked processes. Although many doctors understandably see treating overtly sick individuals as their core task, future health care provision will become increasingly concerned with earlier-stage individual and population-level interventions.

In Europe, public health policy objectives, in part, generally reflect the perceived requirement for decision makers to increase the productivity of their countries. This may be achieved by curbing the incidence of disabilities due to NCDs where possible and by increasing the rights and capacities of older people to work productively and/ or to live independently without an undue need for relatively costly forms of care and support.

The 'return to the apothecary' school of future pharmacy development believes that community pharmacy services could play an important part in chronic disease management. There is robust evidence that more could be done to limit the incidence and impacts of events such as myocardial infarctions and strokes due to common causes such as raised blood pressure and tobacco smoking. In the cardiology arena there are also important opportunities for raising the quality of treatment available for individuals and families affected by disorders such as atrial fibrillation and hyper-cholesterolemia, in part by improved case identification in the community setting.

Reducing obesity-linked health risks in middle and later life is a related public health goal. The time span over which such efforts can be expected to contribute tangible returns is in many instances relatively long. Yet they should eventually reduce not only musculoskeletal disabilities but also the incidence of type 2 diabetes and some forms of dementia and (even if just marginally) cancer. Similar points apply in the context of preventing and effectively treating respiratory illnesses like chronic obstructive pulmonary disease (COPD) and asthma, and infections such as urinary tract infections (UTIs). As with improving the support for people living with, for instance, heart failure, innovative forms of primary and community care allied with enhanced medicines use should reduce avoidable hospital admission rates. The prevention and better handling of emergencies through anticipatory care where possible, and rapid responses when necessary, could also relieve health care system pressures and costs.

Awareness of the need to address more effectively the treatment and support of people with chronic diseases dates back to the beginning of this period, and the publication of public health policy documents such as *Prevention and Health – Everybody's Business* in 1976. So too does the aspiration to improve community pharmacy's positive contributions to the public's health status. Understanding why, in practice, responses to these challenges have not been as successful as some policy makers may have originally hoped could help promote faster progress in the future.

## COMMUNITY PHARMACY: FROM PHARMACEUTICAL SUPPLY TO PHARMACEUTICAL CARE?

### UK COMMUNITY PHARMACY

The present British debate on the future of community pharmacy and pharmacists' roles in pharmaceutical/health care dates back to the start of the 1980s. Dr Gerard Vaughan (a child psychiatrist who became a member of Parliament and was appointed Health Minister in Prime Minister Margaret Thatcher's first administration) told the 1981 British Pharmaceutical Conference that 'one knew there was a future for hospital pharmacists, one knew there was a future for industrial pharmacists, but one was not sure that one knew the future for the general practice [community] pharmacist'. Although mild in terms of today's political discourse, this statement sent shock waves through the community pharmacy world. (In much the same way, the then Secretary of State Patrick Jenkin's low-key publication of the previous Labour government-commissioned Black Report on *Inequalities in Health* over a bank holiday weekend in 1980 had shortly before outraged sections of the public health community.)

The Vaughan intervention was followed in 1986 by the publication of the Nuffield Foundation report: *Pharmacy*. A cascade of subsequent initiatives and new publications followed over the ensuing decades, ranging from the then Royal Pharmaceutical Society of Great Britain's *Pharmacy in a New Age* campaign in the 1990s through to, for instance, the 2002 publication *The Right Medicine: A Strategy for Pharmaceutical Care in Scotland* and the 2008 English White Paper *Pharmacy in England: Building on Strengths – Delivering the Future.* The latest documents in this long line of plans and analyses include the Royal Pharmaceutical Society (RPS)/ Nuffield Foundation's 2013 report *Now or Never: Shaping Pharmacy for the Future* and its 2014 follow-up *Now More than Ever: Why Pharmacy needs to Act.*

There are also numerous examples of UK policy and practice initiatives linking public health and community pharmacy development. These include the establishment by the Department of Health and partner organizations of the Pharmacy and Public Health Forum in 2011 and the associated 2014 publication by Public Health England of the *Developing Pharmacy's Contribution to Public Health* progress report. This has recently been complemented by detailed work on the management of COPD in the community pharmacy setting, which builds on other pilot studies conducted in areas such as pain, weight and alcohol-use management.

There has also been a substantive effort made in developing the healthy living pharmacy (HLP) concept. This was first pioneered in Portsmouth, and has since been developed nationally. There were in the order of 800 accredited HLPs at the start of 2015.

It would be unfair to conclude that nothing of significance has been achieved as a result of these and other well-intended efforts, or via the linked introduction of (for example) the revised Community Pharmacy Contractual Framework and the funding of Medicines Use Reviews (MURs) in England in 2005, the Scottish Chronic Medication Service in 2010 and the English New Medicine Service in 2013. It would also be inappropriate to expect measures of this sort to have a short-term impact on public health data and observable medication use outcomes, and foolhardy not to acknowledge that presently most pharmacists are working hard to fulfil the basic pharmacy function of safely supplying what is now close to one billion NHS prescription items a year in England alone.

However, having acknowledged this, it is reasonable to argue that, given the background described elsewhere in this book, it is disappointing that in the period since the original 1986 Nuffield report (published in 1986) the fundamental nature of community pharmacy practice as a dispensing volume-driven activity has remained largely unchanged. The fact that there is little substantive evidence that the public has come to see community pharmacists primarily as health professionals as distinct from retailers of medicinal and allied product is also disturbing.

The recent *Now or Never* and *Now More than Ever* publications from the RPS and the Nuffield Trust reflect such concerns. So to an extent do documents such as NHS England's 2014 *Five Year Forward View*. At heart, the Nuffield analysis concludes that as a profession, pharmacy in the UK (and elsewhere) is weakly led. This may be because of a fundamental divide between the commercial imperatives underlying the interests of both corporate and independent pharmacy owners and the health care delivery aspirations of a proportion of the currently growing pharmacy workforce. It is of note in this last context that Simon Stephens, the ex-Tony Blair administration adviser who is now the CEO of the English NHS, recently and somewhat ominously commented that 'There is something paradoxical in that we have a surfeit of pharmacists as a result of the number coming through training and yet we also have a surfeit of strategies down the years describing how "If only we could get pharmacies more involved in primary care that would be a win–win for everybody"'. In early

2015, plans were announced for employing up to 3,000 pharmacists in English GP practices.

Financial return drivers have in the past tended to confine pharmacy involvement in care processes to fairly mechanistic 'tick box'-type interventions, rather than pushing into areas requiring free communication and the complex psycho-social interactions fundamentally needed to address serious health and medicine taking-related problems. Without a movement into more 'professional' work levels, pharmacists are unlikely to gain increased authority over the use of medicines as the social (as opposed to simply pharmacological) objects at the centre of their expertise. (See also Chapter 12.)

Suggestions that the NHS should in future contract with individual community pharmacists (as was originally the case with GPs) rather than with pharmacy owners have highlighted relevant tensions, albeit that similar problems exist in other areas of modern British health care. The close association between the State and the NHS, coupled with the latter's dual commitment to the at times conflicting goals of optimizing public health and providing good, as distinct from simply adequate, quality care for individuals has led to the institutions of independent professionalism coming under more focused pressure from the UK government than has been the case in most other OECD nations. This has on occasion led to disputes as to the extent to which professional bodies exist to discipline their members and support the interests of public or private employers and/or care funders, as opposed to protecting practitioners' freedoms and/or pursuing 'genuine' health care excellence.

At this level of analysis, it is by no means clear that shifts in policy articulation are being matched by concomitant changes in mainstream community pharmacy practice, or that either satisfactorily reflect changing consumer preferences and needs. In this sense, Gerrard Vaughan's challenge remains essentially unanswered more than three decades after it was first made. From the improving public health perspective underpinning this chapter, a core question to ask is 'over and above what is already being achieved, what more can community pharmacists, with or without the support of other primary care and hospital colleagues, most cost effectively do to further reduce death, disability and distress rates from infections, vascular diseases, cancers, psychiatric and neurological disorders and other causes of illness over the next 10–20 years?'

## WORLDWIDE COMMUNITY PHARMACY TRENDS

Within Europe, there have been considerable variations between, for instance, the 'Scandinavian pharmacy model' involving relatively high numbers of individuals (5,000–10,000) served by each dispensing pharmacy (backed by additional prescription supply facilities with the extensive use of qualified prescriptionists/dispensers) and the traditional southern European model, employed in countries such as France, Spain and Greece. In the latter, pharmacies typically serve populations of closer to 2,000, and also have higher pharmacist-to-patient operating ratios. The UK sits about midway on this spectrum, although in some ways its approach to pharmaceutical services development has been uniquely proactive.

It is beyond the scope of this chapter to attempt to describe each European nation's community pharmacy system (more information is presented in Chapter 4). However, the following general points are worth emphasis:

• Countries such as Sweden, Denmark, Germany, France, Portugal and the Netherlands can provide a wide variety of examples of community pharmacy practice developments that parallel progress in the UK nations, in areas such as pharmaceutical care standard setting, conducting MURs, supplying emergency contraception, patient/service user health counselling, repeat medication and chronic condition management, IT infrastructure, medication and wider health record building and improvements in access. In this sense, there appears to be a common direction of travel. Yet it is also true to say that throughout Europe, relatively little has been achieved in terms of changing the working relationships between community pharmacists and doctors and nurses practicing in the community in ways that offer clear advantages to health service users and/or yielding care process savings for service funders.

• In the past, southern European countries tended to have relatively low innovative medicines prices, but high overall pharmaceutical costs. Such combinations are typically associated with high prescribing volumes and, more importantly in financial terms, the frequent use of relatively costly 'branded generic' versions of older pharmaceuticals. In countries that lack research-based pharmaceutical companies and publicly funded research institutions capable of competing internationally, local non-innovative producers have often exercised a dominant influence on policy. Some fear this has, on occasion, served to maintain community pharmacy incomes, but also to distort wider resource allocations. However, the post-2008 recession has, in some settings, forced reductions in medicine outlays which to an extent have cut pharmacy returns to an extent. Most notably, Greek pharmaceutical outlays have recently decreased by about 1% of gross domestic product (GDP). The Netherlands has also seen marked reductions in pharmacy-level returns since the start of this century. European pharmacy remuneration systems are becoming more focused on encouraging low-cost medicines supply and recovering manufacturers' discounts for service funders. Yet from a pharmacy perspective, it is still the case that very little income is derived from fees other than those associated with dispensing or other forms of product supply. The situation in England is unusual in that transfers of money from non-transparent discounting to pharmacies into overt payments for providing services such as MURs have been comparatively easy to track.

• Community pharmacies in Germany and similar countries tend to supply relatively high volumes of not only herbal remedies but also what in other parts of Europe are normally classified as 'hospital treatments'. This has to a degree encouraged developments in areas such as 'mail-order' pharmaceutical supply, although in Europe generally community pharmacies have not as yet been strongly affected by such trends. Likewise, mechanized dispensing and the use of large 'dispensing warehouse'-type systems has to date had less impact on community pharmacy in Europe than in the United States, although it is being actively considered in, for instance, the Scottish environment.

Turning to the situation in North America, the health care funding system and the ownership rules surrounding community pharmacies differ significantly from those in most of Europe. The United States can reasonably claim to be the home of pharmaceutical care, and there has been relatively rapid movement towards offering an extended range of clinical and allied services through medication therapy management and allied initiatives. Although developments are, as elsewhere, 'patchy', American pharmacists have been relatively progressive in forming partnerships with physicians and nurses. These have typically been aimed at delivering enhanced preventative care via, for instance, pharmacy-based lipid management and smoking cessation programmes and the provision of immunizations for all age groups.

As in the UK, US community pharmacists and their pharmacy staff colleagues have demonstrated capacities to manage respiratory diseases and conditions such as osteoporosis. One factor that may have encouraged innovative practices in the American setting is the current pressure on medical staff numbers and employment costs. Another may have been the existence of active competition between alternative health care funders seeking to improve affordable access to, and uptake of, primary care services. However, there is evidence that many western European health care consumers are more satisfied with the health services available to them than their US peers.

Overall health care and medicine outlays are high in the American market settings. (More information on the US health care system is provided in Chapter 5.) While older generic medicines are available at low cost, the prescribing of newer patented (or otherwise intellectual property right [IPR]-protected) products is greater than in other countries. The focus on innovation (in areas like new anti-cancer therapy development the American public carries about half of global public and private research and development costs) is linked to a variety of other cultural differences which make valid US/EU comparisons more difficult than is sometimes assumed. However, once again, there seems to be a broad movement of pharmacy in the direction of clinical practice. This is likely to strengthen if, as seems inevitable, the medicines supply element of the pharmacy workload becomes increasingly automated.

Other illustrations of 'developed' nation community pharmacy system and role evolution can be drawn from countries ranging from South Korea and Japan (where a clear separation between medical prescribing and pharmacist dispensing was comparatively late to emerge) to Australia and Canada. Both of the latter have relatively small populations occupying large physical spaces. While contracting for community-supplied pharmaceutical services is undertaken at the federal level in Australia, the Canadian approach is more devolved.

As in England, community pharmacies in Australia offer medicines reviews via the MedsCheck programme, along with services such as home medication reviews for vulnerable people and health promotion services. (See Chapter 5 for further information regarding the place of pharmacy in the Australian health care system.) In Canada, following initiatives such as the publication of the 2002 Romanow report entitled *Building on Values: The Future of Health Care in Canada*, there has been a series of similar developments, albeit with greater provincial variations. In Alberta and British Columbia, community pharmacists already have access to complete medical/health records. Notwithstanding opposition from some doctors, Canadian pharmacists have limited prescribing rights and can monitor and authorize 'refills' of existing prescriptions, and prescribe and dispense in emergencies (the place of pharmacy in the Canadian health care system is outlined in Chapter 5).

Once again, such provisions largely mirror those that have emerged in the UK countries, but the available data indicate that Canada spends almost twice as much of its GDP on community pharmacy product and service supply than do England, Scotland and Wales. Australia is in an intermediate position. A key driver in this context appears to be Canada's desire to support local generic manufacturing, as distinct from the UK's use of low-cost generic medicines purchased in the global free market by pharmacists and other agents.

## Community Pharmacy Outside Countries of the OECD

The numbers of community pharmacies and pharmacists are, relative to populations served, much lower in poorer countries than in wealthier ones (see also Chapter 7). Just as innovative medicines are normally expensive to purchase in less-advantaged communities, so too are highly trained health professionals costly to employ. A key difference is that after IPR expiry, medicines become much more affordable. By contrast, as they individually and collectively mature, professionals tend to become more expensive.

These realities are to a degree reflected in the fact that in less-developed settings doctors often dispense medicines as well as prescribe them, and that both they and their patients are less likely to recognize pharmacists' authority in relation to determining the appropriate use of medicines than is the case in more affluent settings. To the extent that they are available in less-developed countries, qualified pharmacists are typically concentrated in wealthier urban localities and in tertiary (teaching) hospitals. Although they may express concerns about the quality of medicines available from street sellers, relatively few choose to work in poorer urban or remote rural locations. Even in hospitals, pharmacists in many less-developed countries have often been confined to acting as limited-status 'store keepers' (in Latin, the word *apotheca* originally meant 'storehouse') rather than as experts on medicines.

Some observers may conclude that this makes pharmacists part of the problem of medicines supply in less-affluent communities rather than the solution. However, the view taken here is that if they are willing and able to use their skills to organize and manage robust local medicines supply schemes and regulate prescribing, rather than seeking to apply dispensing practice models developed to meet long-established twentieth century European and North American market needs in radically different environments, there should be no doubt about the value of the roles that pharmacists can play.

In countries with growing economies, such as China and India, there are greater numbers of qualified professionals available. Even so, problems with persuading appropriately trained health care professionals to work in areas of high need are persistent. So also are the challenges inherent in providing minimal-cost therapies to very poor populations, even when bulk drug supplies are easily accessible. Without publicly funded primary care facilities staffed by people paid sufficiently to eliminate the need for them to accept inappropriate fees, progress can be very difficult to achieve.

In China, there is often undue reliance on 'big city' hospital care. Hospital pharmacies are often managed by medically qualified individuals, and in many instances there is little confidence in community-based pharmacists' capacities to act as reliable modern health care providers. Likewise, in India, the quality of modern pharmaceutical care available in poorer localities is often limited, despite recent attempts to improve performance. For instance, government attempts to improve low-cost drug provision via Jan Aushadhi pharmacy stores have to date met with little success. This has been in part because of manufacturers' unwillingness to supply minimally priced 'true generics' and in part because of professional resistance to the model being promulgated.

While India has led the world in areas such as challenging patents on innovative anti-cancer treatments developed mainly in the US and the EU, its domestic record on supplying effective, low-cost mature medicines to poor populations has been less impressive. In addition, both India and China are among the world's largest tobacco product makers and consumers. This has also helped block efforts to improve health. Avoidable forms of vascular disease are now the major causes of death and disability in these and many similar nations.

Nonetheless, progress is being achieved. Infant, maternal and child mortality is falling in most relatively poor regions. Furthermore, in countries such as Brazil, significant efforts have been made to reduce tobacco smoking, while affordable essential medicines distribution has been improved via the establishment of Farmácia Popular in areas of higher need. The fact that the Brazilian government has had both a robust vision for pharmaceutical care and the political will to implement funded service innovations goes a long way towards explaining the success of this last initiative, as compared to the record of the Jan Aushadhi pharmacies in India.

## KEY ISSUES IN PUBLIC HEALTH AND PHARMACY DEVELOPMENT

Population ageing in countries such as the UK has not been the major health care cost driver it is sometimes said to be. Nor is the increasing number of people living with multiple diagnoses as fundamental a challenge for the mature industrialized nations as is on occasion claimed. By and large, older populations are in age-standardized terms healthier populations, and although living with several long-term conditions complicates medication regimens, it does not in itself normally increase disability risks via synergistic interactions between disorders. As the age at which death occurs is pushed back, so (depending in part on social and economic as well as biological factors) the age at which loss of independence commences tends to rise.

Modern pharmacy education should incorporate a robust understanding of these realities, as well as other socio-economic and bio-medical insights needed to facilitate appropriate health care delivery. Arguably, being an expert on the 'scientific' properties of medicines without an adequate understanding of the context of their use and the social determinates of their value in practice is unlikely to enable future pharmacists to play an optimally useful role.

However, having acknowledged that neither individual nor collective ageing should be viewed unduly negatively, many of today's central health care tasks are linked to the shift from infectious and allied acute disorders in younger people towards increased chronic disease burdens in later life. In public health terms, it is important to prevent or at least delay the onset of the latter whenever possible, and when such conditions occur, to help affected individuals live with them as well as possible, through the complementary provision of all forms of health and social care. Effective medicine taking can contribute to both prevention and improved treatment outcomes. The opportunities this situation creates for community pharmacists are summarized diagrammatically in Figure 2.4.

Four topics linked critically to the future of pharmacy and its capacity to further enhance national and global public health are briefly considered below, starting with a brief analysis of the increasing importance of self-care promotion and support. It is worth emphasizing that most individuals in their 60s, 70s and 80s require no more help in using pharmaceutical treatments than younger members of the population. Indeed, they may be better able to take drugs and other treatments appropriately than their 'working age' contemporaries. Data suggesting this is not the case have on occasion been distorted by factors such as failures to correct for medicine afford-ability effects in differing national settings.

However, if individuals' intellectual capacities start to decline, it becomes increasingly likely that their use of medicines will become disordered, especially if they need to take complex combinations of drugs. In such circumstances, the available evidence on interventions, such as supplying dispensed items in multi-compartmental containers, suggests that they are often relatively ineffective for maintaining appropriate drug use. This is not to deny their potential utility to

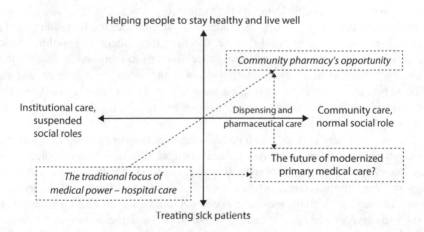

**FIGURE 2.4** Population ageing and allied factors will increasingly focus the work of pri-mary care doctors and nurses on supporting people with serious and complex health and allied care problems. Community pharmacy has an opportunity to support this transition and to extend its role to include self-care support, screening and case finding, risk factor manage-ment and health care provision for common conditions provided in settings such as 'healthy living pharmacies'.

carers and their convenience value to some relatively able consumers. But at worst, such interventions increase costs while leaving those most in need of effective help little better off.

In this context, the Australian example of funding domiciliary medicine-taking assessments is of potential interest, providing this leads to early diagnoses of illnesses, such as dementias, and more adequate community support arrangements being put in place as and when they are needed. There is evidence from countries such as the UK that although the staff responsible for delivering medicines to vulnerable individuals living alone may know who is having problems with taking them, pharmacists themselves are either often not aware of such information or may fail to make appropriate use of it. If community pharmacy is to prosper in the long-term, it must demonstrate capacities to contribute cost-effectively to improving outcomes. When, for example, non-adherence in medicine taking for long-term conditions is of primary importance as a marker of increasing personal care needs, it should be understood as such, in order to elicit appropriate professional responses.

## SELF-CARE IN HEALTH CARE: THE IMPORTANCE OF INDIVIDUAL AUTONOMY IN MODERN COMMUNITIES

The care transition process described in this chapter classically begins with trends towards the increasing formalization of what were originally personal and family care processes. Towards its later stages, when populations have aged and become more educated and gender-related role changes have become established, pressures favouring new patterns of supported self-care emerge. Hand-in-hand with this, establishing and retaining a capacity for independent living tends to become progressively more valued in post-transitional communities, not only for 'healthy' individuals of all ages, but also for people living with mental and physical disabilities.

In some instances, promoting informed self-care, in addition to helping individuals at every stage in life avoid disease and disability wherever possible, reduces health system costs. However, as in all other areas of 'quality management', there is a danger that if expenditure reduction rather than meeting new patterns of public demand becomes seen as the central purpose of such initiatives, they will lose their focus on addressing service users' most important needs. If this occurs, they will ultimately fail.

This is also likely to be so when professional practitioners and service managers underestimate the extent of the behavioural changes needed in order to successfully move away from traditional, overtly directive, care towards facilitative patterns of support aimed at optimizing self-care contributions to health and welfare improvement. Although such challenges were recognized a decade ago in, for example, the 2004 *Choosing Health* public health White Paper and the subsequent *Choosing Health through Pharmacy* publication, it is still arguably the case that their implications have not as yet been fully recognized in either pharmacy education or pharmacy practice in the UK, or elsewhere.

The underlying message for both policy makers and pharmacy service providers is that efforts to improve public health through the promotion of well-informed self-care are most likely to be successful when: first, they are transparently motivated by a desire to enhance individual and wider public well-being, rather than to save money or cut services; and second, they are based on a genuine respect for consumer sovereignty. This is not to say that health care providers such as pharmacists should not seek to provide the populations they serve with knowledge or to create proactively a balanced emotional and intellectual awareness of health hazards and protection opportunities in the minds of individual service users. But simplistic attempts to impose 'responsible behaviour' on unwilling people (or indeed prescribers) are unlikely to succeed.

## DISPENSING ROBOTIZATION AND PHARMACY'S FUTURE

Similar concerns arise in areas such as introducing 'patient-held digital health platforms' and mobile applications aimed at supporting 'healthy' behaviours and appropriate medicine taking, and on the pharmacy supply side introducing robotized dispensing systems. With regard to personal health technologies (including, for instance, talking medication dispensers), there is reason to believe that these help some individuals achieve better outcomes. Yet the extent to which they can substitute for personal care delivered by well-educated people should not be overstated. Naïve failures to resist the 'over-selling' of health-related information and communication technology applications might on occasion impair health care quality.

In the case of dispensing technologies, there is evidence that when appropriately used at a local or a larger regional scale, automated systems can reduce labour costs and/or release pharmacy staff for the delivery of clinical care and 'healthy living' support. In the relatively near future, it is likely that existing legislation will be changed to permit independent pharmacies to invest collectively in automated dispensing. However, the gains to be generated by such innovations should not be exaggerated. When the ongoing costs of safety checking, dispensed drug distribution, acute and emergency prescription item supply and patient support have been accounted for, the maximum net level of cash saving achievable without undermining NHS community pharmacy service standards to a publicly unacceptable degree is likely to be relatively modest. That is, the cost reductions realisable are more likely to be in the order of 10% than, say, 30%. However, if used effectively and in conjunction with other ICTs, they could make significantly greater contributions to raising the cost-effectiveness of pharmacies and pharmacists by enabling them to function like 'walk-in high street preventive health care practices'.

## WORKING RELATIONSHIPS WITH GPS AND OTHER PRIMARY CARE PROFESSIONALS

Awareness of such possibilities opens up a series of questions as to the future working relationships between GP practices and community pharmacies (these arc also considered in Chapter 15). As recent English NHS policy documents like the *Five Year Forward View* indicate, a range of alternatives exists in relation to the future of primary care. Depending in part on what NHS users will come to prefer and demand, the available options include the formation of new types of multi-speciality community diagnostic and treatment centres through to the extension of local federations of practices that could build on existing service structures in ways that enable them to deliver better-integrated services without radically changing the established (and reasonably well-recognized) 'front doors' to health care.

If existing trends continue, the earnings to be made from dispensing prescription items will fall back closer to 'commodity' levels. At the same time, other returns on supplying NHS medicines of all types are likely to be further 'managed down'. In such circumstances, future pharmacists seeking employment in the community are likely to have to choose between working as either employees (or perhaps partners) in GP practices or other primary care centres, or developing extended clinical roles within independently sited corporate or independently owned community pharmacies.

Across the world, there are varying degrees of tension between pharmacy and medicine relating to factors outlined in this chapter. It is likely that in different settings, different solutions as to how best pharmacy and medicine can together evolve to serve public interests will emerge. In the UK, the option of working directly alongside practice-based doctors and nurse practitioners is likely to prove attractive for an increasing number of pharmacists. It also appears to be favoured by growing numbers of GPs. But this should not be allowed to obscure the potential value to the public of further developing separately located community pharmacies as alternative 'first-stage' care and illness prevention support access points.

At root, the available evidence indicates that patients and the public want to combine the advantages of care continuity and being personally known by 'their' doctors and other health professionals who they trust with the benefits of rapid service access in times of emergency and the assurance of being able to consult with specialists with high levels of technical expertise in situations when it is most likely that suboptimal therapy will cause harm. Health service planners and decision makers are likely to share such goals. Yet in systems like the NHS, managers may be more strongly motivated (for public health optimization, cost minimization or other reasons) than service users to trade away the advantages of small-scale competition and service provider familiarity in favour of greater organizational size and for what patients and the public may experience as the mechanistic use of anonymous labour.

In inherently imperfect markets, such as that of health care, such problems may be inevitable. However, pharmacists and their leaders should at least be aware of the reasons why they exist, and in forming new working partnerships and/or competitive relationships with other practitioners seek to serve the needs of individual clients as well as possible, while at the same time respecting the importance of protecting public health as a whole. Defending high as opposed to merely adequate care standards may not always be popular with service funders or taxpayers' elected representatives. However, from a professional perspective, it may nevertheless be the correct thing to seek to achieve.

## PAYING FOR FUTURE 'PUBLIC HEALTH' SERVICES

The NHS and other publicly and statutory/obligatory insurance-based universal health care systems exist to overcome the limitations of free market health (and social) care supply and the public health problems that typify pre-transitional communities that have not yet developed such sophisticated communal provisions. The payment arrangements underpinning the latter are central to maintaining good health and health care in advanced societies. There is robust evidence that from a community-wide perspective, well-managed taxation and universal insurance-funded health care systems are significantly more cost-effective than out-of-pocket payment-based health care funding arrangements.

Across the globe, the financial systems in place to support pharmacy services and the supply of medicines have adapted and are continuing to adapt in order to reflect such understandings and changing health care needs. Yet as communities continue to advance in the wake of demographic and epidemiological transition, it is becoming apparent that the availability of tax raised and allied funds may not be adequate to meet all legitimate health-related consumer expectations. Political and allied pressures could create conditions in which at least a proportion of people may in future wish to 'top up' their publicly funded health care entitlements with private purchases or additional insurance coverage for preventative programmes and/or items such as diagnostics and genetics-based and other risk testing and lifestyle support packages. Consumer-funded demand for high-quality 'personalized screening' services to protect individuals and groups from conditions such as prostate cancer may also rise in future decades.

If this proves to be the case, community pharmacists and pharmacies might well be able to build on their existing roles in areas such as the supply of self-purchased treatments and items such as pregnancy tests and nicotine replacement therapies to supply additional products and services. In overall terms, advocates of such approaches argue this might increase the percentage of GDP spent on health care in general and on public health improvement in particular. However, while this possibility deserves recognition, so do its hazards.

There is a danger, for example, that developments along these lines could in future serve to increase health and other inequalities in ways which will negatively impact not only on minority group well-being but also on societies' overall capacities to foster economic growth and health improvement. There is also a risk that unless community pharmacy payments can be shifted towards receiving fees for providing health care generally, as distinct from selling specific products and services, this will perpetuate perceptions of their being retailer-orientated traders as distinct from 'true' primary care/health professionals. Considerations like these suggest that whenever possible community pharmacists in the UK should continue to seek public funding to underpin cost-effective extensions in their roles, and that when it is needed, private service supply should be subject to regulation via professional values and structures, as well as by state-imposed controls.

## CONCLUSION

The year 2015 marked the 200th anniversary of the passing into British law of the 1815 Apothecaries Act. This sought to improve the standards of education and training for apothecaries and improve the general public's access to safe treatments at around the end of the Napoleonic wars. In so doing, it opened the way in the middle of the nineteenth century to the establishment of the unified medical profession. To permit this, the Guild of Apothecaries split into those who specialized in pharmaceutical chemistry (who were the progenitors of today's pharmacists) and those more centrally concerned with patient care.

In the UK, the origins of general medical practice lie with this last group of practitioners. One option for the future of pharmacy in Britain is that it could once again divide, this time into those most occupied with high-volume medicines dispensing and supply on the one hand and those concerned with health promotion, personal care and the appropriate use of medicines to limit the progression of non-communicable diseases on the other.

For some observers, the possibility of a new split may threaten the long-term survival of pharmacy as an independent health profession, separate from medicine and yet to a degree protected from the direct control of 'profit- and cash flow-driven' managers. Yet for others, it might appear the only practically viable way of overcoming the long-standing barriers that have to date largely blocked the way to pharmacists acting as clinicians in the community.

Similar fundamental choices exist elsewhere in the world. The history of British and in particular English pharmacy is unique. However, the problems and opportunities relating to sustaining health improvement and using medicines and other interventions to optimum effect in preventing conditions such as vascular diseases, type 2 diabetes and dementias, and in reducing the occurrence and harm caused by events such as heart attacks and strokes, are increasingly global. In answer to the question posed earlier in this chapter about what (public) health gain goals community pharmacy should most seek to achieve in the next 10–20 years, the analysis presented here favours, in particular, the further reduction of vascular disease risks. Cutting these will generate multiple benefits relating not only to heart disease burden reductions, but also in areas ranging from cancer prevention to neurological protection.

As computer-based clinical decision making and medicine-dispensing technologies evolve and medicines themselves continue to progress, these too will in all probability drive practice convergence across the world's regions, although the power of cultures to modify and tailor common lines of development to generate special local responses should not be underestimated. It would not therefore be meaningful for this chapter to attempt to detail a single way forward for community pharmacy that will ensure that efforts to strengthen its 'public health' role are successful.

Rather, it is appropriate to conclude that what is ultimately important for any group active in the health sector is to be able to demonstrate that it is not only already playing a useful part, but that it has the potential, in future, to save more lives and prevent more cases of disability and distress than is presently possible. Seen from a broad perspective, there is good reason to believe that this remains as true for pharmacy as it has ever been, provided the profession's members can adequately appreciate the nature and consequences of the continuing health-related transition processes affecting the societies in which we live and are willing to adapt to meet the changing requirements of the individuals and communities they have the opportunity to serve. In the final analysis, this is most likely to involve twenty-first century community pharmacists, if they are to survive as future health professionals, playing extended clinical roles while fulfilling reduced drug supply functions.

## FURTHER READING

Anderson, S.C. 2007. Community pharmacy and public health in Great Britain 1936 to 2006: How a phoenix rose from the ashes. *Journal of Epidemiology and Community Health*, **61**, 844–848. Available at http://www.ncbi.nlm.nih.gov/pmc/articles/PMC2652958/pdf/844.pdf.

Anderson, S.C. 2008. From 'bespoke' to 'off-the-peg': Community pharmacists and the retailing of medicines in Great Britain 1900 to 1970. *Pharmacy in History*, **50**(2), 43–69.

Eades, C.E., Ferguson, J.S. and O'Carroll, R.E. 2011. Public health in community pharmacy: A systematic review of pharmacist and consumer views. *BMC Public Health*, **11**, 582. Available at http://www.biomedcentral.com/1471-2458/11/582.

Gidman, W., Ward, P. and McGregor, L. 2012. Understanding public trust in services provided by community pharmacists relative to those provided by general practitioners: A qualitative study. *British Medical Journal*, **2**, e000939.

Goundrey-Smith, S. 2014. Examining the role of new technology in pharmacy: Now and in the future. *Pharmaceutical Journal*, **293**(7817).

*Harbingers of Change in Healthcare: Implications for the Role and Use of Medicines IMS Institute Report*; London, September 2014.

*Healthy Lives, Healthy People: Our Strategy for Public Health in England*. Department of Health; London, November 2010.

Houle, K.D., Grindrod, K.A., Chatterley, T. and Tsuyuki, R.T. 2014. Paying pharmacists for patient care: A systematic review of remunerated pharmacy clinical care services. *Canadian Pharmaceutical Journal*, **147**, 209–232.

Jones, E.J.M., MacKinnon, N.J. and Tsuyuki, R.T. 2005. Pharmaceutical care in community pharmacies: Practice and research in Canada. *Annals of Pharmacotherapy*, **39**, 1527–1533.

Laliberté, M.-C., Perreault, S., Damestoy, N. and Lalonde, L. 2012. Ideal and actual involvement of community pharmacists in health promotion and prevention: A cross-sectional study in Quebec, Canada. *BMC Public Health*, **12**, 192.

McMillan, S.S, Wheeler, A.J, Sav, A. et al. 2013. Community pharmacy in Australia: A health hub destination of the future. *Research in Social and Administrative Pharmacy*, **9**, 863–875.

Patwardhan, A., Duncan, I., Murphy, P. and Pegus, C. 2012. The value of pharmacists in health care. *Population Health Management*; **15**, 157–162.

## REFERENCES

*Developing Pharmacy's Contribution to Public Health: A Progress Report from the Pharmacy and Public Health Forum*, London, June 2014.

*Five Year Forward View*, NHS England, 2014.

Mossialos, E., Naci, H. and Courtin, E. 2013. Expanding the role of community pharmacists: Policymaking in the absence of policy-relevant evidence? *Health Policy*, **111**, 135–148.

# 3 Hospital Pharmacy

## Michael Wilcock and Joanna Lawrence

## CONTENTS

### KEY POINTS

- Hospital pharmacy service standards are regulated to ensure the safe and effective use of medicines.
- Initiatives to reduce dispensing errors include electronic prescribing, patient bedside medication lockers, one-stop dispensing and medicine administration systems.
- Hospital pharmacists are increasingly adopting techno-vigilance: using electronic prescribing data to monitor patient safety.

## INTRODUCTION

The scope of hospital pharmacy practice is broad, with a remit to ensure the safe, effective and efficient management of all aspects of medicines usage and with a focus on the patient and delivering value for money (Healthcare Commission 2007). In general, a typical hospital pharmacy department will have staff involved in a variety of roles (Box 3.1).

## STANDARDS FOR HOSPITAL PHARMACY

There is a wide and demanding regulatory framework surrounding the use of medicines within hospitals. In addition to working towards delivery of numerous national recommendations, hospitals are also now required to register with the Care Quality Commission and meet its required medicines management standards. Other 'regulators' that may inspect hospital pharmacy departments include the NHS Litigation

## BOX 3.1    HOSPITAL PHARMACISTS' ROLES

- Procurement of medicines and management of arrangements for supplies via homecare.
- Dispensing and supply of medicines for inpatients and outpatients.
- Manufacture and quality control of medicines (e.g. some treatments, such as chemotherapy and parenteral nutrition, require preparation under aseptic conditions).
- Advisory (see the 'Clinical Pharmacy' section in this chapter) with the pharmacy team working closely with medical and nursing staff on the wards to ensure patients receive the most appropriate treatments and providing help and advice to patients in all aspects of their medicines.
- Independent prescribing activities: some specialist pharmacists will act as independent prescribers, possibly running their own clinics in certain areas such as renal medicine or rheumatology, or may prescribe on particular wards, such as intensive care or medical admissions units.
- Medicines information: pharmacists and technicians may use a range of reference sources to provide detailed information and support to health care professionals and patients about all aspects of medicines usage. Medicines information may also be involved in the writing of medication-related guidelines and the development of a hospital and/ or health community formulary.
- Management: pharmacists may combine their professional role with some form of managerial responsibility, such as managing a particular aspect of the pharmacy service or other members of the pharmacy team. This may include monitoring and reporting on expenditures from the budget for medicine usage within hospital or the monitoring of contracts and arrangements with providers of home care services or outpatient dispensary partners.

Authority (and their equivalents in devolved countries), the General Pharmaceutical Council and, for controlled drugs, the Home Office. In addition, the culture of the National Health Service (NHS) is changing, subsequent to the Francis and Berwick Reports. Pharmacists need to demonstrate the correct values and behaviours to work in a NHS where patient care is at the forefront and all professionals feel empowered to challenge a lack of care or compassion.

The Royal Pharmaceutical Society's Professional Standards for Hospital Pharmacy Services were developed to help organizations across Great Britain to ensure patient safety – making health care safer by the development of quality services. These standards provide a broad framework to support pharmacy departments to improve services and to shape future services and pharmacy roles to deliver quality patient care. The standards underpin the patient experience and the safe, effective management of medicines within organizations. They will help patients experience a consistent quality of service that will protect them from incidents of avoidable harm and help them to get the best outcomes from their medicines.

Similarly, the European Association of Hospital Pharmacists has released statements which express commonly agreed objectives which every European health system should aim for in the delivery of hospital pharmacy services (The European Summit on Hospital Pharmacy 2014). Although the nature of how hospital pharmacy is delivered and the types of services provided do vary across European countries, the opening statement summarizes succinctly the broad aim of hospital pharmacy – the overarching goal of the hospital pharmacy service is to optimize patient outcomes through working collaboratively within multidisciplinary teams in order to achieve the responsible use of medicines across all settings.

## MEDICATION SYSTEMS

The systems and processes used to prescribe, supply, store and administer medicines in a hospital setting can have a substantial impact on medication errors. The types of errors that can occur can be divided into two categories: errors of commission and errors of omission. The former include, for example, prescribing or supplying (via dispensing or direct administration to the patient) the wrong medicine or wrong dose. The latter include, for example, omitted doses or a failure to monitor, such as the international normalized ratio for anticoagulant therapy. Various national medication safety and quality initiatives have been introduced in NHS hospitals to help understand and reduce the number and severity of these errors, though it is known that hospitals have implemented these core medication systems in different ways. These include the use of electronic prescribing and medication administration systems, the use of patients' own drugs during hospital inpatient stays, one-stop dispensing supplies (which are hospital inpatient medications labelled with administration instructions for use at discharge as well as during the inpatient stay) and patient bedside medication lockers. More recently, there have been recommendations for health care organizations to have medication safety officers and multi-professional groups to review medication error incidents and improve medication safety locally (NHS England and MHRA 2014). Pharmacy teams, with their expert knowledge on medicines and safe systems of practice, would contribute extensively to such groups.

## CLINICAL PHARMACY

There are various definitions of clinical pharmacy, with the American College of Clinical Pharmacy defining it as the area of practice in which pharmacists provide patient care that optimizes medication therapy and promotes health, wellness and disease prevention (American College of Clinical Pharmacy 2008). A clinical pharmacy presence on the wards, be it a pharmacist or pharmacy technician, enables communication and discussion with patients and professionals, in addition to ensuring the safe and appropriate supplies of medicines. The pharmacy team when on the ward will typically be involved in medicines reconciliation (i.e. taking a medication history from patients and resolving any discrepancies, as published work suggests that pharmacists are able to take more accurate medication histories than medical staff). This key task of undertaking medicines reconciliation for patients on admission to hospital has been endorsed by the National Institute for Health and Clinical Excellence and the National Patient Safety Agency (National Institute for Health and Clinical Excellence 2007), which recommended that pharmacists should be involved in medicines reconciliation as soon as possible after hospital admission, noting that this is a cost-effective intervention.

In addition to medicines reconciliation at admission, the pharmacy team plays an important role in medicines safety during the inpatient stay. A report from the General Medical Council in the UK showed that 8.9% of orders in a selection of UK hospitals contained an error when written. The majority of these errors are intercepted before actual harm occurs to patients by the intervention of clinical pharmacy staff (Dornan et al. 2009).

The pharmacy team, in conjunction with microbiology departments, also has a leading role in antimicrobial stewardship and ensuring the correct and appropriate use of antibiotics. A great deal of work in hospitals has focused on reducing health care-acquired infections, with pharmacists working as part of multidisciplinary teams to ensure that the choice of antimicrobial agent and treatment plan follows national standards and local microbiology expertise.

## FUTURE DEVELOPMENTS

### Technology: Electronic Prescribing and Automated Dispensing

In 2003, the Department of Health in the UK issued a report authored by the Chief Pharmacist entitled *Building a Safer NHS for Patients: Improving Medication Safety* (Smith 2003). This highlighted potential benefits in helping to reduce medication errors by the introduction of electronic prescribing and robotic dispensing. With computerization, it should be possible to routinely assess the performance of the many steps in the medication use process. Hence, the term 'techno-vigilance' has appeared in the literature and refers to how the pharmacy team can make use of routinely gathered electronic data as a warning system for missed doses of prescribed medicine and for making improvements to patient safety. For example, an electronic system could be programmed to trigger a series of emails if, for example, a patient missed more than two doses of antibiotics or other critical medicines. Such a system, using real-time data, can also prompt the pharmacy team to review, in conjunction with medical staff, those patients who are prescribed high-risk medicines.

Although computers and automated dispensing systems can help with reducing medication errors, technology does have its limitations and will not replace the direct contact between the pharmacy team and patients that is necessary for patients to fully understand their medicines. Any technological changes put in place should also free up time for the pharmacy team to focus even more on the delivery of clinical care.

### Seven-Day Service

It is reported that the number of patients coming through hospital doors has increased year on year: a cumulative rise of 37% over 10 years (Royal College of Physicians

2013). As a result of these gradual increases in the number and complexity of emergency admissions, recommendations have been made for hospital services to deliver high-quality treatment and care seven days a week. Currently, there is variability in the consistency of the services delivered by pharmacy departments outside of normal working hours. This limited availability, particularly at weekends, has been reported as resulting in:

- An increase in missed doses
- Prescription errors
- Lack of medicines reconciliation
- Delayed discharge due to waiting for discharge medication

Hence, a future challenge to hospital pharmacy will be the effective delivery of a seven-day service.

## CONCLUSION

Pharmacy as practised in a hospital revolves around the supply of medicines and the provision of clinical, pharmaceutical expertise to the staff and patients of hospital. Hence, an integral part of hospital pharmacy is being part of the health care team and working closely with all other health care professionals to provide advice and support on medicines usage.

## FURTHER READING

McLeod, M., Ahmed, Z., Barber, N. and Franklin, B.D. 2014. A national survey of inpatient medication systems in English NHS hospitals. *BMC Health Services Research*, **14**, 93. http://www.biomedcentral.com/1472-6963/14/93.

Royal Pharmaceutical Society. 2014. *Seven Day Services in Hospital Pharmacy Giving Patients the Care they Deserve*. London: Royal Pharmaceutical Society.

## REFERENCES

American College of Clinical Pharmacy 2008. The definition of clinical pharmacy. *Pharmacotherapy*, **28**, 816–817.

Dornan, T., Ashcroft, D., Heathfield, H. et al. 2009. *An In Depth Investigation into Causes of Prescribing Errors by Foundation Trainees in Relation to their Medical Education. EQUIP Study*. London: General Medical Council.

Healthcare Commission 2007. *The Best Medicine. The Management of Medicines in Acute and Specialist Trusts. Acute Hospital Portfolio Review*. London: Healthcare Commission.

National Institute for Health and Clinical Excellence 2007. *NICE Patient Safety Guidance 1. Technical Patient Safety Solutions for Medicines Reconciliation on Admission to Hospital*. London: National Institute for Health and Clinical Excellence, National Patient Safety Agency.

NHS England and MHRA. 2014. Patient Safety Alert. Stage 3: Directive. Improving medication error incident reporting and learning. http://www.england.nhs.uk/wp-content/uploads/2014/03/psa-med-error.pdf.

Royal College of Physicians 2013. The Future Hospital Commission Report. Available at http://www.rcplondon.ac.uk/sites/default/files/future-hospital-commission-report.pdf.

Smith, J.M. 2003. *Building a Safer NHS for Patients: Improving Medication Safety*. London: Department of Health.

The European Summit on Hospital Pharmacy 2014. The consensus statements of hospital pharmacists, healthcare professionals and patients. *European Journal of Hospital Pharmacy*, **21**(5), 256–258.

# 4 Community Pharmacy in Europe

*J. W. Foppe van Mil*

## CONTENTS

---

**KEY POINTS**

- There is wide variability in the availability of medicines across Europe.
- Payment systems for medicines vary, ranging from wholly privatized health care to state-organized systems.
- Across Europe, there is considerable variation in the size of the population served by community pharmacies, with French and Spanish pharmacies each serving fewer than 3,000 people, compared with 18,000 in Denmark.
- Pharmaceutical care has yet to be fully assimilated in Italy, Greece, Turkey, France and some of the Eastern European countries.

- Community pharmacies in Austria, Denmark, France, Germany, Greece, Poland, Portugal and Switzerland do not routinely label dispensed medicines.

## INTRODUCTION

In Europe, pharmacies are places where the public can get medicines and where pharmacists are the responsible persons. This, however, is the only common denominator. In the past, pharmacy revolved around the manufacture and provision of medicines, rather than around those who consumed them. However, in the latter half of the twentieth century, extemporaneous preparations largely disappeared from pharmacies in many European countries, such as Denmark, Greece, Portugal and Sweden. In the Netherlands, they currently constitute 3% of all dispensed medicines, and most of these medicines are now centrally prepared. In the 1960s and 1970s, the focus of pharmacists' activities shifted towards an increased emphasis on the effects of medicines, namely clinical pharmacy. This change happened throughout Europe, although the pace of change differed between countries.

Pharmacies in Europe differ considerably in terms of size, staffing and the services provided, reflecting the independent development of health care across Europe. Before discussing these elements, this chapter will explore some of the factors which serve to explain these international variations. There are a few European organizations in the field of pharmacy that impact on community and hospital pharmacy practice. In the Pharmaceutical Group of the European Union (PGEU), the European pharmacist organizations exchange their views on their professional needs and try to influence European developments. The Europharm Forum is a cooperative platform between some European pharmacist associations and the World Health Organization. In this organization, the focus is on the implementation of pharmaceutical care, quality management and their indicators. The Pharmaceutical Care Network Europe (PCNE) is a European research platform for pharmacy practice and pharmaceutical care research, and the European Society for Clinical Pharmacy is an educational network for practicing clinical pharmacists in hospitals and the community. The European Association of Hospital Pharmacists (EAHP) represents and supports hospital pharmacy.

The availability of medicines varies throughout Europe, due to differences in the registration procedures and policies of their pharmaceutical industries. However, the introduction of the European Agency for the Evaluation of Medicinal Products – now called the European Medicines Agency (EMA) – in 1993 increasingly reduced this variation between countries belonging to the European Union, although national authorities still have some authority under national and the so-called 'decentralized' procedure. The EMA's current system for the licensing of medicinal products was introduced in 1995, though a pharmaceutical company may, for commercial reasons, still decide not to market a certain medicine in a particular country despite it having received regulatory approval.

In most European countries, only physicians, dentists and veterinary practitioners are permitted to prescribe medicines. However, Irish and UK pharmacists have (limited) prescribing rights; in the UK, pharmacists can prescribe within their limits of professional competence. In some countries, midwives, nurses and other health professionals may also have prescribing rights.

## PHARMACY EDUCATION

Although there have been attempts to promote international cooperation and convergence in Europe under the European Association of Faculties of Pharmacy, the content and duration of pharmacy courses still vary between countries. In most countries, there has been a shift within the curriculum away from chemistry and biology to a more clinical and social emphasis. The Scandinavian countries, the UK and the Netherlands were the first to incorporate clinical pharmacy into their pharmacy curricula, Germany has included clinical pharmacy in its official pharmacy curriculum since 2000. There are, however, still countries within Europe whose pharmacy education does not or hardly encompasses clinical pharmacy, such as Turkey. Many faculties now also teach social pharmacy, including communication skills, as a separate subject area.

The duration of pharmacy courses varies between four and six years, with the average age of pharmacy graduates being between 22 and 26 years. Subsequently, graduates undertake a further six months to four years of training before they are fully licensed as pharmacists. In some countries, not all involved in the supply of medicines are university educated. For example, some Scandinavian countries have receptars, who do not receive a full university education but have approximately the same rights as pharmacists. Receptars receive 2.5 years of training, which includes nine months' placement in a pharmacy. They can therefore be compared with the Dutch assistant pharmacists. In the Netherlands, these assistant pharmacists undertake a three-year non-university education which includes a placement in a pharmacy. They may only practice under (indirect) supervision of a pharmacist. Other countries have licensed technicians, but their educational levels vary.

### CONTINUING EDUCATION

In most countries, being a community pharmacist is subject to a licensing/registration system, but significant differences exist as to the ways licenses can be renewed. In about half of the European countries, undertaking continuing education is now required in order to retain a license to practice as a community pharmacist.

## HEALTH CARE SYSTEMS

In 2011, the national drug budgets in Europe varied between 5.1% (Denmark) and 19.6% (France) of the national health care costs. The high percentage costs in countries such as France, Portugal and Spain (around 16%) can be explained by their relative low expenditures on health care in general. This also explains why some governments are more active in controlling drug costs than others. Nevertheless, the drugs budget is an important area of cost containment in most European countries. The cost of drug consumption per capita in 2012 varied between 224 euros in

England and 600 euros in Switzerland. These differences are only partially due to different pricing systems.

Although the majority of European countries have a health care system wherein the rich support the poor, the systems for paying for medicines vary widely. In Switzerland and the Netherlands, the health care system has been totally privatized; in other countries, the system is organized totally or partially by the state. This results in differences in the access of the population to medicines, depending on individual wealth and insurance systems. The UK is alone within Europe in having a National Health Service (NHS), which enables health care costs – of which the drug budget is a part – to be controlled (see also Chapters 1 and 2). Most other countries have a form of NHS for people with a low income, usually called a sick fund, and a private insurance system for people having a higher income. However, in some countries, the state supports the insurance companies by paying part of their expenses. The method of remuneration in different countries is reflected in the administrative burden placed on pharmacies. Co-payment systems vary throughout Europe. A co-payment is that part of the drug price paid by the patient. This can be a certain percentage, a stepped scale or a fixed sum. Co-payments for all health care services, including dispensing medicines, are increasing across Europe as a way to force the population to 'consume' less health care and decrease the health care budget. Whatever the patient has to pay to a pharmacist to obtain a medicine is regarded as the co-payment.

Pharmacies are usually either independent or part of a chain, now also Sweden, where the pharmacy system used to be different from the rest of Europe. All Swedish pharmacies were previously owned by a 'company', Apoteket (called Apoteksbolaget up until 1999), but the monopoly ended a few years ago under pressure from the European Union. In Denmark, Italy and Spain, only pharmacists may own a pharmacy. Ownership in other countries is less restricted. In some countries (such as Sweden), however, it is explicitly stated that medical doctors may not own a pharmacy.

## OTHER PROVIDERS OF MEDICINES

In a few European countries, such as the Netherlands, Switzerland and the UK, physicians may supply medicines to patients, usually in sparsely populated areas. The reason for this is that pharmacies in those areas are not supposed to be commercially viable, and physicians are the most ready sources of expertise about medicines. They are often supported by pharmacists who compound preparations and occasionally supply drugs to the physician's pharmacy. However, in Switzerland, dispensing doctors can also be found in cities, and they compete with pharmacists for their share of the drug market.

Veterinary medicines are also sometimes dispensed through community pharmacies, such as in Finland, Iceland and Luxembourg. In other countries, veterinarians dispense these drugs.

Although some attempts have been made to establish mail-order pharmacy in different European countries, this form of dispensing has not (yet) become popular, probably because Europe is relatively densely populated compared with the US. Internet pharmacies have also not yet significantly penetrated the European market, although there are signs that some Europeans are starting to buy their medicines from Internet companies. This especially applies to lifestyle drugs and alternative remedies, rather than to prescription medicines.

## AVAILABILITY OF OVER-THE-COUNTER MEDICINES

Although prescription-only medicines (POMs) are routinely supplied from pharmacies, the outlets for over-the-counter (OTC) medicines are varied. For a long time, OTC medicines were only available from pharmacies, with the exception of the Netherlands and Germany, where druggists (a person with a license obtained after a 2-year part-time non-university education) were allowed to sell a limited assortment of medicines. The increasing pressure from the pharmaceutical industry in the 1990s has changed this situation. In many European countries, many OTC medicines are now available (often in small packs only) through outlets such as supermarkets and petrol/gas stations. In a smaller number of European countries, the public still does not have this option, with all medicines being sold through pharmacies. However, change is imminent under pressure from the European Union. In order to reduce drug costs, there has been a move to make some previous POMs available for sale: the POM to OTC switch. Consequently, the sale of OTC medicines from pharmacies and other outlets in some countries has increased.

## PROFESSIONAL PROTECTION

In the past, throughout Europe, only pharmacists could own a pharmacy. This is now changing, since governments want to introduce more competition in the distribution process for medicines in anticipation of costs being reduced.

In some countries, the government or pharmacy's professional body regulates the establishment/registration of a pharmacy. In the Scandinavian countries and the Netherlands, the latter system in the past resulted in relatively large pharmacies. In the Netherlands, Norway, Sweden and Iceland, this system has now been abandoned. In Iceland and Norway, this has resulted in more and smaller pharmacies, though in the Netherlands and Sweden, no similar effect has been observed. In Denmark, the number of pharmacies is still restricted, and becoming a pharmacy owner involves a rather complicated selection procedure, which ultimately benefits elderly pharmacists. However, that system is under political pressure as well, not only locally, but also from within the European Union.

## THE SIZE OF PHARMACIES IN EUROPE

The size of pharmacies in Europe shows large differences (Table 4.1). In some countries, pharmacies serve relatively small populations (i.e. there are a large number of pharmacies serving a relatively small population). For example, those in France and Spain, on average, serve less than 3,000 people, while in Greece, an average pharmacy serves only 1,900 people. By contrast, the average Danish pharmacy serves a population of nearly 18,000, though in Denmark there are satellite pharmacies which are an organizational part of the main pharmacy. Although there is a clear correlation between the number of clients and the average size, calculated as surface area

**TABLE 4.1**
**Average Size and Population Served by Community Pharmacies**

| Country | Average Population | Average Size in m² |
|---|---|---|
| Austria | 7,841[a] | 200 |
| Croatia | 3,956 | 100 |
| Denmark | 17,783 | 470 |
| Finland | 6,599[a] | 104 |
| France | 2,667[a] | 80 |
| England | 4,452 | n/k |
| Germany | 3,915 | 165 |
| Greece | 1,143[a] | 47 |
| Hungary | 4,000 | 80 |
| Iceland | 5,455 | 200 |
| Ireland | 2,700 | nn |
| Italy | 3,281 | 60 |
| Luxembourg | 5,429[a] | 120 |
| The Netherlands | 8,467 | 240 |
| Norway | 6,755 | 270 |
| Poland | 6,094[a] | 150 |
| Portugal | 3,600 | 85 |
| Spain | 2,200 | 70 |
| Sweden | 7,297 | 300 |
| Switzerland | 4,500 | 217 |

*Note:*   n/k: not known.
[a]   Data from 2000.

of the pharmacy, it is remarkable that this average surface area also shows a large variation (Table 4.1).

The amount of time devoted to each customer in a pharmacy also shows variation between countries. If one only considers the prescriptions dispensed to clients per licensed staff member, then a staff member in Finland dispenses on average 24 prescriptions daily, while in Great Britain this number is 76, and in Spain, a staff member dispenses 140 prescriptions per day. These data are, however, from around the year 2000, and newer data are not available. These numbers are a reflection of the internal organization of pharmacies. In Finland, for instance, the pharmacist often sits behind a desk when assisting the client. Packages are opened and tablets counted. All medicines are dispensed with an individual label. In many other countries, packages are never opened, nor are labels made, and the stock in (small) pharmacies is limited. There are indications that the number of prescriptions dispensed is increasing.

## THE STAFFING OF PHARMACIES IN EUROPE

Depending on its size, a pharmacy may have one or as many as 10 pharmacists. Where there are many pharmacists, a few non-trained staff are also employed.

In many countries, pharmacy staff members must be licensed, with the exceptions being Greece, Spain, France and the UK. These non-pharmacist staff members can perform some of the dispensing tasks in a pharmacy. Their education, however, shows broad variation. Whereas in the Netherlands assistant pharmacists are allowed to dispense drugs without the necessity of a pharmacist being present on the premises, in almost all other countries, the pharmacist must be present and must supervise and control the dispensing process carried out by assistants or technicians. This supervisory role does not require the pharmacist to control all activities of a trained assistant; rather, the pharmacist must have overall control of the pharmacy, and is the first responsible person when mistakes are made.

## THE RANGE OF PRODUCTS AVAILABLE FROM EUROPEAN PHARMACIES

In Europe, the dispensing of prescribed medicine comprises approximately 80% of a pharmacy's financial turnover. However, in Switzerland, this figure is only 50%.

In some countries, pharmacies are heavily dependent on the sale of non-medical items such as cosmetics and food. In Croatia, Italy and Ireland, such items add more than 20% to a pharmacy's turnover. Cosmetics are particularly important in Portugal, Great Britain and Ireland, where they account for more than 10% of their turnover. OTC medicines constitute a large proportion (around 30%) of pharmacies' turnover in countries such as Sweden and Switzerland. In a number of European countries, even toys are sold by pharmacies (e.g. England, Iceland and Italy). Reading glasses can be obtained in pharmacies in most Western European countries, except the Netherlands.

The place of alternative medicines (herbal medicines and homeopathic preparations) in pharmacies varies, partially as a result of the historical developments in a particular country. In Germany and the Eastern European countries, for example, they are much more prominent than in the Scandinavian countries, where they have a minimal place in health care. In Sweden and Malta, homeopathic products cannot be found in pharmacies.

## THE SERVICES PROVIDED IN EUROPEAN PHARMACIES

### Clinical Pharmacy Services

As pharmacists have embraced clinical pharmacy as a concept, their concerns about adverse effects and drug interactions have increased and they have found a new role in the protection of patients from undesirable drug effects and drug-related problems. In most countries, this role is poorly structured and involves performing retrospective drug use evaluations (see also Chapter 20). Prospective drug use evaluation, or medication surveillance, is not yet standard in Europe, although it certainly is part of the Good Pharmacy Practice concept in most countries. In the UK and Ireland, prescribing pharmacists can be found, although this prescribing is only seldom really independent and usually not part of pharmacy services. In other European countries, this concept has not taken root, and the fundamental legal and ethical separation between prescribing and dispensing still exists. However, repeat prescribing is now increasingly being initiated in the pharmacy to improve adherence.

Reliable medication surveillance can only be performed using a computer and when key patient-related data, such as indications and contraindications, are accessible. Although the majority of community pharmacies in Europe are computerized, these systems were not originally developed for a clinical pharmacy function, but rather to enable billing for the medicines dispensed and for the labelling of medicines. Additionally, in most Scandinavian countries, privacy laws hinder pharmacists from keeping patient data for an extended period of time on a computer.

Well-developed computerized medication surveillance can be found in the Netherlands, but even there only some major indications for drug use are available to the pharmacist. In Iceland and Denmark, concurrent drug use evaluation is always carried out when patients present a prescription in the pharmacy. However, in these countries, essential patient data are also missing and, unlike in the Netherlands, patients in Iceland and Denmark do not always go to the same pharmacy. In Austria, Croatia and Poland, no medication data are kept in the pharmacy (see Chapter 20 for further details on medication surveillance methods).

## Pharmaceutical Care

Around 1990, in many European countries, the focus of the pharmacist's activities started to shift from the drug to the patient. This was due in part to the introduction of the pharmaceutical care philosophy, developed first by Hepler and Strand in 1990 in the US. Currently, most European countries are trying to incorporate pharmaceutical care into their pharmacy systems, stimulated by the national pharmacists' organizations, the PCNE and the International Pharmaceutical Federation. In Europe, pharmaceutical care is considered to be 'the pharmacist's contribution to the care of individuals in order to optimize medicines use and improve health outcomes', according to the 2013 PCNE definition (Alleman et al. 2014). In practice, many barriers to the implementation of pharmaceutical care are still apparent throughout Europe, as shown in Box 4.1. Universities and national pharmacists' organizations are continuously trying to address these barriers.

Pharmaceutical care has not yet been fully assimilated across Europe. No clear change in pharmaceutical practice can yet be noted in Italy, Greece, Turkey, France and some of the former Eastern European countries. The opportunities for pharmaceutical care appear to be greatest in countries with large, well-equipped pharmacies

---

**BOX 4.1   THE MAJOR BARRIERS TO
IMPLEMENTING PHARMACEUTICAL CARE***

- Lack of resources
- Lack of pharmacist's time
- The attitudes and opinions of other health professionals
- Inadequate communication skills of pharmacists
- The health care structure in general

---

* As identified in a study of the pharmaceutical care network Europe conducted by the University of Groningen in 1998–1999.

such as those in Scandinavian countries and the Netherlands, where tasks can be divided among team members.

Another major barrier exists when patients do not always visit the same pharmacy. In most countries except Greece, Iceland, the Netherlands, Norway and Switzerland, less than 80% of people visit the same pharmacy when they need medicines. Because care is, by definition, a process that takes place over time, this is an important consideration.

According to a recent survey by a Portuguese academic institute, extended services which have been implemented in one or more countries are: smoking cessation, medication reconciliation, medication review and counselling. Some disease-specific programmes have been implemented in a number of countries, such as supporting programmes for patients with diabetes, asthma and chronic obstructive pulmonary disease (COPD). The structures for such programmes are usually provided by the national pharmacists' associations.

## Diagnostic Testing

Although the performance of blood and urine tests in pharmacies was quite common at the beginning of the twentieth century, in most countries, these activities are now performed by specialized laboratories. Urine tests, for example, are performed by almost all pharmacies in Denmark, Germany, Iceland, Spain and Switzerland, but not elsewhere. In the same countries plus Portugal and Italy, patients can go to almost any pharmacy for a blood pressure test. Spain is the only European country in which the majority of pharmacies offer glucose testing. In Belgium, Ireland, the Netherlands, Norway and Sweden, clinical tests are not routinely performed in community pharmacies.

## Drug Information to the Public

Most pharmacies in Europe provide drug information to the public, although this has not always been the case. In many countries, physicians have long claimed the right to provide patients with drug information, as they feared patients would become confused if they received such information from different sources. However, when the pharmaceutical industry began to inform the patient (because of liability issues), the situation changed. Patients often became upset when reading information leaflets supplied in packages of medication, and sought other sources of information. In the 1970s, pharmacotherapy was included in the pharmacy curriculum in most countries, and consequently, pharmacists have the knowledge to provide appropriate drug information to the public. Additionally, pharmacists now learn skills for counselling in their university education in almost all European countries.

The spontaneous provision of information from pharmacies is still limited. For instance, in Austria, Denmark, France, Germany, Greece, Poland, Portugal and Switzerland, medicines are not labelled when dispensed. In most countries, medicines are dispensed with special patient information leaflets, either from the pharmaceutical industry or from the pharmacy. However, this is still not routinely the case in Finland, France, Iceland, Ireland, Norway and Portugal.

## Drug Information to Other Professionals

In some countries, pharmacists also provide drug information to other health professionals, especially general medical practitioners. This activity is still developing and depends on the quality of the relationship between pharmacist and physician (see also Chapter 15). In Croatia, Germany, Greece, Ireland, Italy, Poland, Portugal and Switzerland, pharmacy organizations have reported that the relationships between the general practitioner and pharmacist are 'not so good'. However, governments are looking for pharmacists to influence prescribing patterns to achieve cost containment. In the Netherlands, for example, there are regular pharmacotherapeutic meetings between general practitioners and community pharmacists. All pharmacists and general practitioners attend regional or local meetings at least once every two months. Prescription data are used to analyse and influence general practitioners' prescribing behaviour (de Vries et al. 1999). In Norway and Sweden, attempts are being made to introduce a similar system. However, with increasing competition for health care funds, the relationships between these professionals in many European countries have also become more strained.

## CONCLUSION

Most community pharmacies in Europe are moving towards a pharmaceutical care practice philosophy, as is apparent from the 2013 definition of the PCNE. The patient is increasingly becoming the focus of pharmacists' attention. The PCNE stresses the importance of a regular medication review involving the pharmacist, general practitioner and patient, combined with appropriate and timely counselling as the cornerstones of that care. Concomitantly, clinical pharmacy and pharmacology have become increasingly important, as has the provision of information to other health professionals. The demands put on pharmacists have also changed. Continuing professional development is increasingly required, often coupled with licensing requirements.

It is clear that throughout Europe, pharmacies are under financial pressure, even though medicines are usually the cheapest treatment option available in health care. Governments are seeking to reduce their health care budgets, and in particular, their drugs budget seems to be an easy target. Well-educated pharmacists and influential pharmacists' organizations are required to inform these developments and facilitate the future changes and development of pharmaceutical service delivery across Europe.

## ACKNOWLEDGEMENTS

Some of the data in this chapter are derived from the dissertation of van Mil (2000). More recent data come from two important studies conducted in 2013–2014 by the Instituto Superior de Ciências da Saúde Egas Moniz in Lisbon, Portugal, and the University of Leuven in Belgium. The results of both studies will be published.

## REFERENCES

Allemann, S.S., van Mil, J.W., Botermann, L., Berger, K., Griese, N. and Hersberger, K.E. 2014. Pharmaceutical care: The PCNE definition 2013. *International Journal of Clinical Pharmacy* **36**, 544–555.

de Vries, D.S., van den Berg, P.B., Timmer, J.W., Reicher, A., Blijleven, W. and Tromp, T.F. 1999. Prescription data as a tool in pharmacotherapy audit (II). The development of an instrument. *Pharmacy World Science* **21**, 85–90.

van Mil, J.W.F. 2000. *Pharmaceutical Care, the Future of Pharmacy. Part III. Pharmaceutical Care in World-Wide Perspective* [Dissertation]. University of Groningen.

# 5 Pharmacy in North America

*Qian Ding, Albert I. Wertheimer and Joaquima Serradell*

## CONTENTS

### KEY POINTS

- The health care system in the United States is complex and includes regulators, facilities, health care providers, multiple payers and patients/consumers.
- Financing of health care services involves multiple payers and complex mechanisms of payment.
- Conventional health care cost reimbursement is based on a retrospective fee-for-service basis, paid by patients or indemnity health insurers.
- The government runs Medicare, Medicaid and alternative programmes offering medical and health-related services insurance to certain sections of the population.
- Managed care organizations have contracts with doctors and hospitals; patients insured with them use only those services nominated by the insurance company.
- In managed care, physicians are limited in what they can prescribe and pharmacists are constrained regarding pricing and the items for which they can expect to be paid.

- Formularies are employed to contain costs and eliminate access to inappropriate drugs.
- There are two categories of pharmaceuticals in the United States: prescription and over-the-counter medicines.
- In the United States, pharmacists have a role in dispensing medicines, medication therapy management, quality of care and patient safety.
- The growth of technologies and automation in health care systems has improved efficiency.
- Canada has a single-payer, largely public-funded health care systems.
- Mexico has a complex system: a social security system provides care for the poor, an alternative system provides care for government employees and there is a rapidly growing privately funded sector.

## INTRODUCTION

The United States has the most expensive health care system in the world. In 2012, US health care expenditure reached $2.8 trillion, or $8,915 per person (Centers for Medicare and Medicaid Services; National Health Expenditures 2012). The share of health spending to gross domestic product (GDP) in the United States was 18% in 2011 – remaining well above the Organisation for Economic Co-operation and Development (OECD) average of 9.3% among 34 advanced member countries (Organisation for Economic Co-operation and Development 2013). On a per-capita basis, the United States spent $8,508 on health care – the biggest spending country – which was more than double the $3,322 average of all OECD countries in 2011 (Organisation for Economic Co-operation and Development 2013).

The health care system in the United States has developed into a complex system with components of regulators, facilities, health care providers, multi-payers and patients (consumers). Fundamentally, there are two types of health care system: the privatized health care system and the government schemes. In 2012, 84.6% of the US population (263.2 out of 311.1 million) had some type of health insurance, with 63.9% of the population (198.8 million) covered by a private health insurance plan through employment-based or direct purchase (DeNavas-Walt et al. 2013). In the traditional privatized health insurance systems – in terms of both for-profit (e.g. Aetna) and not-for-profit (e.g. Blue Cross/Blue Shield) organizations – a premium is paid based not on the ability to pay, but on the services required and the probability of being sick. With insurance schemes, a health premium is paid to an insurance company and the individual is free to go to any doctor or hospital for treatment. Insurance companies pay the bill. This has the disadvantage of high costs for the insurance company, as there is no direct control on the provider of health care. In health maintenance organizations (HMOs), the health insurance company and the provider of health care have a contract with each other. The individual is restricted to the doctors and hospitals nominated by the insurance company. HMOs have subsequently become managed care organizations (MCOs). The other system, covering 32.6% of the population (101.5 million people), received coverage through the US Government in 2012: Medicare (48.9 million), Medicaid (50.9 million) and/or Veterans Affairs or other military care (13.7 million) (people may be covered by more than one government plan) (DeNavas-Walt et al. 2013). In the Medicare system, free inpatient medicines and hospital treatment are provided to those aged 65 and over and the disabled. It excludes several types of treatment, such as medically unnecessary private-duty nursing and nursing homes. The Medicaid program provides medical and health-related services for poor people aged younger than 65 years who cannot afford to pay insurance premiums. In 2012, 15.4% of people (48.0 million) in the United States had no health insurance (DeNavas-Walt et al. 2013).

Although the United States spends more on health care than other industrialized countries, the system does not produce the best health care for Americans. The American health care still retains severe problems by not providing health insurance to 48 million uninsured people. The 2001 Institute of Medicine (IOM) report *Crossing the Quality Chasm: A New Health System for the 21st Century* recommended that all health care organizations, as well as professional groups and purchasers of health care, pursue six major aims of health care improvement: safety, timeliness, effectiveness, efficiency, equity and patient-centredness (Institute of Medicine Committee on Quality of Health Care in America 2001). However, the latest 2014 Commonwealth Fund international surveys report from patients' and primary care physicians' perspectives indicated that the United States ranks last in terms of the health outcomes access related to cost, efficiency, equity and healthy lives among the following 11 industrialized countries: Australia, Canada, France, Germany, the Netherlands, New Zealand, Norway, Sweden, Switzerland, the UK and the US (Davis et al. 2014). The data in this report were collected before the full implementation of the Patient Protection and Affordable Care Act in 2014. As of May 2014, approximately 20 million Americans had gained insurance coverage under the Affordable Care Act and the percentage of uninsured Americans dropped from 18% in the third quarter of 2013 to 13.4% in May 2014 (Blumenthal and Collins 2014).

Pharmacy, as a subsystem, plays an important role in the overall health care systems by providing prescription drugs to prevent acute diseases, provide relief from pain, control chronic diseases and hence improve the quality of life of Americans. Growing expenditure on pharmaceuticals over the last decades has motivated employers, insurers and MCOs to manage this cost better. Between 1990 and 2000, prescription expenditures grew by an average of 11.6%: much faster than spending for hospital (5.2%) and physician and clinic (6.2%) care during the same period (National Center for Health Statistics 2014). The total prescription drug expenditures reached $263 billion, accounting for 10% of all national health expenditures in 2011 (National Center for Health Statistics 2014).

Financing of the health care services in the United States involves multiple payers and complicated mechanisms of payment. The conventional reimbursement method is based on fee-for-service, a retrospective payment system in which the charges for health care services are billed after the health care service has been provided. Third-party payers usually have an agreement, also called the reimbursement formulary, with the health care providers on what and how much will be paid to the providers. Here, a branded drug product is usually prescribed, free from any formulary or other controls. The patient pays for such medication out of their own pocket, or in some cases is partly or wholly reimbursed by an indemnity health insurer. A second market is the government as payer for health insurance for Medicare, Medicaid or alternative programmes, including hospitals, long-term care facilities, governmental facilities, the military and veterans care centres. Most often, these large buyers make purchase decisions based upon annual tenders or solicited bids and use generic (non-branded) products wherever possible. A third market is the managed care market, in which branded and generic products are used based upon negotiations between manufacturers and MCOs regarding price, rebates and market share requirements. The managed care market includes HMOs, preferred provider organizations (PPOs) and other alternative insurance plans. If an HMO was able to guarantee that a particular product would maintain 90% of its therapeutic category sales, that HMO would be able to purchase that product for its patients at a lower price than an HMO guaranteeing a market share of 60%. A PPO is a network of health care providers who agree with the payers to provide health care services at a lower/discounted price in return for a large volume of patients. Patients are encouraged to use these providers in the network by lower co-payments, as well as deductibles, and are discouraged with higher co-payments and fewer deductibles for using the providers outside of the network.

## THE US HEALTH CARE SYSTEMS

The health care systems in the United States comprise three major players: patients or consumers, health care providers and third-party payers or multi-payers. Third-party payers including private health insurance companies and the government play a major role serving as an intermediary for managing the financial risk between patients and health care providers. The individual patient pays the premiums to third-party payers under the individual policy (HMOs or PPOs) in exchange for some amount of medical insurance coverage. Employers in the United States usually pay the majority of the premiums as part of the benefits package for their employees, and the employee pays the remainder of the premiums. Third-party payers will pool all the resources and allocate medical service resources to the individual who is sick. As part of the health insurance plan, the patients or consumers may first pay a certain sum of money before getting medical service coverage as a deductible and a fixed amount of co-payment per service, or a fixed percentage of the cost as co-insurance for each service. Health care providers provide medical services to the patients, bill the claims to third-party payers and receive reimbursement under a fixed-payment or variable-payment system. When a fixed payment is reimbursed to the health care providers, regardless of how many resources were used or services were delivered to the patients, the financial risk is transferred from the patients to the health care providers by third-party payers. Under a variable-payment system, such as fee-for-service, health care providers may face relatively less risk, but may produce unnecessary resource waste and expense.

In the real world, a number of components existing simultaneously throughout the US health care systems do not routinely communicate with each other. This may lead to inefficiencies, duplication and, ultimately, increased costs. The UK, where an overwhelming majority of care is provided and paid for by a single organization (the National Health Service), ranks at the top in terms of health outcomes, effectiveness, safety, patient-centred care, access related to cost and efficiency among the 11 industrialized countries in the 2014 Commonwealth Fund international surveys report (Davis et al. 2014).

The founders of the United States escaped religious and other persecution and believed in 'small government' that would do only what people could not do for themselves. The various religious groups established their own hospitals to care for their own communities as well as to provide for the poor. This was accomplished independently of what was happening or being planned by other religious denominations. The military services created a health care system of ambulatory sites and hospitals to take care of their members and dependents. The Veterans Administration established a network of hospitals and clinics to serve those no longer in the military services. Medical faculties provided care at major university sites to generate revenue, to provide patients for teaching and research purposes and to offer their expertise in difficult and complex situations. Cities and counties have established hospitals, originally for treatment of the poor, in order to compete with other urban areas and to attract industry, jobs and people interested in having such services nearby. Prisons have health services, as do student health facilities at colleges, nursing homes and mental health care centres. There is also another huge establishment: the 'for-profit' chains of hospitals, long-term care facilities and emergency care centres.

In 1966, the Medicaid and Medicare programs were enacted by the US government (Centers for Medicare and Medicaid Services 2006). The Medicaid program is designed for low-income and disabled people. Although it is financed jointly by the states and federal government through taxes, states administer the Medicaid program by determining the eligibility and medical benefits covered. People who are aged 65 or older, those under the age of 65 with certain disabilities and those having end-stage renal disease (permanent kidney failure requiring dialysis or a kidney transplant) at all ages are eligible for the Medicare program, which is compulsory with free premiums for most enrolees and covers hospital care, skilled nursing facility care, nursing home care (not custodial or long-term care), hospice care and some home health care. Medicare Part B (medical insurance), which is voluntary with premiums of $99.90 per month in 2012, covers doctors' services, outpatient care, emergency room services and some other medical services that Part A does not cover, such as some of the services of physical and occupational therapists and some home health care. Medicare Part C, also referred to as Medicare Advantage plans, consists of Medicare-approved private health insurance plans that provide all Medicare Part A, Part B and medically necessary services for individuals who are still in the Medicare program. As additional benefits, many Medicare Advantage plans include Medicare Part D prescription drug coverage. The Medicare Prescription Drug, Improvement, and Modernization Act was enacted into law by President George W. Bush on December 8, 2003, and introduced Medicare Part D, also known as Medicare Prescription Drug Plans, to everyone covered by Medicare in 2006. The patients who were enrolled in Medicare Part D needed to pay a $310 deductible, 25% of total drug costs between $310 and $2,850 and 100% of drug costs between $2,850 and $6,455 in total drug costs, equal to $4,550 in out-of-pocket expenses, known as the donut hole, in 2014 (Medicare.gov). After reaching the $4,550 out-of-pocket limit, the enrollees will automatically get catastrophic coverage to pay 95% of further drug costs. Co-payments are $2.55 for generic and $6.35 for brand name drugs (Centers for Medicare and Medicaid Services 2014).

The Children's Health Insurance Program (CHIP), signed into law by President Bill Clinton in 1997, is a public health insurance programme designed for children under 18 years old from low-income families who are ineligible for Medicaid but cannot afford private insurance. Like Medicaid, CHIP is jointly funded by the federal government and states, but administered by the states. As of 2011, 46 states and the District of Columbia cover children up to or above 200% of the federal poverty level (FPL) ($44,700 for a family of four in 2011), and 24 of these states offer coverage to children in families with incomes at 250% of the FPL or higher (The Center for Medicaid and CHIP Services [CMCS]). The Children's Health Insurance Reauthorization Act of 2009, signed into law by President Barack Obama in 2009, is designed to extend and expand coverage of CHIP by supporting continued coverage, expanding the enrolment eligibility of children, covering pregnant women and removing the 5-year waiting period for lawfully residing immigrant children and pregnant women. The Patient Protection and Affordable Care Act, also known as 'Obamacare', was signed into law by President Obama on 23 March 2010, and went into effect in January 2014. Under the Affordable Care Act, low- to moderate-income families between 100% and 400% of the FPL are now eligible for financial assistance in obtaining coverage, but they must purchase plans from the marketplaces in the HealthCare.gov website to get these funds.

## PHARMACEUTICALS

There has been food and drug legislation in the United States since 1906, when it originally dealt with adulteration and mislabelling of products. It has gradually evolved into the Food and Drug Administration (FDA) that today regulates food, drugs, cosmetics, medical devices and radiation-emitting equipment. A pharmaceutical medicine is referred to as a substance with a single active chemical ingredient or a combination of other pharmacologically active substances, which is recognized by an official pharmacopoeia or formulary and is intended to be used in the diagnosis, cure, mitigation, treatment or prevention of disease (US Food and Drug Administration). There are two categories of pharmaceuticals in the United States:

1. Prescription medicines: those which require a prescription from a duly licensed practitioner (physician, dentist, veterinarian, osteopath or optometrist) to purchase. Some pharmaceuticals (i.e. controlled substances) are controlled more carefully than others.
2. Over-the-counter (OTC) medicines: those which are sold directly to the general public without a prescription from a health care provider.

Prescription medicines include brand name medicines and generic medicines. A brand name medicine is a medicine marketed under a proprietary, trademark-protected name. A generic medicine contains the identical amounts of the same or therapeutically equivalent active ingredient(s) as the brand name product, but does not have trademark protection.

The OTC group may be sold in any type of store or vending machine, door to door or by mail order and are typically found at gasoline stations, hotel gift shops and convenience grocery markets. Because OTC medicines have a relatively lower risk and can be adequately labelled with indications, consumers can use them for self-diagnosed conditions without any professional supervision. OTC medicines include antihistamines for allergies and as hypnotics, topical steroid creams and ointments, topical antibiotic agents, $H_2$ receptor antagonists for ulcers, hair restorers, phenyl-propanolamine as a decongestant and dieting aid and dextromethorphan as a cough suppressant. In addition, there are many thousands of preparations that have been available OTC for many years, such as aspirin, some non-steroidal anti-inflammatory drugs, antacids, wart removers, laxatives, vitamins and minerals.

A pharmaceutical product usually experiences a life cycle of preclinical testing (laboratory synthesis and animal testing), Investigational New Drug application, clinical trials (Phase I, II and III), New Drug Application and clinical testing: post-marketing Phase IV. The FDA's Center for Drug Evaluation and Research evaluates the safety and efficacy of all prescription and OTC medicines. The FDA approves the label and, in particular, the claims made for the product. It is not necessary to ask for advance approval of marketing and advertising materials since the manufacturer knows the limits of what claims have been approved. The phenomenon of direct-to-consumer pharmaceutical advertising in the United States has grown rapidly in the past decades. A manufacturer might advertise to the public, prompting patients to consult a physician to seek medical advice. The FDA also monitors the media and has the ability to stop advertising that does not portray a fair balance between benefits and risks, or activities that exceed the approved claims. Price is a separate matter for the manufacturer to determine and for the marketplace to evaluate, and the government has no role in this.

Pharmaceutical manufacturers sell their brand name medicines primarily to wholesalers at 20% or more lower than the average wholesale price (AWP), or list price suggested by the manufacturer. The wholesalers sell the drugs to the retail and mail-order pharmacies at the wholesale acquisition cost, generally 2%–4% above their purchase price. The profit margins of generic medicines are larger than brand name medicines because the wholesalers can obtain the lowest priced generic medication by price bidding among various generic pharmaceutical manufacturers. In the 1970s, the pharmacy benefit management companies (PBMs) were developed in the pharmaceutical prescription market with rebate negotiations with pharmaceutical manufacturers, formulary management, drug utilization reviews, generic drug substitution and disease management programmes. More and more private payers contract with PBMs to manage prescription drug benefits for their enrolees. In 2008, the American big three PBMs (Caremark/CVS, Express Scripts and Medco) dominated 42% of the US prescription drug market (Abrams 2009).

Until the mid-1960s, a pharmacy transaction was a two-party interaction. The first party – the patient – brought a prescription to the pharmacy. The second party – the pharmacist – dispensed medication and charged a fee to the patient, who paid that bill. Sometimes, that patient would have indemnity private or public health insurance and would submit the receipt for the prescription to the insurance company for eventual reimbursement. The insurers or PBMs would negotiate with the pharmacies and pharmaceutical manufacturers for discounts, thereby lowering the amount paid by consumers and reimbursed by an insurance company.

It is said that 'he who pays gets to call the shots'. This is certainly true with a drug benefit. Certain events occur in the United States that may not be permitted in other countries. The payer establishes a network of retail pharmacies which agree to discount the dispensing fee. A typical scenario would be where the usual and customary pharmacy dispensing fee is $5 and where an insurer visits pharmacies, saying that the workers of Zoom Motorworks will have a new medical insurance plan that includes prescribed medicine. They are to print a directory of pharmacies where these prescriptions may be dispensed at a co-payment fee of only $2 per prescription. Your shop can be in that directory if you agree to accept a dispensing fee of $3. In such a case, you collect the $2 from the patient and $1, plus the ingredients cost, from the health insurance company (Navarro and Wertheimer 1996). The pharmacist appreciates that $3 is lower than the customary payment, but may agree on the basis that an increased number of customers will visit the shop, some of whom may also purchase additional merchandise while waiting for the prescription to be dispensed.

## MANAGED CARE

In order to provide high-quality, cost-effective health care services, there are two essential aspects of every activity in health care delivery that must be managed: the unit cost and the utilization rate of each product or service (Navarro and Hailey 2006).

In 1973, some health insurers evolved into HMOs, a highly controlled staff model plan, which operated medical facilities and employed health care providers. They managed care as well as costs, established utilization review procedures, case management and cost control efforts and made contracts with physicians, hospitals and pharmacists that would offer discounts based on their bargaining power. Just as they set up their own network of community pharmacies, they sought discounts at local hospitals and sent all of their patients to those one or two hospitals offering them the lowest prices. For instance, they might ask for bids from ophthalmologists for cataract removal procedures. If the going rate was $2,000, they would accept an offer of $1,500 from one clinic for a two-year contract for all of their patients requiring cataract removal. In two years, the bidding process would begin again, and those ophthalmologists who were excluded for the past two years would be expected to be aggressive bidders, perhaps opening offers at $1,200 this time around.

HMOs subsequently became MCOs. They were able to compare the cost of prescribing, number of patients seen, etc., for different locations. Just as they limited the number of ophthalmologists, they also limited the number of pharmacies, and controlled the variety and selection of drugs they would pay for. This was accomplished through the use of a formulary for which the MCO would pay, a list of prescription medicines that today is only found online.

HMOs had privileges in controlling the cost, but offered less freedom of selection in health care providers and services. Unlike HMOs, another type of MCO is a PPO, which provides greater freedom of choice in an expanded network of health care providers. In the PPO plan, patients are encouraged to choose within the contracted network of health care providers for a provider of choice. However, the patients are allowed to choose services from the non-contracted out-of-network health care providers for a higher cost and lower rate of reimbursement.

## Managed Care Pharmacy

MCOs place limitations on each of the participants in the health system. Patients have some incentives and disincentives that influence their choices and have to face some limitations. Physicians have limitations on what they can prescribe and pharmacists have constraints on their pricing and on what items they can expect to be paid for. Especially when prescription expenditures grew faster in the past decades, managed care pharmacy developed formularies and co-payment tiers and other dispensing limitations. As a result, many professional opportunities are open to pharmacists, such as medication therapy management (MTM) services, clinical pharmacy services, health outcomes research, pharmacy and therapeutics committees and PBMs. Let us examine these instruments of cost containment and quality assurance.

## Formularies

The formulary is a continually updated list of medications that represents the clinical and cost-effectiveness judgements of a group of pharmacists and physicians who are experts in diagnosis and disease management. The third-party payers and PBMs use drug formularies as a basis for reimbursement to promote the most cost-effective medicines. Clinical trial data on efficacy, price effectiveness and safety are the primary criteria for the formulary decision. Increasingly, health outcomes research in real-world settings provides evidence in comparative effectiveness study, health-related quality of life and health care utilization, which are important in reimbursement assessment and payer decision making.

There are two basic types of formularies: positive and negative. Positive formularies are vastly more popular for a number of reasons. They are inclusive and specify which drugs are eligible for reimbursement. For example, if the practitioner does not find the beta blocker required in the formulary, the beta blocker section will present acceptable alternative agents in that category. The positive formulary gives control to the publisher. If it is not listed, it is not paid for. This type of formulary uses tier co-payments (tier I, II, III and IV) to encourage the prescription of lower-cost generics or preferred brand formulary products. The tier I of preferred generics contains the lowest co-payment. The high-tier medicines are non-preferred brand medicines that require high co-payment. A negative formulary is exclusive and lists drugs not covered. There is a constant battle to list each new product as it is marketed, so it can be excluded until more information is available or until such time that the formulary committee can discuss it and make a decision. Generally, new drugs are not considered in the formulary for at least a few months after launching due to safety concerns. Prior authorization is used as an interim step. Often it is used as a utilization management tool until a formal formulary decision is made. Providers might have to telephone the MCO and describe the rationale for the new or authorization-requiring drug. The mere fact that a telephone call is required usually serves as a deterrent to its use. Prior authorization is seen as reasonable for drugs with a high liability due to off-label or unconventional usage. A negative formulary is a never-ending endeavour and must be revised almost constantly.

Formularies serve several purposes. They may be used as instruments to eliminate inferior, less effective or more dangerous drugs. They can be tools to contain costs by including only the least costly items in each category or those found to be optimally cost effective. In addition, they may be used as a revenue source. Some MCOs ask a fee from manufacturers to have drugs listed in the formulary. There are business negotiations undertaken routinely in which an additional discount is offered to MCOs if a specified product achieves a certain market share.

## Co-Payments

A co-payment is a fixed amount of fee charged to the patient at the time of dispensing if the patient is enrolled in a health insurance plan. Patients are encouraged to use cost-effective drugs and preferred brand name drugs through the four-tier programme to differentiate co-payments among generic medicines (tier I), preferred brand name medicines (tier II), non-preferred brand name drugs and preferred speciality drugs (tier III) and speciality drugs (tier IV). Tier I has the lowest co-payment and tier IV has the highest co-payment. Some programmes contain five tiers by dividing generic medicines into two tiers: preferred generics and non-preferred generics. A typical co-payment for a preferred generic drug varies from $4 to $10 for a 30-day supply. Increasingly, many pharmacy stores, such as Walmart, Target and K-Mart, offer the lowest co-payment of $4 for a 30-day supply of preferred generic drugs. The co-payment for brand name and non-formulary drugs varies from $20 to $50 or more and would serve as a strong incentive for the patient to authorize the dispensing of the cheaper medication.

A patient brings his or her plan membership card and the prescription to any pharmacy participating in the network of community pharmacies. The pharmacist enters the patient identification information, health insurance plan and the prescription data into the computer and instantly receives a message from the PBM or directly from the MCO. Health care providers can now transmit electronic-based prescriptions directly to the patient's preferred pharmacy from the point of care through a computer network system. Patient eligibility is checked, the co-payment rate is provided to the dispensing pharmacist and a drug utilization review process is initiated. If the drug is contraindicated with other drugs used by that patient dispensed at any other network pharmacy, a message is sent to the dispensing pharmacist, alerting the pharmacist to the situation. Similarly, if both warfarin and aspirin are prescribed to the same patient, it would be called to the attention of the pharmacist.

Not visible to the pharmacist or patient are the data-gathering functions of the computer system. It is typical for PBMs to track the percentage formulary compliance of the physicians, percentage generic drug use, cost per patient, average cost per prescription and total cost for prescribed drugs compared with other physicians within the same category and location.

## Drug Distribution Systems

Drug distribution systems comprise pharmaceutical manufacturers, wholesalers and pharmacies. There is a drug supply chain through which medicines are delivered from manufacturers to the patients. Pharmaceutical manufacturers are the providers of the prescription drugs in the drug supply chain. After mergers and acquisitions in the past decades, relatively few large global manufacturers are responsible for a large proportion of the revenue of the brand medicines today. The ten largest pharmaceutical corporations accounted for 56% of the total global sales of $817 billion in 2013: Johnson and Johnson ($67.2 billion), Novartis ($57.9 billion), Roche ($52.5 billion), Pfizer ($51.6 billion), Sanofi ($45.4 billion), Merck and Co ($44.0 billion), GlaxoSmithKline ($43.9 billion), Bayer ($40.2 billion), Fresenius ($28.0 billion) and AstraZeneca ($25.7 billion) (Current Partnering – life science intelligence for deal makers).

Simply put, pharmaceutical manufacturers sell a large quantity of drug products to the wholesalers or large purchasers, such as retail pharmacy chains, hospital chains or government purchasers, at a slightly lower price than the AWP or list price suggested by the manufacturer. There used to be hundreds of small local wholesalers, but the three big nationwide wholesalers have bought out most of their smaller competitors. In 2012, the total revenues of the drug distribution divisions were $289.8 billion from the big three wholesalers – McKesson Corporation ($116.9 billion), AmerisourceBergen Corporation ($95.1 billion) and Cardinal Health, Inc. ($77.8 billion) – generating 85% of all revenues from drug distribution in the US (Fein 2013). The wholesalers sell medicines to the retail and mail-order pharmacies at a few percentages above their purchase price. The vast majority of prescription medicines are dispensed to the patients/consumers from community pharmacies, with a growing percentage through large corporate chains, pharmacies located in supermarkets and mail service pharmacies. The informational labelling, approved by US FDA, and electronic bar-coding technology on the drug package ensure the safety of the drug supply chain and prevent errors in dispensing. Few drugs are distributed directly from pharmaceutical manufacturers to patients/consumers. According to the State of the Industry 2014 report, the corporate chains dominate, with Walgreens, the largest drug chain having 8,221 drug stores, followed by CVS Caremark (7,660), and Rite Aid (4,587), in the top three (Redman 2014). On the revenue side, Walgreens led the field in total sales ($72.2 billion), followed by CVS Caremark ($65.6 billion, retail drug store sales only) and Rite Aid ($25.5 billion) (Redman 2014). Recently, Internet-based pharmacies have emerged, though these generally use a mail service pharmacy to deliver drugs. While their market share is currently small, it is expected to grow rapidly due to its convenience and price advantages.

## Pharmacy Personnel

Traditionally, there was only the Accreditation Council for Pharmacy Education (ACPE)-accredited baccalaureate degree in four-year or five-year pharmacy programmes. The transition to the Doctor of Pharmacy (PharmD) as the sole professional practice degree (six-year programme in the United States) was initiated in 1997, with the implementation requirements for entering professional classes in the academic year 2000–2001, and completed in the academic year 2004–2005 with the graduation of the last student from an ACPE-accredited baccalaureate in pharmacy programme (Accreditation Council for Pharmacy Education 2011). PharmD programs usually comprise two years in general studies with completion of the pre-pharmacy requirements, followed by four years at pharmacy school. After completion of the highly structured curriculum in a PharmD program, graduates are eligible to sit for the North American Pharmacist Licensure Examination. Each of 50 states conducts its own examination. According to data from the American Association of College Pharmacy, as of autumn 2013, there were 62,743 students enrolled in the first professional year of PharmD programs (American Association of College Pharmacy 2013). In the past decade, rapid growth in new pharmacy schools and student enrolment has eased pharmacist workforce shortages in the United States. PharmD graduates may also undertake two postgraduate years (PGY1 and PGY2) in a residency programme in clinical pharmacy practice settings, community pharmacies and MCOs. The residency programme further trains pharmacists specializing in a particular disease area such as psychiatry, geriatrics, oncology, pediatrics and pharmacotherapy.

Traditionally, the role of the pharmacist is to dispense medicines to the patients. It is also common to see that the pharmacist is assisted by a certified technician or assistant. Technicians are most widely used in hospitals and in the mail service pharmacy areas. State laws usually regulate the maximum number of assistants who may be supervised by one pharmacist. Automations such as ScriptPro dispensing workstations have been widely used in community pharmacies to improve efficiency. The growth of health information technologies has significantly impacted the medication delivery systems in hospital pharmacies in the last decade. The American Society of Health-System Pharmacists national survey in 2011 showed that among the total 562 hospital respondents, 89% of hospitals used automated dispensing cabinets (ADCs) in their medication distribution systems, 67% used an electronic medication administration record system and 50% had barcode-assisted medication administration systems to verify patient identity and electronically check doses administered by nurses (Pedersen et al. 2012). Today, besides verifying the accuracy and appropriateness of prescriptions and dispensing, pharmacists have progressively undertaken further professional services for patients, including MTM services, patient counselling and health economic outcomes research.

The IOM published *To Err Is Human* in 1999, highlighting the safety concerns in medication delivery systems (Institute of Medicine 2000). A cross-sectional study in 2009 showed that dispensing errors occurred in 22 of 100 prescriptions (22%) at 100 community chain pharmacies in large metropolitan areas of Florida, Georgia, New Jersey and New York, with 43 shoppers (43%) receiving verbal counselling and 68% of warfarin shoppers purchasing aspirin without the pharmacist verbally warning them of possible consequences (Flynn et al. 2009). The results show that there is great scope for pharmacists to improve the quality of medication services to patients.

## CANADA AND MEXICO

Canada has a single-payer, mostly publicly funded health care system that is operated through each of the provinces and territories under the guidelines set by the federal government. Essentially, every Canadian citizen is covered by a group of socialized health insurance plans. In 2011, Canada spent 11.2% of GDP on health care and was the second placed country in terms of pharmaceutical expenditure per capita among the OECD countries, spending \$701 on pharmaceutical expenditure per capita, following the United States (\$985) (Organisation for Economic Co-operation and Development 2013). The Health Canada Act, as federal legislation, ensures Canadians receive comprehensive and universal health care services. All insured Canadians have access to the basic services, including primary care physicians and hospitals. If the insured resident moves to a different province, territory or country, the insurance is portable to the resident from their home province. As a supplement to primary health coverage, Canadians also have the option to choose the private health insurance plans usually offered as part of employee benefit packages by employers for services such as dental services, optometrists, prescription medications and specialized services. Fees are established centrally, and there is a combination of public and private institutions which work side by side. Benefit design varies slightly from province to province. The provincial governments determine their own formularies. Virtually all Canadian residents are included in the plan. The same drugs as in the US are marketed by the same multinational firms within the Canadian market. The personnel practising at Canadian pharmacies must have a bachelor's or doctor of pharmacy degree and complete the national board examination through the Pharmacy Examining Board of Canada.

Mexico is more difficult to characterize since three systems operate independently and in parallel. A large social security system operates that provides care for the poor. Another huge system provides care for government employees and some employees of government-owned firms. Both of these groups have formularies and other utilization controls. There is also a robust and rapidly expanding private sector made up of fee-for-service care and the newly emerging managed care and indemnity health insurance market places. Mexico spent 6.2% of GDP on health care and less money on pharmaceutical expenditure (\$295) per capita in 2011 (Organisation for Economic Co-operation and Development 2013). Unlike its sister North American nations, one may walk into a Mexican pharmacy and purchase nearly all drugs OTC, except for narcotics and scheduled abusable products. The personnel at pharmacies are usually minimally educated lay people. Mexico shares one positive feature with Europe not seen in the United States or in Canada: pre-packaged unit of use medicines (original packs). In the United States, the pharmacist dispenses a prescription for 36 or 45 or 90 tablets by counting that number of tablets from a bottle of 500 or 1,000 tablets.

## CONCLUSION

Pharmacy is practised very differently in North America from Europe and Asia, reflecting different social, political, economic, historical and financial traits, customs and traditions. All three systems of the United States, Canada and Mexico are largely different in terms of their health care delivery characteristics and yet they appear to function adequately in every region of North America. As out-of-pocket payments per capita and the uninsured population have increased substantially in recent years, the United States has undertaken a number of successful and unsuccessful efforts to improve the coverage and the quality of health care for Americans. The US health care system now consists of multiple systems that operate largely through private stakeholders and in collaboration with high levels of funding but a distinctively low level of involvement from government, with Medicare and Medicaid programs only arriving in the mid-1960s. More than 60% of Americans receive their coverage from private health insurance and 30% of the population is covered by government public health insurance. One in six Americans is uninsured and the population with no insurance is expected to gradually reduce with insurance coverage after the implementation of the Affordable Care Act in 2014. The United States is one of only two countries that permits the advertising of prescription drugs directly to patients and is one of only a small number of countries in which the manufacturer sets the drug price without any government involvement. The Canadian government regulates the price of pharmaceuticals and provides publicly funded health care systems. With advantages and disadvantages for each system, it is impossible to say which systems are 'right'. Likewise, it would be overly simplistic to state which systems are the 'best'. Some are more efficient or more controlled, but the basic question is whether the drugs/pharmacy sector can satisfy local expectations and remain compatible with changes and improvements in the overall health care delivery systems.

It appears that counterfeiting in the United States and Canada is minimal because of the tight controls and rules by the government on regulating the quality of pharmaceutical products. It remains an intriguing question as to whether all of the rules, regulations and controls make the United States or Canada safer for pharmaceutical users compared with many countries in which there are nearly no rules or laws that are followed, and whether certain system features might have universal benefit and be applicable elsewhere.

## FURTHER READING

Brown, T.R. 2006. *Handbook of Institutional Pharmacy Practice* (4th Ed.). Bethesda: American Society of Health-System Pharmacist.

Santerre, R. and Neun, S. 2012. *Health Economics: Theories, Insights and Industry Studies* (6th Ed.). Mason, OH: South-Western, Cengage Learning.

Smith, M.I., Wertheimer, A.I. and Fincham, J.E. 2013. *Pharmacy and the US Health Care System* (4th Ed.). London: Pharmaceutical Press.

Wertheimer, A.I. and Smith, M.C. 1989. *Pharmacy Practice: Social and Behavioral Aspects*. Baltimore: Williams and Wilkins.

## REFERENCES

Abrams, L.W. 2009. *Express Scripts' Unspoken Plan for its Wellpoint PBM Acquisition*. Retrieved from: http://www.nu-retail.com/The_Express_Scripts_Wellpoint_PBM_Deal.pdf.

Accreditation Council for Pharmacy Education 2011. *Accreditation Standards and Guidelines for Professional Programme in Pharmacy Leading to the Doctor of Pharmacy Degree*. Available at: https://www.acpe-accredit.org/pdf/FinalS2007Guidelines2.0.pdf.

American Association of College Pharmacy 2013. Profile of Pharmacy Students Fall 2013. Available at: http://www.aacp.org/resources/research/institutionalresearch/Documents/Fall_13_Introduction.pdf.

Blumenthal, D. and Collins, S.R. 2014. Health care coverage under the Affordable Care Act – A progress report. *New England Journal of Medicine*, **371**(3), 275–281.

Centers for Medicare and Medicaid Services 2006. Key milestones in medicare and medicaid history, selected years: 1965–2003. *Healthcare Financing Review*, **27**(2), 1–2. Retrieved from: http://www.cms.gov/Research-Statistics-Data-and-Systems/Research/HealthCareFinancingReview/downloads/05-06Winpg1.pdf.

Centers for Medicare and Medicaid Services 2012. National Health Expenditures 2012. Highlights. Available at: http://www.cms.gov/Research-Statistics-Data-and-Systems/Statistics-Trends-and-Reports/NationalHealthExpendData/Downloads/highlights.pdf.

Centers for Medicare and Medicaid Services 2014. Announcement of Calendar Year (CY) 2015 Medicare Advantage Capitation Rates and Medicare Advantage and Part D Payment Policies and Final Call Letter. Available at: http://www.cms.gov/Medicare/Health-Plans/MedicareAdvtgSpecRateStats/Downloads/Announcement2015.pdf.

Current Partnering – life science intelligence for deal makers. Top Pharmaceutical Companies. Retrieved from: http://www.currentpartnering.com/insight/company-tracker/top-50-pharma/.

Davis, K., Stremikis, K., Squires, D. and Schoen, C. 2014. *Mirror, Mirror on the Wall: How the Performance of the U.S. Health Care System Compares Internationally, 2014 Update*. New York: The Commonwealth Fund.

DeNavas-Walt, C., Proctor, B.D. and Smith, J.C. 2013. *US Census Bureau, Current Population Reports, P60-245, Income, Poverty, and Health Insurance Coverage in the United States: 2012*. Washington, DC: U.S. Government Printing Office.

Fein, A.J. 2013. *2013–14 Economic Report on Pharmaceutical Wholesalers and Specialty Distributors*. Philadelphia, PA: Drug Channels Institute.

Flynn, E.A., Kenneth, N.B., Berger, B.A., Lloyd, K.B. and Brackett, P.D. 2009. Dispensing errors and counseling quality in 100 pharmacies. *Journal of the American Pharmacists Association*, **49**(2), 171–182.

Institute of Medicine. 2000. *To Err Is Human: Building a Safer Health System*. Washington, DC: The National Academies Press.

Institute of Medicine Committee on Quality of Health Care in America 2001. *Crossing the Quality Chasm: A New Health System for the 21st Century*. Washington, DC: The National Academies Press.

National Center for Health Statistics 2014. *Health, United States, 2013: With Special Feature on Prescription Drugs*. Hyattsville, MD.

Navarro, R. and Hailey, R. 2006. Evolution of the management of U.S. health care: Managing costs to care management. In Brown, T. R. (Ed.), *Handbook of Institutional Pharmacy Practice* (4th Ed.). Bethesda, MD: American Society of Health-System Pharmacists, 85–98.

Navarro, R. and Wertheimer, A.I. 1996. *Managing the Pharmacy Benefit*. Warren, NJ: Emron.

Organisation for Economic Co-operation and Development 2013. Health at a Glance 2013: OECD Indicators. Available at: http://dx.doi.org/10.1787/health_glance-2013-en.

Pedersen, C.A., Schneider, P.J. and Scheckelhoff, D.J. 2012. ASHP national survey of pharmacy practice in hospital settings: Dispensing and administration – 2011. *American Journal of Health-System Pharmacy*, **69**(9), 768–785.

Redman, R. 2014. The Top 10 Drug Store Retailers. Available at: http://www.chaindrugreview.com/front-page/newsbreaks/the-top-10-drug-store-retailers.

The Center for Medicaid and CHIP Services (CMCS). CHIP Eligibility Standards. Retrieved from: http://www.medicaid.gov/Medicaid-CHIP-Program-Information/By-Topics/Childrens-Health-Insurance-Program-CHIP/CHIP-Eligibility-Standards-.html.

The Official U.S. Government Site for Medicare. *Drug Coverage* (Part D). Retrieved from: http://www.medicare.gov/part-d/index.html.

U.S. Food and Drug Administration. *FDA Glossary of Terms*. Retrieved from: http://www.fda.gov/drugs/informationondrugs/ucm079436.htm.

# 6 Pharmacy in New Zealand and Australia

*Pauline Norris, Alesha Smith and Rhiannon Braund*

## CONTENTS

---

### KEY POINTS

- Health care is organized in Australia on a federal system involving both national and state governments. In New Zealand, it is organized by central government.
- New Zealand and Australia have five broad classifications of medicines.
- Australia has 18 schools of pharmacy and there are two in New Zealand.
- New Zealand has a declining number of community pharmacies, while these have increased in Australia.
- Community-based pharmacists with advanced clinical knowledge are able to provide advanced services.

---

## HEALTH CARE SYSTEM

Australia and New Zealand health care systems are often recognized as first rate, due to their universal coverage and affordability for both health services and pharmaceuticals. The similarities and differences between these two jurisdictions are outlined below. Many of the differences are due to Australia being a federal system, with both national and state governments being involved in aspects of the health service.

93

The New Zealand health system is primarily funded through taxation. Each year, the government decides how much of its tax revenue (from income tax, sales tax, company tax, etc.) to allocate to health services. Most of this money is allocated to the 20 District Health Boards (DHBs), which are responsible for providing appropriate health services to people in their geographic region. Most hospital care is provided free of charge to patients in publicly owned hospitals. There are some private hospitals, but they do not provide a full range of health services, concentrating mainly on non-urgent surgery. Most primary care is provided in the community by private sector practitioners contracted to the DHB. For example, general practitioners (GPs) work in privately owned practices, usually in small groups. The DHB contributes towards the cost of GP visits, but patients also pay a charge for each visit. DHBs also contract with community pharmacists to dispense medicines and to provide pharmaceutical services to patients. Until recently, pharmacists have been paid per item for dispensing medicines, but in 2012, the introduction of a new community pharmacy services agreement, which included a long-term conditions service (IT Health Board 2014), aimed to increase the professional service fee paid to pharmacists for actively assisting those patients with long-term conditions and a need for extra support regarding medication use. This was accompanied by a corresponding decrease in the traditional 'dispensing' fee.

The Australian health care system is funded through three different mechanisms: taxes, a Medicare levy (based on income) and private health insurance financing. The Commonwealth-based Medicare and Pharmaceutical Benefits Schemes (PBSs) cover all Australians and subsidize payments for private medical services, such as GP or specialist visits and pharmaceuticals, respectively. Patients are required to pay the remaining cost of these fees, if applicable, as out-of-pocket payments, which can vary based on the medical services provided or the discretion of the provider.

The Commonwealth and state governments also jointly fund public hospital services. However, the responsibility for the delivery of services falls to the individual state and territory governments. These services are provided free of charge to people who choose to be treated as public patients, approximately 60% of all hospitalizations in 2011–2012.

Private health insurance can cover private and public hospital charges (public hospitals charge only patients who elect to be private patients in order to be treated by the doctor of their choice) and a portion of medical fees for inpatient services. Depending on the level of cover chosen, private health insurance can also cover allied health services (e.g. physiotherapy, paramedical services and complementary health services, such as massage/acupuncture and some aids/appliances, including spectacles) (Australian Government [A] Department of Human Services 2014).

## MEDICINES REGULATION

The quality, safety and efficacy of medicines in New Zealand is regulated by Medsafe (the New Zealand Medicines and Medical Devices Safety Authority), a business unit of the Ministry of Health. Medsafe approves medicines for marketing in New Zealand, decides on how medicines should be classified (e.g. prescription only), ensures appropriate post-marketing surveillance and decides how to act on reports of adverse reactions to medicines.

The Therapeutic Goods Administration (TGA) is part of the Australian government Department of Health. Its role is very similar to that of Medsafe in New Zealand. The TGA is responsible for regulating the supply, manufacturing and advertising of therapeutic goods, including prescription medicines. The TGA schedules medicines based on different levels of risk to patients; medicines with a higher risk (usually prescription medicines) are assessed by the TGA for quality, safety and efficacy; medicines with a lower risk (usually over-the-counter [OTC] medicines; e.g. complementary medicines) are only assessed for quality and safety. Once available for supply in Australia, the TGA monitors all products and has a comprehensive adverse event reporting programme.

In recent years, there has been discussion and some movement towards establishing a regulatory body which will license medicines for both New Zealand and Australia (Medsafe 2013a,b). In 2013, the TGA and Medsafe established a parallel early warning system in Australia and New Zealand for the early advising of potential safety concerns associated with medicines or medical devices.

## FUNDING OF MEDICINES

In New Zealand, most medicines are funded by the government through DHBs. The Pharmaceutical Management Agency (PHARMAC) negotiates prices for medicines with pharmaceutical companies. PHARMAC uses a range of strategies, such as reference pricing across therapeutic groups and contracting for the sole supply of single medicines (like paracetamol). These strategies have led to very low medicines prices by international standards (Cumming et al. 2010). PHARMAC also plays a role in encouraging appropriate medicines use, such as a campaign about antibiotic use.

Patients pay a small co-payment (currently N.Z.$5) per prescription item for most medicines. Some medicines are only partially subsidized, because PHARMAC and manufacturers have been unable to agree on prices. In this case, the patient pays the difference between the subsidy that PHARMAC is prepared to pay and the price demanded by the manufacturer. Patients (or families) should only pay for 20 items per year before they are exempt from prescriptions charges. However, some people do not know about or receive this exemption. There is evidence that even this small co-payment can prevent some people accessing prescription medicines (Jatrana et al. 2010).

Once a medicine has been approved for supply in Australia, the manufacturer can apply to have it listed on the PBS. The Pharmaceutical Benefits Advisory Committee (PBAC) is an independent expert body appointed by the Australian government; membership includes health professionals, health economists and consumer representatives. The primary role of this committee is to recommend new medicines for listing on the PBS. When recommending a medicine for listing, the PBAC takes into account the medical conditions for which the medicine was registered for use in Australia and its clinical effectiveness, safety and cost effectiveness compared with other treatments (Australian Government [B] Department of Health 2014).

Once recommended for listing, the Commonwealth government negotiates a price with the supplier and makes the medicines available to all Australians at a subsidized cost. Patients then pay the lowest value of either the total cost of the medicine or the co-payment fee, which is set each year by the government; in 2014, this was set at

AUS$36.90 for general patients and AUS$6.00 for concession patients. The patient safety net threshold is currently AUS$1,421.20 and AUS$360 for general and concession patients, respectively. When a person and/or their family's total applicable co-payments reach this amount, they may apply for a safety net concession card and pay the concessional co-payment (for general patients) or receive free pharmaceuticals (concession patients) for the rest of that calendar year. Patients are required to pay more than the co-payment for prescriptions if they choose to use a particular brand of medicine listed on the PBS which costs more than another brand of the same medicine (brand premium). If a medicine is not listed on the PBS, patients pay the full cost (Australian Government [C] Department of Health 2015).

## MEDICINES CLASSIFICATION

Both New Zealand and Australia have five broad classifications of medicines (Box 6.1). Australia has a further four classifications (schedules), though medicines are not normally listed in these, and will therefore not be discussed.

---

**BOX 6.1   NEW ZEALAND AND AUSTRALIA BROAD CLASSIFICATIONS OF MEDICINES**

1. Controlled medicines: mainly narcotics and certain psychotropic agents which have the potential to be misused.
2. Prescription-only medicines: these require a prescription from an authorized prescriber. In New Zealand, this includes doctors, nurse practitioners, midwives, dentists, pharmacist prescribers, endorsed optometrists and prescribing dieticians (special foods only). In Australia, this includes doctors, dentists, endorsed optometrists (restricted list of medicines only), endorsed midwives (restricted list of medicines only) and nurse practitioners.
3. Pharmacist-only medicines (sometimes referred to as restricted medicines) can only be sold in pharmacies by pharmacists and the details of the sale must be recorded (New Zealand only). Pharmacists should provide advice and professional input into the sales of these medicines.
4. Pharmacy-only medicines may only be sold in a community or hospital pharmacy or a shop in an isolated area that is licensed to sell that particular medicine. The sale may be made by any salesperson.
5. General sale: most other medicines can be sold in any shop, although there are some restrictions on pack size. For example, paracetamol is sold in supermarkets, convenience stores (dairies) and petrol stations, but only in small pack sizes.

Medsafe 2013b. Classification Categories and Criteria. Available from: http://www.medsafe.govt.nz/profs/class/classificationCategoriesAndCriteria.asp (accessed October 2014).

---

As in other countries, it is becoming increasingly common for people in New Zealand and Australia to purchase medicines from websites. Many of these websites appear to be from developed and well-regulated countries, but in fact they sell products of dubious identity and quality (US Food and Drug Administration 2014). Neither country has a land border with other countries, so all medicines are likely to come in by air, either in the mail or with passengers. Pharmacists are employed to advise border control officials on medicines identified at the border.

## PHARMACY EDUCATION

Schools of pharmacy in both Australia and New Zealand are accredited by the Australian Pharmacy Council. There is an indicative curriculum for pharmacy education, so there is considerable consistency in the programmes provided by Australian and New Zealand schools.

There are two schools of pharmacy in New Zealand: one at the University of Otago in Dunedin and the other at the University of Auckland. In order to register as a pharmacist in New Zealand, students must successfully complete both a bachelor's degree in pharmacy (four years of study) and a one-year internship organized by the Pharmaceutical Society.

At the University of Otago, most students complete a one-year course called Health Sciences First Year, which includes biochemistry, chemistry, physics, physiology and epidemiology. Entry into pharmacy is competitive and based on the grades students have achieved in their previous study. Because of high health needs among Māori and Pacific communities in New Zealand and shortages of Māori and Pacific pharmacists, students from these communities are preferentially selected. Approximately 150 students enter the school of pharmacy each year, and this usually includes about 30 international students, most of whom are studying in New Zealand as part of schemes sponsored by their home governments.

At the University of Auckland, most students enter pharmacy directly after secondary school. Entry into pharmacy is competitive and based on the grades students have achieved in their previous study and an interview.

Both the universities of Otago and Auckland also provide postgraduate courses for pharmacists to continue to develop their knowledge and skills. These include a new course to equip pharmacists to become prescribers.

There are 18 schools of pharmacy in Australia and 24 approved programmes of study. These are spread across all states and territories and offer three types of courses as pathways to becoming a pharmacist: a bachelor's degree of four years, a master's degree of two years and a joint bachelor's and master's degree of 4.5 years. Upon graduation, all students must then complete a 1-year intern training programme to become a registered pharmacist. Intern training programmes are offered by a number of providers, including universities, the Pharmaceutical Society of Australia and the Pharmacy Guild of Australia (Australian Health Practitioner Regulation Agency 2014). In 2014, there were 1,846 provisionally registered (intern) pharmacists in Australia, with the majority of these training in Queensland and New South Wales (Table 6.1).

Admission into a pharmacy degree in Australia is generally grade based and a competitive process. With the three different types of programmes on offer, students

**TABLE 6.1**

**The Number and Type of Pharmacy Programmes on Offer in Australia**

| State | Number of Schools | Number of Programmes | Approximate Student Numbers (as of 2014) |
|---|---|---|---|
| New South Wales | 5 | 4 × Bachelor's<br>3 × Master's | 638 |
| Queensland | 4 | 4 × Bachelor's<br>1 × Master's<br>1 × Bachelor's and Master's | 427 |
| Victoria | 3 | 3 × Bachelor's | 366 |
| Western Australia | 2 | 1 × Bachelor's<br>2 × Master's | 181 |
| South Australia | 1 | 1 × Bachelor's | 133 |
| Tasmania | 1 | 1 × Bachelor's | 48 |
| Australian Capital Territory | 1 | 1 × Bachelor's<br>1 × Master's | 34 |
| Northern Territory | 1 | 1 × Bachelor's | 19 |
| *Total* | *18* | *24* | *1846* |

can enter as school leavers, as graduates of a degree or transfer from another degree and complete an accelerated or fast-track course depending on each university's specific requirements. There is a mixture of domestic and international students training throughout Australia and most of the universities offer either scholarships or fee-free places to indigenous and/or rural students.

There is also a mix of research higher degrees (e.g. PhD or coursework-based postgraduate study options) throughout Australia. These provide continuing professional development aimed at enhancing clinical knowledge and skills.

## COMMUNITY PHARMACY

In New Zealand, the number of community pharmacies has decreased somewhat over the last 20 years, while the population has increased. In 1995, there were 1,049 pharmacies (one pharmacy per 3,534 people), but by 2010, there were 916 pharmacies (one pharmacy per 4,796 people). Some small rural towns have lost their community pharmacy as well as other shops and services, leading to potential problems with accessing medicines and pharmacists' advice (Norris et al. 2014). In some rural areas, a depot system operates, by which prescriptions are faxed to a community pharmacy in a larger town, dispensed by that pharmacy and transported to a shop which is licensed to act as a depot. Patients then pick up their prescriptions from the depot. This addresses some of the problems of access to medicines (although not usually to OTC medicines), but it does not address the problem of access to pharmacists' professional advice.

Community pharmacies must be owned by a registered pharmacist(s) and no pharmacist can own more than five pharmacies (Chesney and Ram 2012). Patients are free to visit any community pharmacy they wish, except to pick up repeat prescriptions, for which they must go back to the pharmacy where they took the original prescription.

All of the staff working within the pharmacy are legally under the supervision of the pharmacist. The staffing composition is generally considered to be in two sections: the dispensary and the front of shop. The front-of-shop staff range in their level of training and experience, but all must be familiar with the level of privacy expected within a health care setting. Some front-of-shop staff may be trained in basic information gathering needed to obtain the necessary patient history and recommend a treatment (general sale or pharmacy-only medication), but this must only occur under the direct supervision of a pharmacist.

Within the dispensary, the majority of the mechanical aspect of dispensing (packaging, preparation, labelling, etc.) is done by pharmacy technicians. Unlike some European countries, medicines are not dispensed in their original packages. Packs are opened and a specific label is prepared for each patient, with instructions and precautions. Pharmacy technicians must have completed – or be in the process of completing – a nationally recognized technicians' course. All prescriptions must be double checked by a pharmacist. Intern pharmacists (graduates who are completing their pre-registration year) have the same authority as a pharmacy technician.

In New Zealand, most community pharmacies sell OTC medicines, cosmetics and skin care products. Many also sell complementary medicines and some sell gift items. However, they do not stock grocery items, as many North American pharmacies do.

In Australia, the number of pharmacies continues to increase each year, and in 2014, there is estimated to be 5,500 community pharmacies that generate revenue of over $15 billion a year. The majority of pharmacies (>80%) are located in urban areas and in the Eastern Seaboard States of New South Wales, Victoria and Queensland. In all states, the average number of people per urban pharmacy is far less than the number of people per rural pharmacy. The Australian Community Pharmacy Authority regulates the number and location of pharmacies and only qualified pharmacists can own a pharmacy (IBISWorld 2012).

Core pharmacy services provided in Australia are medication management information, advice on minor ailments and OTC medicines and preventative care services. Community pharmacies are also the primary distribution points for prescription and scheduled OTC medicines. In addition, community pharmacies sell general retail products including a variety of therapeutic substances and aids (including vitamins and minerals), baby needs, beauty products, optical products, giftware and film development services. In 2011/2012, prescription items accounted for 65% of sales, non-prescription medicines accounted for 15% of sales and general retail accounted for 20% of sales (IBISWorld 2012).

In New Zealand, prescriptions for chronic conditions are usually written for three months' supply, provided to the patient as a 1-month supply with two repeats for non-stat, or three months' supply for stat (or all-at-once) dispensing. Whether a particular medication is on the stat or non-stat list is determined by a combination of the cost of the medication (low-cost medications can be given all at once) and the potential for harm (dangerous medications in overdose are generally given non-stat). The patient must return to the same pharmacy for repeats. In Australia, the doctor indicates how many repeats the patient is to be supplied with (up to five), and the patient can visit any pharmacy for the number of times indicated. The prescription and repeats are valid for 12 months from the original prescription date (Australian Government Department of Health 2014a).

Since the 1990s, there have been opportunities for community-based pharmacists with advanced clinical knowledge to provide a more clinically focused service to patients. In the early 1990s, there were Pharmaceutical Review Services, and in the late 1990s, there was Comprehensive Pharmaceutical Care. In 2006, the introduction of the National Pharmacy Services Framework provided a defined and stepwise approach to levels of pharmaceutical care based in the community. The first level of service is medication use reviews and adherence support, which involves an accredited pharmacist providing medication reviews and individualized assistance with adherence. The next level is medicines therapy assessment, which is intended to improve medication optimization and utilization. Comprehensive medicines management aims to improve medication optimization and utilization, but with more autonomy for the pharmacist. Legislation to allow pharmacists to prescribe was recently introduced, and in 2013 and 2014, the first two groups of pharmacists (16 in total) achieved registration as pharmacist prescribers (Ministry of Health New Zealand 2014, Pharmacy Council of New Zealand 2012). Twelve of these are prescribing in a hospital setting or at the interface of primary and secondary care. Specialities include mental health, paediatrics, renal medicine, surgical pre-admission and emergency care.

Alongside these defined clinical roles, pharmacy has grown a suite of other services, such as anticoagulant monitoring and immunizations. Under the 5th Community Pharmacy Agreement between the Australian government and the Pharmacy Guild, there have been a number of federally funded initiatives introduced to improve access to pharmacy services and to enhance the quality use of medicines. One such programme is a medication management initiative. Accredited pharmacists can conduct a comprehensive medicines review in residential aged care homes (residential medication management review [RMMR]) or patients' homes (home medicines review [HMR]), not in the pharmacy, after a referral from the patient's GP or hospital. The payments for these services are indexed and capped annually; in 2014, pharmacists received AUS$208.22 and AUS$105.29 per HMR and RMMR, respectively (Australian Government Department of Health 2014b).

## HOSPITAL PHARMACY

Thirteen percent of pharmacists (approximately 470) in New Zealand and 18% of pharmacists (approximately 3,762) in Australia work in hospital practice (Health Workforce Australia, Pharmacy Council of New Zealand 2012). In New Zealand and Australia, clinical pharmacy services are provided in each hospital and most wards are visited daily by a pharmacist. Clinical interventions of various types are carried out during ward visits and recorded for monitoring purposes and to identify recurring issues (Millar 2008, Plant et al. 2006). Pharmacists are involved in multidisciplinary team meetings and ward rounds and in services such as medicines information, medicines utilization review and aseptic production. In the larger hospitals, pharmacists may specialize in one clinical area (e.g. oncology, surgery, paediatrics, older people's health, mental health or clinical trials). However, in the smaller hospitals, they usually work in more than one speciality. Medicines reconciliation is carried out by pharmacists or technicians in many hospitals. Electronic medicines reconciliation systems and/or electronic prescribing systems have been established in a few hospitals, with continuing pharmacist input. Some newer roles for pharmacists are in emergency departments, antimicrobial stewardship, medication safety, surgical pre-admission clinics and 'medical admission pairing'.

## ACKNOWLEDGEMENT

We are very grateful to June Tordoff, Adele Print and Lorraine Welman for their help in the preparation of this chapter.

## USEFUL WEBSITES

The New Zealand health system: http://www.health.govt.nz/new-zealand-health-system
The Australian health system: http://www.health.gov.au/
Medsafe: www.medsafe.govt.nz
Therapeutic Goods Administration (TGA): http://www.tga.gov.au/
PHARMAC: www.pharmac.govt.nz
Pharmaceutical Benefits Scheme: www.pbs.gov.au
Pharmacy Council of New Zealand: www.pharmacycouncil.org.nz
Australian Pharmacy Council: http://pharmacycouncil.org.au/content/

## REFERENCES

Australian Government [A] Department of Human Services. 2014. Medicare. Available at: http://www.humanservices.gov.au/customer/subjects/medicare-services.

Australian Government [B] Department of Health. Therapeutic Goods Administration. 2014. Available at: http://www.tga.gov.au.

Australian Government [C] Department of Health. 2015. About the PBS. Available from: http://www.pbs.gov.au/info/about-the-pbs.

Australian Government Department of Health 2013. *Classification Categories and Criteria*. Therapeutic Goods Administration.

Australian Government Department of Health. 2014a. *Pharmaceutical Benefit Scheme (PBS)*. Available at: http://www.pbs.gov.au/.

Australian Government Department of Health. 2014b. 5th Community Pharmacy Agreement: Medication Management Initiatives. Available at: http://5cpa.com.au/.

Australian Health Practitioner Regulation Agency. 2014. Approved Programs of Study. Available at: http://www.ahpra.gov.au/.

Chesney, K. and Ram S. 2012. *Pharmacy Law Guidebook*. Wellington, New Zealand: Thomson Reuters.

Cumming, J., Mays, N. and Daube, J. 2010. How New Zealand has contained expenditure on drugs. *British Medical Journal* **340**, c244.

Health Workforce Australia. 2014. Available at: http://www.hwa.gov.au/.

IBISWorld, IBISWorld Industry Report G525a Pharmacies in Australia. 2012. Available at: http://www.ibisworld.com/.

IT Health Board 2014. Community Pharmacy Services Agreement. Available at: http://ithealth-board.health.nz/our-programmes/medicines/community-pharmacy-services-agreement.

Jatrana, S., Crampton, P. and Norris, P. 2010. Ethnic differences in access to prescription medication because of cost in New Zealand. *Journal of Epidemiology and Community Health*, **65**, 454–460.

Medsafe 2013a. Medicines Classification Committee – General Principles of Trans-Tasman Scheduling Harmonisation. Available at: http://www.medsafe.govt.nz/profs/class/harmon.asp.

Medsafe 2013b. Classification Categories and Criteria. Available from: http://www.medsafe.govt.nz/profs/class/classificationCategoriesAndCriteria.asp.

Millar, T., Sandilya, R., Tordoff, J. and Furguson, R. 2008. Documenting pharmacist's clinical interventions in New Zealand hospitals. *Pharmacy World and Science*, **30**(1), 99–106.

Ministry of Health New Zealand 2014. Pharmacist Prescriber [cited 2014 October]. Available from: http://www.health.govt.nz/our-work/health-workforce/new-roles-and-initiatives/established-initiatives/pharmacist-prescriber.

Norris, P., Horsburgh, S., Sides, G., Ram, S. and Fraser, J. 2014. Geographical access to community pharmacies in New Zealand. *Health and Place*, **29**, 140–145.

Pharmacy Council of New Zealand 2012. *2012 Annual Report*. Wellington, New Zealand.

Plant, E., Norris, P. and Tordoff, J. 2006. Workforce and service delivery analysis across New Zealand hospital pharmacy departments. *Journal of Pharmacy Practice and Research* **36**(4), 271–274.

U.S. Food and Drug Administration 2014. The Possible Dangers of Buying Medicines over the Internet. Available from: http://www.fda.gov/forconsumers/consumerupdates/ucm048396.htm.

# 7 Pharmacy in Developing Countries

*Felicity Smith*

## CONTENTS

### KEY POINTS

- Many developing countries increasingly have patterns of morbidity and mortality commonly associated with developed countries.
- Although medicines exist for many prevalent ailments in developing countries, they are not always available when needed.
- Health insurance schemes funded through governments and social insurance are increasingly common in developing countries.
- The World Health Organization initiative for a policy framework providing for an adequate supply of safe and effective medicines of established quality at an affordable price that are properly prescribed has had some, but limited success in developing countries.
- Traditional medical practices and/or indigenous healers often operate alongside Western medical practices in developing countries.

- The production and distribution of counterfeit medicines, which have a huge impact on health outcomes, is a problem in many developing countries.
- There is an inverse relationship in those parts of the world with greater health needs and the availability of health professionals.

## INTRODUCTION

There are different ways in which the countries of the world are grouped (e.g. geographical regions, level of industrialization, economic measures and social and cultural characteristics). Traditionally, the United Nations distinguished developed (industrialized) countries and developing countries. While there has been no established convention for the designation of 'developed' and 'developing' countries, approximately 20% of the world's population has been considered to live in industrialized countries (Japan in Asia, Canada and the United States in North America, Australia and New Zealand in Oceania, and countries of Europe) and the remaining approximately 80% living in developing regions. However, the world is changing and new classifications have emerged. In particular, the World Bank classifies countries as low, middle and high income based on gross domestic product/capita. In recent decades, as the economies of many formerly designated developing countries have expanded and diversified, this has led to some new groupings (e.g. BRIC countries [Brazil, Russia, India and China] and, more recently, the MINT countries [Mexico, Indonesia, Nigeria and Turkey]). There are many countries which possess some features typical of developed countries and other characteristics typical of developing countries. In particular, some rapidly developing countries, while now richer, have wide variations of wealth within their populations (e.g. Nigeria, India and South Africa).

Although complex and to some extent flawed, these broad classifications correspond to many important national features of the political, social and economic profile of a country. These features are also reflected in mortality and morbidity patterns, resources available for health care and the provision and delivery of health services. Many of the poorest developing countries (often referred to as the least developed countries [LDCs]) are hampered in their endeavours to improve the economic, social and health status of their populations because of both debts to, and having to operate in international markets designed by, the industrialized world.

Since 2000, the international development agenda has been driven by the Millennium Development Goals (MDGs). United Nation member states formally adopted eight goals and associated targets to be achieved by 2015. These covered eradication of poverty and hunger, education, gender equality, child and maternal health, infectious disease, environmental sustainability and global partnerships for sustained development. During this time, these goals have provided (and continue to provide) the framework for public health interventions and health service development, including those to improve access to, and responsible use, of medicines.

The World Health Organization (WHO) has identified particular problems in developing countries in relation to the supply and use of medicines. In the 1980s,

> **BOX 7.1   WHO/INTERNATIONAL NETWORK FOR RATIONAL USE OF DRUGS PRESCRIBING INDICATORS: FOR MONITORING OF PRESCRIBING PRACTICES**
>
> - Average number of medicines per patient encounter
> - Percentage of medicines prescribed by generic name
> - Percentage with an antibiotic
> - Percentage with injection prescribed
> - Percentage prescribed from essential medicines list or formulary
> - Percentage of prescriptions in accordance with clinical guidelines
>
> Adapted from World Health Organization 2003. *Drugs and Therapeutics Committees: A Practical Guide.* Geneva: World Health Organization, 81–84.

the WHO set up an action programme to promote rational use of medicines and highlighted the potential role of pharmacists in contributing to health care by being more active in promoting the safe and appropriate use of medicines (World Health Organization 1988) (Box 7.1). More recently, the WHO is pursuing policies to support the 'responsible use of medicines', recognizing that barriers to this exist at all levels, such as: availability/affordability of medicines for large populations; questionable practices in the prescribing and supply of medicines; inappropriate use by patients; and inadequate systems to support policy makers and health professionals (World Health Organization 2012).

This chapter will discuss the use of medicines and pharmacy services in the context of the political, economic and social outlooks of developing countries, patterns of health problems and wider health service policy objectives and provision. The roles of pharmacists and the practice of pharmacy should reflect the specific health needs and health care problems of developing countries. Although there are differences between developing countries, there are also many similarities which result in common issues for pharmacy services (see also Chapter 2).

## HEALTH IN DEVELOPING COUNTRIES

### Patterns of Morbidity and Mortality

There are striking differences in the morbidity (prevalence and incidence of diseases in a population) and mortality patterns (death rates and causes) between the poor and the rich nations. In low-income countries, infectious disease (diarrhoea, malaria, human immunodeficiency virus [HIV], tuberculosis and other tropical diseases) and malnutrition persist as major health problems. However, many of these countries have been experiencing significant changes in morbidity and mortality towards patterns generally associated with developed countries: across the globe, the rising prevalence of chronic diseases, especially those associated with more affluent and sedentary lifestyles (e.g. diabetes and cardiovascular disease), have become priorities.

Alongside these changing disease patterns, the world is also experiencing significant demographic transition. While developing countries generally have younger population age structures, population ageing is a global phenomenon. Neurological diseases (e.g. dementia) have become new priorities as their prevalence is rapidly rising and these diseases present a huge burden for patients, families and health services. Mental health problems are projected to be one of the greatest contributors to disease burden within the next decade. Mental health services worldwide, but perhaps most markedly in developing countries, are very under-resourced. The patterns of morbidity and mortality in any country or region will be important determinants of the health needs, medicines required and indicators of priorities for pharmacy services.

## DETERMINANTS OF HEALTH

The relationship between poverty and health, both between and within countries, is widely acknowledged. Many people believe that poor health and poverty are so closely linked that major improvements in the health status of the world's poorest people cannot be realized without addressing the underlying political, economic and socio-economic factors. The MDGs recognized that to improve the lives of the large number of the world's poor, concerted actions were needed across all sectors. The low levels of economic development and the lack of finance is reflected in the extent and quality of infrastructure, education, housing, transport, social support, enforcement of law, nutrition, etc., all of which affect health status, and the ability of governments and health professionals to provide appropriate services to address the health needs of their populations.

For a large proportion of the world's poor, the WHO identified that health needs were often basic and the most appropriate response was an approach to health care which emphasized low-technology, preventative services rather than high-technology curative care, with community-based provision, based on local resources and services, targeted at local priorities and needs. The WHO, in promoting primary health care to address the extreme health problems in developing countries, recognizes that these problems are a result of a complex interaction between political, social, economic, environmental and lifestyle factors; and that they needed to be tackled as such. For example, the lack of access to clean water is a major health hazard for many people. In many developing countries, especially in Africa, there is a high prevalence of water-borne infectious disease. Schistosomiasis (bilharzia) is transmitted as a result of faecal or urinary contamination of the water in which people bathe. Dehydration from diarrhoea as a result of gastrointestinal infestation is a common cause of death among young children. A call to renew this emphasis on primary health care was launched in 2008. However, many LDCs still experience huge barriers to providing basic health services for their people. Primary health care continues to be seen as the most effective approach to addressing the health care needs of the populations in the poorest regions of the world.

In many developing countries, mortality and morbidity rates, health status and health care provision vary significantly between urban and rural areas. In general, access to amenities such as clean water, sanitation facilities and health care are better in urban areas. Appropriate political processes and priorities within countries to address these internal imbalances need to be supported.

Health status and access to medicines are inextricably linked to the role and opportunities of women in society. Gender equality and education of girls was central to the MDGs. Investment in the education of women is seen as an important factor, both as a mark of and to promote political, economic and social development in society. The lower status accorded to women in many societies is a barrier to their seeking health care and access to medicines. In most households and societies, informal health carers are predominantly women. Thus, the increased emphasis on the education of girls and women contributes to health care indirectly though promoting socio-economic development, and directly as a result of informal carers being in a position to understand more about health problems and the use of medicines and other therapies. It is to women that information about health and medicines should principally be targeted. Illiteracy, especially among women, has major implications for the provision of pharmacy services and in ensuring the correct use of medicines in developing countries.

Many health problems in developing countries are rooted in poverty and low levels of development, and it is clear that problems cannot be addressed by the health sector alone. Problems are often compounded by a lack of high-quality facilities and professional services (including pharmacy services) where they are most needed. Medicines exist for many of the most prevalent health problems in developing countries. However, as a result of wider problems, these medicines are often not available when needed, and although pharmacists could assume an important role in providing guidance on their use, they too are often in short supply.

## HEALTH SERVICES IN DEVELOPING COUNTRIES AND THE PLACE OF PHARMACY

Health care worldwide is a mixture of public and private provision. In many of the poorest countries, publicly provided health care is often inadequate to meet the basic needs of the population, even though a high proportion of the population may depend on it for their care. This results in health care being paid for by individuals by out-of-pocket payments as the need arises. People in developing countries are far more likely to have to pay for their health care in this way than those in richer countries where relatively high standards of care and comprehensive provision is funded through governments and social insurance.

The introduction of health insurance schemes that are common in developed countries is seen as a solution to this. How these schemes operate varies between countries. Many of these, when they commence, may focus on particular population groups (e.g. public sector workers) or be confined to particular regions or services. All governments aim in the longer term to make health care available to their entire populations and to gradually increase the range of services included. In the last decade, many schemes in low- and middle-income countries have been successfully expanding to include higher proportions of their populations and more extensive ranges of services.

However, in many low-income countries, a private health care market, funded by private individuals (or voluntary insurance contributions) and provided by private practitioners or institutions, remains prominent in health care provision. As in any market, the services provided in the private sector are generally those for which purchasers are able and willing to pay. Thus, the services provided in the private sector are largely geared to the perceived needs of the richer population groups.

Medicines account for a significant proportion of health expenditure, and this (as a proportion of total health expenditure) tends to be greater in low-income countries. Many developing countries are unable to find sufficient funds to ensure continuous supplies of essential medicines to remote areas.

A system of co-payments was the basis of the Bamako Initiative of the United Nations Children's Fund (UNICEF). The proposal was that UNICEF would provide essential funds for medicines in primary care clinics on the condition that charges would be made for medicines and services. Not surprisingly, the proposal was controversial. It was criticized on both ethical grounds (e.g. charging sick and poor people for essential medicines) and for its difficulties in deciding payment levels. Charging for health care, including medicines, may deter people in need of services or therapy from using them. This may be particularly detrimental when long-term medicines use is important for successful therapy, when symptoms may subside before the end of a course of therapy and for people with very low incomes. However, co-payments for medicines became incorporated into pharmaceutical policy at a primary care level in many developing countries and were acknowledged to provide the health sector with a much-needed source of finance.

Within developing countries, there are often huge discrepancies in wealth, health and access to health care, which often follow an urban–rural divide. Hospitals, better-equipped clinics, private health facilities and health workers are generally more accessible in urban areas. The WHO is campaigning for 'universal coverage'. One of the greatest challenges is the availability of health care personnel. Of particular note is the lack of midwives or skilled birth attendants. Many women in low-income countries, especially in rural areas, do not have access to antenatal, perinatal or post-natal care. Maternal mortality rates are high. Health personnel often want to work where facilities, amenities and quality of life is higher. There is also significant migration of health workers from low- to high-income countries, and within countries, there is a preference to work in urban areas, where opportunities and amenities are greater.

Pharmacy services, as with other health care services, exist in the public and private sectors. It is common for pharmacists in the public sector, or those employed by a hospital or health care organization, to receive a salary. Pharmacists in the community, however, are generally private practitioners. Pharmacists' incomes are usually largely obtained directly from the public through the sale of pharmaceuticals and other products. Additional services which may be provided (e.g. administration of injections, consultation and interpretation of medical reports) are often not remunerated. There has been much debate on the advantages and disadvantages of different methods of payment. Many people believe that remuneration should seek to achieve optimal professional practice (and many payment systems in industrialized countries have been devised and modified to achieve specific health care objectives). In a system in which pharmacists' incomes are derived from the sales of medicines, they have a financial incentive to sell expensive products, irrespective of whether or not this is the most appropriate response to an individual's health needs. Although evidence is limited (Smith 2009b), more formal integration of and remuneration through newer health insurance systems may enable pharmacists to contribute more effectively to public health policies and priorities in collaboration with these agencies.

As with other private health care facilities in developing countries, pharmacies are generally concentrated in urban areas, where there is a market for medicines and hence an income for pharmacists and their staff. Thus, the urban–rural divide in many developing countries extends to pharmacy services (professionals being more numerous in cities) and the availability of medicines (usually a wider range and more dependable supplies in urban areas). However, problems of access to medicines and their rational use in urban areas in developing countries are also well documented.

Fees for private primary medical care are determined by doctors. The costs of care and patients' perceptions of their health needs will influence the extent of their use of medical services. To avoid the costs of a medical consultation, many people are believed to go directly to a pharmacy for medication. Thus, pharmacies may fulfil a health need for people who cannot afford to see a doctor, or where there is no medical practitioner available.

## MEDICINES USE AND POLICY

It is easy to assume that patterns of medicines use will reflect a country's health needs. However, differences in availability and use of medicines between (and within) countries are subject to a wide range of political, economic and other factors. For example, medicines policy (e.g. whether or not a country has a national medicines policy in operation) and its regulation will influence which products are on the market. The availability of medicines will be affected by the country's infrastructure and transport system. The health care system will determine whether or not consultations with professionals, as well as drug therapy, are free at the point of use and to whom; people's ability to pay may determine their consumption. The accessibility of health professionals to the public will have an impact on the extent of self-medication and the appropriateness of medicines use. Education and practices of professionals will affect the quality of prescribing, advice giving and non-prescription drug recommendations. Health beliefs and health literacy will influence how patients manage their illness and use medicines. In many developing countries, 'Western' medicine exists alongside other traditions of care. These social and cultural contexts will also affect health-seeking behaviours and medicines use (see also Chapter 8). In its report *The Pursuit of the Responsible Use of Medicines*, the WHO highlights how problems in access to medicines and their irrational use are important barriers to optimal use in many low- and middle-income countries (World Health Organization 2012).

### WHO AND ACCESS TO MEDICINES

Little or no regular access to essential medicines by large numbers of people in developing countries (especially India and Africa) was the trigger to the WHO's Action Programme for Essential Medicines. Access to medicines may refer to the development or availability of medicines that are relevant to the population health needs, geographical factors and distance people may need to travel, continuity of supplies (especially for long-term conditions), quality of products and affordability for health facilities and/or the population.

The Action Programme on Essential Medicines was introduced in 1981 to promote the development of national medicines policies including essential medicines lists. The WHO advocates that every country should have a national medicine policy that provides a framework for an adequate supply of safe and effective medicines of established quality at an affordable price, which are properly prescribed and used. The programme was established to provide operational support to countries developing national medicines policies (World Health Organization 1992). The WHO recognizes that problems such as a lack of resources, poor infrastructure, shortages of skilled personnel, difficulties of planning and enforcing policy and the economic crisis have resulted in the limited success of some programmes.

In an effort to improve access to medicines, as part of this Action Plan, there was a specific focus on 'essential medicines'. The WHO estimated that approximately 200–300 drug products should be sufficient to address the health care needs of the majority of the populations in developing countries. The WHO drew up an 'Essential Medicines List', which is updated every three years (Box 7.2). It is intended as a guide from which individual countries draw up their own lists to comprise medicines which 'satisfy the health care needs of the majority of the population and should therefore be available at all times in adequate amounts and in appropriate dosage forms' (World Health Organization 1998).

---

### BOX 7.2   ACHIEVING OPTIMAL USE OF MEDICINES: ACCESS AND RATIONAL USE*

| Requirement | Value of medicines lost if these: |
| --- | --- |
| Drug innovation should align with health care needs and address pharmaco-therapeutic gaps. | ...are not developed. |
| General availability, affordability and access to medical care and medicines are a precondition for responsible use. | ...are not available/ affordable. |
| When presenting to a health professional, a medicine has to be prescribed, dispensed, recommended and supplied as fits treatment requirements. | ...appropriate medicines not provided. |
| Patients need to understand and be supported/ empowered to use medicines to ensure they improve his/her well-being. | ...not appropriately taken by the patient. |
| Health system capabilities, data and evidence base should support all stakeholders to enable evaluation of interventions at the patient and system level. | ...not used with the right capabilities in place. |

Adapted from World Health Organization 2012. *The Pursuit of Responsible Use of Medicines.* Geneva: World Health Organization.

The WHO advised countries to draw up their own lists of 'essential medicines' and to focus on ensuring that these

- Address the health care needs of the majority of the population
- Are in suitable dosage forms
- Are of good quality
- Are based on non-proprietary names
- Are affordable
- Are available at all times in adequate amounts in all communities
- Are prescribed and supplied according to guidelines

The WHO also devised monitoring criteria so countries could assess the extent to which standards were achieved in their health facilities. Many developing countries – including over 80% of African countries – developed a national medicines policy in which an essential medicines list was an important part. In recent years, the WHO has been focusing on the access to essential medicines for children. Many products are not available in appropriate formulations. Although large numbers of people (estimated 47% of people in African countries) are still without regular access to essential drugs, the situation has improved (World Health Organization 2011b).

These medicines policies have largely focused on health services in the public sector (hospitals and clinics). However, in low- and middle-income countries, many medicines are sourced from private providers. These include pharmacies, licensed chemical sellers and unlicensed (including itinerant) suppliers. Licensed chemical sellers have only limited training, but their roles can be vital in helping ensure some access to medicines in communities where there is no professional service.

Access to medicines for malaria and HIV was a focus of the MDGs. Malaria interventions between 2002 and 2012 are estimated to have saved the lives of 3 million young children. However, in 2012, there were about 207 million cases of malaria worldwide and over 600,000 deaths, mostly of children aged less than five years (Millennium Development Goals 2014). In many regions of the world, progress has been made. Key interventions that have contributed to these successes are the more widespread use of bed-nets, the use of rapid diagnostic tests to confirm cases early on and promoting artemisinin-based combination therapies, which are the most effective treatments for severe forms of the disease. Since 2000, the availability of artemisinin combination therapies for confirmed malaria and intermittent treatment during pregnancy were important components of international strategies for malaria control. The success of these programmes depends on the involvement of all outlets in both the public and private sectors.

Over the same period, there has been concerted international effort to ensure access to anti-retroviral therapies for people living with HIV. The number of new cases of HIV infection has declined, but it is still too high. In 2012, it was estimated that almost 600 children died every day of acquired immune deficiency syndrome-related causes (Millennium Development Goals 2014). The proportion of people with HIV who have access to medicines has risen considerably. However, while access to anti-retroviral therapy has improved, there are still many disparities and population groups for which access is poor (e.g. children and adolescents, sex workers, people who inject drugs and men who have sex with men).

## MEDICINE DONATIONS

Many developing countries, in an effort to meet the needs of their populations, have received medicine donations from other countries. However, concerns have been expressed about the suitability of these products. Many instances have been reported of donations of products of poor quality (sometimes unacceptable for use in the donor country) and products that have expired or are near to their expiry date or are inappropriate to the needs of the population. Processing small quantities of products that may have a short shelf-life and distributing (or sometimes disposing of) products that do not fall into a country's formularies can be burdensome and costly. The WHO has identified core principles for medicine donations (see Box 7.3), as well as a more specific set of guidelines (World Health Organization 2011a):

- All donations should benefit the recipient.
- There should be respect for the wishes and authority of the recipient.
- There should not be a double-standard in quality.
- There should be effective communication between the donor and recipient.

## MEDICINES, PHARMACY AND NON-GOVERNMENTAL ORGANIZATIONS

In low-income countries, particularly in times of crisis, non-governmental organizations (civil society: charities and other voluntary, not-for-profit organizations) have an important role in meeting the health and medicine needs of populations. Health infrastructure will often be compromised and local circumstances can result

---

### BOX 7.3   WHO GUIDELINES FOR MEDICINE DONATIONS

- Be based on expressed need and relevant to the disease pattern of the recipient country.
- Be approved for use in the recipient country.
- Be of presentation, strength and formulation that are similar to those used in the recipient country.
- Be obtained from a reliable source and comply with quality standards in both donor and recipient countries.
- Not include drugs returned by patients.
- Have a remaining shelf-life of at least 1 year.
- Be labelled in a language easily understood by health professionals in the recipient country.
- Be packed and labelled in accordance with international shipping regulations.
- Be presented in larger-quantity units or hospital packs.

in challenges in ensuring the appropriate medicines in adequate quantities are available to people who need them (see Villacorta-Linaza 2009).

## WHO AND PROBLEMS OF IRRATIONAL USE OF MEDICINES

Worldwide, it is estimated that around half of all medicines are inappropriately prescribed, dispensed or sold, and that about half of patients fail to use their medicines properly (World Health Organization 2012). Many researchers have highlighted the incidence and prevalence of irrational drug use in developing countries. They have explored associated factors and attempted to explain some of the structures of and processes in the delivery of care from the perspectives of both health professionals and consumers that lead to irrational use.

Many features in patterns of medicines supply and use have been found to be common to developing countries. These include inappropriate treatment with unsuitable products, extensive use of polypharmacy (due to both wide use of combination products and multiple prescriptions), frequent injections, inappropriate use of antibiotics and unnecessary supply of vitamins.

Inadequate health services and low availability of professionals leads people to self-medicate without adequate knowledge and information or to rely on advice that may not be optimal. The wide availability of 'prescription' medicines without a prescription has been documented in many developing countries. Products can be purchased from pharmacies when available, but in rural areas, there are often no pharmacists. People are forced to rely on untrained personnel, obtaining drugs from other drug stores or itinerant sellers.

Irrational drug use is not confined to the informal sector. Many studies have examined the prescribing practices of medical practitioners and advice giving and recommendations from pharmacies and found practices to be questionable.

A number of features of pharmacy services contribute to pharmacists' prominence as a source of health advice in developing countries. Although pharmacists are often not accessible to many rural populations, in urban areas, retail pharmacies are often numerous. Pharmacists potentially have an important role in promoting the safe and appropriate supply and use of products. However, many researchers have uncovered poor practices and have been critical of pharmacists and their staff (trained and untrained) for selling pharmaceuticals without questioning or advising clients to ensure the suitability of products (Smith 2009a).

## CULTURAL PERSPECTIVES AND THE USE OF MEDICINES

People's understanding and use of medicines is not only restricted to pharmacological and therapeutic properties, but will also be influenced by their social and cultural circumstances, views and perceptions of their health problems, expectations of health care and beliefs regarding the role and effects of medicines.

Pharmaceutical anthropology is a discipline which seeks to explore the social and cultural contexts in which medicines are produced, exchanged and consumed (van der Geest and Whyte 1991). The promotion of rational drug use will only be successful if policies are devised which take into account relevant political, economic, social

**BOX 7.4   SOCIAL/CULTURAL FACTORS, HEALTH BELIEFS AND THE USE OF MEDICINES**

- There are significant inequities in access to health care and medicines between population groups.
- In low-income countries, there is a high reliance on self-medication for a wide range of health problems.
- Indigenous health beliefs shape health behaviours. They are:
  - Often diverse
  - Context-specific (depend on people's situation, priorities and experience)
  - Negative and positive in terms of potential outcomes
- 'Western' medicines are often used alongside other 'strategies'.
  - Lack of literary (including health literary) information hinders informed decision making.
- Practices of health professionals and marketing are important influences, especially:
  - Health professionals – inadequate advice and poor labelling
  - Aggressive marketing

and cultural priorities and contexts. In addition, within industrialized countries, differences between population groups with different cultural backgrounds and distinct perspectives on health, health care and drug use have been identified.

The use of medicines by individuals is influenced by their own health beliefs and social/cultural norms (Box 7.4). The beliefs of individuals or communities about an appropriate response to symptoms can be very diverse. Health beliefs and understanding will be important determinants in the uptake of care and consequently the use of medicines.

Health beliefs and cultural perspectives (including a lack of information or understanding) can be important barriers to appropriate therapy. For example, poor understanding of the aetiology of epilepsy and stigmatization of sufferers is known to be a barrier to effective care. Mental health problems are prevalent in all communities, but they are often not viewed as a health service priority, and again, stigma is commonly a reason why individuals and families do not seek help. The MDGs also highlighted the place of women in many cultures as an important barrier to a wide range of opportunities, including access to health care.

## PLURALISM IN HEALTH CARE

Just as the co-existence of formal and informal sectors has been identified in the distribution of 'Western' medicines, in many developing countries, traditional and 'Western' medical practices also operate side by side.

In China, traditional Chinese medicine and 'Western' medicine operate side by side within the formal health care system. In India, Ayurvedic medicine continues to be practised, and in Africa, there are many traditional or indigenous healers consisting of both spiritually and non-spiritually based (e.g. herbalist) practitioners.

Many developing countries have experienced periods of colonization by the industrial nations. 'Western' medicine, introduced by the colonial powers for the benefit of immigrant personnel, would exist alongside existing traditions of care, gradually becoming more pervasive. Banerji (1974) traces the development of health services in India from the period prior to British rule. Focusing on political and economic changes, he illustrates how a 'Western' health care system, including education, was imposed to serve the perceived needs of the British immigrants and 'privileged' Indians, and eventually dominated formal health care. He questions whether, at the time of the introduction of 'Western' health care, this was superior to the existing systems.

In many developing countries, 'Western' medicine has remained more concentrated in urban areas, while other traditions of medical care have persisted and are more widely practised in rural areas. It would be expected that when two or more systems operate side by side, each may influence the development of the other. Many authors have described how different health care systems, while remaining distinct, have incorporated practices from other traditions. Regarding the use of medicines, instances in which 'Western' medicines have become part of the armamentarium of traditional practitioners and cases of indigenous remedies being incorporated into 'Western' practice have been documented. Furthermore, people seeking care move between these different health care systems according to factors such as traditions of help seeking in the society, perceived needs, perspectives on the roles of different health personnel or healers, beliefs regarding the appropriateness of particular courses of action, the availability of practitioners and the success of therapy.

The importing and imposition of 'Western' systems in developing countries has had a major impact on patterns of medicines use, pharmacy services and professional education. Approaches to and developments within pharmacy education in low-income countries continue to be influenced by those in the industrialized world.

## THE PHARMACEUTICAL INDUSTRY AND DEVELOPING COUNTRY HEALTH NEEDS

Considerable controversy surrounds the issue of the extent to which the operations of pharmaceutical companies in developing countries are sensitive to the health needs of the populations in low-income countries. Neglected tropical diseases continue to cause significant morbidity and mortality in the developing world, affecting around 1 billion people, including 500,000 children (Drugs for Neglected Diseases Initiative 2014).

The motivation for drug companies to produce new pharmaceutical products is the maximization of profits. The most profitable products will be those for which consumers are able and willing to pay. The pharmaceutical industry has always claimed that, as a result of the financial investment required for successful research and development, new products will be costly to the consumer. Thus, the pharmaceutical industry is less inclined to invest extensively in products for which the market is limited in terms of available finance for purchasing. The term 'orphan drug' is used to refer to products for which there is a health need, but for which, because of the lack of purchasing power of potential consumers, the industry would be unlikely to recoup the research and development costs.

Thus, of the 1,556 new drugs approved between 1975 and 2004, only 21 were specifically developed for tropical diseases and tuberculosis. Over 10% of the global disease burden is attributed to neglected tropical diseases (Drugs for Neglected Diseases Initiative 2014).

In recent years, there have been a number of proposals to address the problem of neglected diseases. To achieve these aims, a range of initiatives have commenced. These include public–private partnerships in the development of new medicines which draw on funds from the public sector, private (for-profit) sector and civil society and philanthropic funds to invest in research and development of drugs for neglected diseases. These initiatives are many and varied, but they enable the combining of basic science and industrial expertise, product development and clinical research. In 2012, a group called Uniting to Combat Neglected Tropical Diseases, involving pharmaceutical companies, donor and endemic countries, private foundations, civil society organizations and others, pledged to control, eliminate or eradicate 17 neglected tropical diseases by 2020 (Uniting to Combat Neglected Tropical Diseases 2014). As a result of recent programmes, there are many examples of improved access to medicines for neglected diseases for populations in low-income countries.

Many authors over several decades have been critical of the operations of the pharmaceutical industry in low-income countries and communities. For example, local production of pharmaceuticals and marketing of products by multinational companies does not necessarily focus on the country's needs, fall in line with their national medicines policies or assist in the provision of essential medicines. Many researchers have uncovered evidence of varying standards in marketing and information provision. Promotional material distributed in developing countries, for example, has been criticized for including wider indications and less comprehensive information regarding side-effect profiles. Many products of doubtful value are both intensely promoted and expensive. For health professionals and pharmacists in developing countries, promotional material from pharma companies is often their main source of product information and a powerful influence on prescribing and sales. A lack of impartial information and material that provides accurate and balanced interpretations of the evidence and enables comparison between treatment options contributes to the inappropriate use of medicines.

Heavy criticism of their practices has led to some improvement in the marketing operations of pharmaceutical companies in developing countries. However, there is still a far heavier reliance on company representatives for product information in low-income countries than in the developed world. To some extent, involvement of the pharmaceutical industry in public–private partnerships and other new initiatives enables them to be seen to be making a helpful contribution to international endeavours to address the important health care needs of the poorest people in the world.

## QUALITY OF MEDICINES AND COUNTERFEITS

Assuring the quality of medicines in low-income settings can be problematic (Box 7.5). In poor communities, there will be a market for cheaper alternatives

**BOX 7.5    SOME PROBLEMS THAT COMPROMISE
QUALITY OF MEDICINES**

- Random and chaotic supply chains
- Weak laws and lack of enforcement
- Lack of resources and infrastructure
- Poor tracking, making recall difficult
- Poor manufacturing practices and quality assurance
- Corruption in health care systems
- High import tariffs in some countries
- Medicines – low bulk and high value

to expensive brand name products. However, the infrastructure for regulation and enforcement to ensure minimal acceptable standards is often inadequate. The marketing of substandard drugs (e.g. with inadequate levels of active ingredients) produced by local companies has been documented in many studies, with a call for the stricter application of the national medicines policy, in particular in regard to the issue of licences and sanctions against companies breaking the law.

Production and distribution of counterfeit medicines is acknowledged to be a problem in many developing countries. Counterfeit medicines have been defined as medicinal products which have been deliberately or fraudulently mislabelled with respect to identity and/or source. They may include products with the correct ingredients, wrong ingredients, without active ingredients, with insufficient active ingredients or with fake packaging. Research studies have uncovered wide ranges in the prevalence of counterfeit medicines in developing countries. There have been reports of counterfeits in the medicine chains in all parts of the world, but problems have been consistently found to be far greater in the least developed regions. Most counterfeits are found in low-income countries. Counterfeit medicines can have a huge impact on health outcomes. Antibiotics are the most commonly counterfeited products. Consequent treatment failures have led to many deaths from potentially curable diseases. Addressing the problem of counterfeit medicines in the supply chain is a health priority for many low-income countries. For example, bar-coding of products with unique identifiers enables users to check their authenticity. New methods of detection are also being more widely used (e.g. devices [including portable devices] that employ spectroscopy and chromatography for local testing of products). Researchers have emphasized the need for continuing vigilance among pharmacists and the benefits of distributing medicines through pharmacies.

## HEALTH WORKFORCE AND PHARMACY

Inadequate numbers and the inequitable distribution of health workers is believed by the WHO to be one of the greatest barriers to health service provision, especially in low-income countries (World Health Organization 2006; International Pharmaceutical Federation 2012). Many of these countries have a health workforce

**TABLE 7.1**

**Health Professionals per 1,000 People in Selected Countries**

| Country | Physicians | | Nurses | | Pharmacists | | Dentists | |
|---|---|---|---|---|---|---|---|---|
| | Number | Density/1,000 People | Number | Density/1,000 People | Number | Density/1,000 People | Number | Density/1,000 People |
| Afghanistan | 4,104 | 0.19 | 4,572 | 0.22 | 525 | 0.02 | 630 | 0.03 |
| Azerbaijan | 29,687 | 3.55 | 59,531 | 7.11 | 1,842 | 0.22 | 2,272 | 0.27 |
| Belgium | 46,268 | 4.49 | 60,142 | 5.83 | 11,775 | 1.14 | 8,322 | 0.81 |
| Brazil | 198.153 | 1.15 | 659,111 | 3.84 | 51,317 | 0.30 | 190,448 | 1.11 |
| Ghana | 3,240 | 0.15 | 19,707 | 0.92 | 1,388 | 0.06 | 393 | 0.02 |
| Somalia | 310 | 0.04 | 1,486 | 0.19 | 8 | 0.00 | 15 | 0.00 |
| Thailand | 22,435 | 0.37 | 171,605 | 2.82 | 15,480 | 0.25 | 10,459 | 0.17 |
| United States | 730,801 | 2.56 | 2,669,603 | 9.37 | 249,642 | 0.88 | 463,663 | 1.63 |
| Zimbabwe | 2,086 | 0.16 | 9,357 | 0.72 | 883 | 0.07 | 310 | 0.02 |

*Source:* World Health Organization 2006. *Working Together for Health: The World Health Report 2006.* Geneva, World Health Organization.

## TABLE 7.2
### Number of Pharmacists in Selected Countries

| Country | Number of Pharmacists | Population (000) | Pharmacists per 100,000 Population |
|---|---|---|---|
| Finland | 7,500 | 5,172 | 145 |
| France | 62,800 | 59,238 | 106 |
| United Kingdom | 43,370 | 59,415 | 73 |
| United States | 201,095 | 283,320 | 71 |
| Australia | 11,485 | 19,138 | 60 |
| Jamaica | 860 | 2,576 | 33 |
| India | 300,000 | 1,008,937 | 30 |
| Malaysia | 3,560 | 22,218 | 16 |
| Russia | 9,340 | 145,491 | 6.4 |
| Albania | 85 | 3,134 | 2.7 |
| Zimbabwe | 335 | 12,627 | 2.7 |
| Tanzania | 850 | 35,119 | 2.2 |
| Eritrea | 53 | 3,659 | 1.4 |
| Gambia | 10 | 1,303 | 0.8 |

Source: Anderson, S. 2004. *Managing Pharmaceuticals in International Health*. Basel: Birkhauser Verlog.

crisis, which is particularly pronounced in their rural regions. The problems of an inappropriately sized and placed health workforce span all health professional groups: physicians, nurses, pharmacists, dentists and others (Table 7.1).

In terms of pharmacists, their numbers per 100,000 of the population differ hugely across the world, and generally follow a pattern of increasing numbers in countries of greater wealth (Table 7.2). Thus, in the parts of the world where health needs are arguably greater, health professionals are fewer. Furthermore, the discrepancy in the distribution is even more marked within these countries. In the poorer countries, health professionals and pharmacists tend to be concentrated in urban areas, with very few in rural locations. The problems are further compounded by the migration of health professionals to other parts of the world where professional opportunities and quality of life are more attractive.

## CONCLUSION

There is huge diversity between regions and countries of the world in terms of health needs, service provision, priorities in the use of medicines and the contribution of pharmacy services. However, developing countries do share many features and problems.

The potential of pharmacy services to contribute more effectively to health care and outcomes in these settings is unclear. However, pharmacies and pharmacists are viewed by many as underutilized resources, with a presence in many communities with huge health needs. In promoting safer, more effective use of medicines, the wider context of patterns of disease, public health programmes, policy priorities and social and cultural contexts all need to be taken into account.

## FURTHER READING

Anderson, S.C., Huss, R., Summers, R. and Wiedenmayer, K. 2014. *Managing Pharmaceuticals in International Health*. Basel: Birkhauser.

International Pharmaceutical Federation website. Available at: http://www.fip.org.

*Lancet 2012, Vol 380 September 8th 2012*: includes a series of articles on Universal Health Coverage.

- Sachs JD, Achieving universal coverage in low-income settings 944–947.
- Lagarmasino G et al., Moving towards universal health coverage: Health insurance reforms in nine developing countries in Africa and Asia. 933–943.
- And several other articles.

Newton, P.N., Green, M.D. and Fernandez, F.K. 2010. Impact of poor quality medicines in the developing world. *Trends in Pharmacological Sciences*, 31, 99–101.

World Health Organization: *World Health Report 2010. Health Systems Financing: The Path to Universal Coverage*. World Health Organization.

World Health Organization website. Available at: http://www.who.int.

- provides information on all diseases and trends
- provides country specific information

World Health Organization: World Health Statistics 2013.

- This comprises tables of data relating to all countries of the world: It includes development and health indicators, prevalence of disease and risk factors, features of health care systems. While comprehensive, it is just tables of data.

## REFERENCES

Anderson, S. 2004. *Managing Pharmaceuticals in International Health*. Basel: Birkhauser Verlog.

Banerji, D. 1974. Social and cultural foundations of health services systems. *Economic and Political Weekly*, **9**, 1333–1346.

Drugs for Neglected Diseases Initiative 2014. Drugs for Neglected Diseases Initiative. Available at http://www.dndi.org.

International Pharmaceutical Federation 2012. Global Pharmacy Workforce Report. Available at: http://www.fip.org/humanresources.

Millennium Development Goals 2014. *The Millennium Development Goals Report 2014*. New York: United Nations.

Smith, F. 2009a. The quality of private pharmacy services in low and middle-income countries: A systematic review. *Pharmacy World and Science*, **31**, 351–361.

Smith, F. 2009b. Private local pharmacies in low-and middle-income countries: A review of interventions to enhance their role in public health. *Tropical Medicine and International Health*, **14**, 362–372.

van der Geest, S. and Whyte, S.R. (Eds.) 1991. *The Context of Medicines in Developing Countries: Studies in Pharmaceutical Anthropology*. Amsterdam: Het Spinhus Publishers.

Villacorta-Linaza, R. 2009. Bridging the gap: The role of pharmacists in managing the drug supply cycle within non-governmental organisations. *International Journal of Health Planning and Management*, **24**, S73–S86.

World Health Organization 1988. *The Role of the Pharmacist in the Health Care System*. Geneva: World Health Organization.

World Health Organization 1992. *Essential Drugs: Action for Equity*. Geneva: World Health Organization.

World Health Organization 1998. *The World Health Report 1998: Life in the 21st Century – A Vision for All*. Geneva: World Health Organization.

World Health Organization 2003. *Drugs and Therapeutics Committees: A Practical Guide.* Geneva: World Health Organization, 81–84.

World Health Organization 2006. *Working Together for Health: The World Health Report 2006.* Geneva: World Health Organization.

World Health Organization 2011a. *Guidelines for Medicine Donations (Revised 2010).* Geneva: World Health Organization.

World Health Organization 2011b. *Essential Medicines Monitor 5.* Geneva: World Health Organization.

World Health Organization 2012. *The Pursuit of Responsible Use of Medicines.* Geneva: World Health Organization.

# Section II

Health, Illness, Well-Being
and Medicines Use

# 8 The Social Context of Health and Illness

*Sarah Nettleton*

## CONTENTS

## KEY POINTS

- Formal 'expert' knowledge, including that of pharmacists, is increasingly being challenged, and people's experiences of trial and error and having 'gone through it' can carry as much authority or legitimacy as professionals' knowledge.
- Lay (i.e. non-professional) health knowledge can contribute to how health and illness is understood, rather than being labelled as 'incorrect' knowledge by professionals.
- The concept of 'health capital' proposes that factors such as fitness levels, immunity, resilience to diseases and positive attitudes can be accumulated to preserve health, but this capital can also be depleted by factors such as smoking, unhealthy diets, work pressures and exposure to environments posing a risk to health.
- Illness has not only physical but also social consequences. When it limits how we normally function, this can threaten the sufferer's

self-esteem, undermining a cultural imperative for maintaining a sense of independence and self-reliance.

- Patients are not simply passive recipients of care; rather, they and their relatives and friends are also providers of that care and as such develop considerable amounts of expertise and knowledge which may even surpass that of the medical profession.
- A consequence of patients being active participants in the processes of health care work is a growing legitimacy of their experience commensurate with a declining faith in 'experts'.

## INTRODUCTION

This chapter explores the changing nature of contemporary society by first highlighting some of the salient features of our current social context. It then focuses more specifically on people's understanding of health and their experiences of illness. Finally, the implications of these for interactions between health professionals and patients are discussed.

There are a number of characteristic features of modern society that are salient to the understanding of health knowledge and health practice. The first of these is the changing nature of the disease burden. The latter half of the twentieth century saw a transformation from predominantly acute, life-threatening infectious diseases to chronic and sometimes non-life-threatening conditions, such as cancer, cardiovascular disease, diabetes and asthma. Life expectancy increased and these chronic conditions are more prevalent in an ageing population. However, although we are living longer, there are signs that we are experiencing increasingly high levels of morbidity. Concomitantly, in addressing ill-health, there has been a shifting emphasis from intervention to treat disease to surveillance of risk factors, and from curing to caring. By definition, chronic conditions are not amenable to successful intervention and so medicine is limited to ameliorative responses.

The changing nature of the disease burden and the amelioration of symptoms has occurred alongside the growing emphasis on the prevention of illness and promotion of health. The causes of many contemporary diseases are related to social factors and are now considered to be largely preventable, hence the emphasis on screening for early intervention and the growing preoccupation with so-called 'lifestyle' factors, such as smoking, diet, stress and alcohol consumption. Health care provision for physical and mental ill health is increasingly community rather than hospital based. These responses to ill health are facilitated by technological changes – not least the growth in information technology, which enables screening and the surveillance of 'at-risk' populations. Technological innovations, most especially in biotechnologies and information communications technologies, which are now integral to contemporary society, are rapid. Indeed, the pace of change is said by some commentators to be one of the key features of modern society (Giddens 2002, 2013). This is especially the case in relation to a process termed 'globalization'. The process is typified by the Internet, wherein time and space become contracted. For example, information on health and illness can be accessed almost instantly by the public and professionals alike (see the hypothetical example in Box 8.1).

A further change in contemporary society is that formal 'expert' knowledge is being challenged. Those hitherto regarded as experts – such as scientists and health professionals – are increasingly subject to challenge. This process has intensified with the 'crises' surrounding bovine spongiform encephalopathy (BSE), debates on genetically modified food and climate change. Although 'experts' have always debated the scientific issues, their arguments now gain considerable media attention. For example, in 2014, the use of statins to treat the risk factors of heart disease was challenged not only in the medical press (e.g. Tresidder 2014), but also in the wider media. Increasingly, experience, trial and error and having 'gone through it' seem to carry as much authority or legitimacy as the codified knowledge of the 'expert'. The pharmacist, the doctor, the counsellor, the social worker, the nurse and the health visitor are not the only sources of advice and information. The fact that professionals have been schooled in a particular way and have a body of codified knowledge is not enough. For example, people may ask the pharmacist about a particular drug regimen, but then turn to the Internet to check out the suitability of a drug and its possible adverse effects. Medical sociologists have argued for some time that the public possess expertise about their own health and illness. Today, however, people are increasingly aware of their own expertise and are willing to share it. The growth of self-help groups, commonly mediated online, is an illustration of this.

The Internet is routinely used to access information on particular medical conditions, or for making contact with other people who have a shared experience. People may use this to access information on topics such as health, illness and how to treat various ailments and diseases, or seek advice about an illness which they are currently suffering from. Sociological studies of websites and online communities have revealed how the proliferation of sources relates to a diversity of patient identities. Fox et al. (2005) and Fox and Ward (2006), for example, observed how patients use a variety of Internet forums to share, inform, purchase and exchange

### BOX 8.1   AN EXAMPLE OF THE PUBLIC'S ACCESS TO HEALTH INFORMATION

At 10.00 a.m. one Monday morning, a woman has a meeting with her consultant. She learns that she has been diagnosed as suffering from multiple sclerosis (MS). After talking to her consultant briefly, she makes an appointment for a longer consultation with her general practitioner (GP) the following morning. She goes home and spends the rest of the day logged onto the Internet, accessing various websites and newsgroups concerned with MS. Not only does she gather much information from a myriad of formal and informal sources, but she also receives advice and support from many people with direct experience of MS from around the globe. By the time of the consultation with her GP the next day, she is far better informed than her GP about her potential condition and is able to question a number of statements made by the doctor.

health advice and for the consumption of pharmaceuticals. For example, users of a web forum *X-Online* exchanged advice and information on a drug Xenical, which they bought for help with weight loss. The 'lay' advice proffered was predominantly couched in medical language. By contrast, members of the forum *Anagrrl*, which provided support for those with anorexia, explicitly resisted medical models of the condition and exchanged information on how to live with the condition and resisted medical approaches. Today, online platforms and social media sites proliferate. Lupton (2013) refers to 'digitally engaged patients' to describe the phenomenon of lay people both consuming and producing information on health and medical topics. While this gives scope to patient participation and empowerment, she also cautions that patient involvement in digitized services gives scope for exploitation. Where lay people and patients submit information about themselves on a large scale, this then generates data for commercial care providers who can use this to profile users and target and market goods and services (Lupton 2014). Thus, notions of health and illness do not simply map onto or mirror formalized medical views. Moreover, lay accounts are influential and professional views and working practices may be challenged. Box 8.2 contains an example of a post from a commercial online platform.

The proliferation of virtual support does not seem to have quelled the appetite for and production of health and fitness magazines and health and lifestyles programmes on television. Moreover, these have emerged in tandem with a diversity of types of health care – with the growth of alternative medicine being perhaps the most obvious example. Thus, patients are not passive recipients of health care and health advice; increasingly, they are discerning consumers and users of health care.

Given the way that rapid social change impinges on everyday life, it is imperative that health practitioners have some appreciation of the social context in which they practice. These changes also point to the fact that all modern-day health care practitioners should have some understanding of the nature and complexity of people's views about health and illness. Sociological studies of ideas about health and illness can throw some light on these.

## LAY HEALTH KNOWLEDGE

### WHY STUDY LAY HEALTH KNOWLEDGE?

The sociological study of lay (i.e. non-professional) health knowledge is of value to health care practice in a number of ways. First, the findings can contribute to an understanding of professional–patient interactions, in that they can provide an insight into lay conceptualizations which might otherwise be treated as simply 'incorrect' knowledge by professionals. Second, an understanding of people's ideas about health maintenance and disease prevention is crucial to the effectiveness of health education and health promotion programmes. Third, the study of health beliefs may contribute to our knowledge of informal health care. Most health care work is carried out by lay people either in the form of self-care or caring for relatives and friends. Finally, lay knowledge is not static: people's knowledge, ideas and beliefs are constantly changing and are shaped by the social milieu of their lives.

## BOX 8.2   AN EXAMPLE OF A POST FROM THE
## ONLINE PLATFORM *CURETOGETHER*

If anyone can give advice or insight...I have been recently diagnosed with migraines after suffering from recurring headaches with aura becoming more and more frequent until I finally completely lost my vision on the left side. At that time I was diagnosed with uveitis which resolved after about 6 weeks of medication but the horrific headache, dizziness, eye pain and visual disturbances have not resolved and an magnetic resonance imaging (MRI) confirmed migraines. I am also having leg weakness and numbness on the right side and vision loss in the left eye, not to mention trouble reading and concentrating or thinking and remembering. The headache has been consistent and unrelenting for 12 weeks now and I am feeling desperate. I have been on Topomax but do not feel any difference yet. Any advice from fellow sufferers is greatly appreciated.

I did not begin to experience migraines until May of 2013, when I had to see the dentist for a large filling on the top right side (#13). In June of 2013 a burning sensation began under my right eye. I saw the doctor fearing I had inhaled a mold spore or something similar was occurring. They stuffed an endoscope up my nose and came to the conclusion that they were just headaches not the result of some sort of localized infection. I saw my dentist who x-rayed the region and determined there was no abscess. I was then treated for migraines for the next nine months. My teeth on the top right side were constantly sensitive to temperature changes from food. I experienced 3–5 migraines of significant intensity per week during that time period. I want to talk briefly about successful migraine treatments then what occurred this year.

Treatment by excedrine was unsuccessful due to rebound headaches. Imitrex also proved a temporary relief until I came onto this site and learned about the drug 'treximet' which is a combination of Imitrex and Aleve (naproxin sodium). I switched from Excedrin to Aleve plus Imitrex with the approval of the neurologist treating me. Those two together provide significant relief from migraines. Other successful treatment included a block of ice in a bag applied directly to my right temple and the area below my right eye. Staying in completely dark conditions also helped. I am one of those migraine sufferers that gains light sensitivity during and after the migraine, and warning of impending migraine by halo experience.

In January of 2014 I had a root canal done on that tooth. The entire nerve was necrotic! The terminal end of the root was in the same spot I had originally complained about a localized burning sensation. Since the root canal I have only had 2 migraines of significant intensity, a dramatic reduction in frequency and severity.

Due to my training in molecular biology I came to the following hypothesis: the bacteria attacking the nerve were triggering signalling up the nerves in my face, inducing migraine. This is outside of my personal field of study (bacterial genetics) but I wanted to contribute this information to the community for doctors who do study this.

Available from http://curetogether.com/migraine/discuss/

## DEFINING HEALTH

It is customary to distinguish between both negative and positive definitions of health and functional and experiential definitions. The medical view of health – the absence of disease – is clearly negative. By contrast, an example of a positive definition is that offered by the World Health Organization: a state of complete physical, mental and social well-being. A functional definition implies the ability to participate in normal social roles (see below), and this may be contrasted with an experiential definition, which takes sense of self (i.e. ideas about who 'I am' as a person) into account. Another approach to defining health is via the examination of people's perceptions of the concept. For example, in a study of elderly people in Aberdeen, Williams (1983) identified, from his interview data, three lay concepts of health: health as the absence of disease; health as a dimension of strength, weakness and exhaustion; and health as functional fitness.

Empirical studies have found that people's ideas are likely to incorporate a number of these dimensions. However, there is evidence to suggest some relationship between types of beliefs and social circumstances. For example, Cornwell (1984) found that the gender-dependent division of labour impacted upon women's responses to illness. While men could take time off work, women could not. As one participant in the study notes:

Men, they are like babies. You don't know what I put up with from him. Women, they get on with it...I'd say woman have more aches and pains than men, but, as I say, when you've got a family, you will find a women will work till she's dropping. But she'll do what she's got to do and then she'll say, "Right, I'm off to bed." Whereas it's alright for a man. If he's ill he's got nothing to do, he just lies there doesn't he?

Moreover, this experience appears to transcend 'race'. In her study of Pathan mothers living in Britain, Currer (1986) reports participants as stating that 'we do not have time to be ill. I have not been ill at all ... whether we are well or ill, happy or unhappy, we do our work'. Clearly, then, definitions of health are related to the structure of people's everyday lives.

Blaxter (2010) proposes the concept 'health capital' to capture subjective lay reasoning on health matters. The idea of capital implies an accumulated stock of health resource that might include factors such as fitness, immunity, resilience, attitude, etc. All of these resources can be augmented, but may also be depleted. Depletion may be associated with behaviours such as smoking, unhealthy eating, work pressures and exposure to particular environments. The gains and losses for some individuals may be associated with luck, but at a population level, they are socially patterned. Fundamentally, the wealthier have greater stocks of social capital, are more likely to live in physical and social environments that are conducive to health and are least exposed to health threats.

## HEALTH MAINTENANCE AND DISEASE PREVENTION

Ideas about the maintenance of health are separated in lay logic from ideas about the prevention of disease. Calnan (1987) states that health and disease are not direct opposites:

> Lay ideas about health maintenance were more coherent than...ideas about disease prevention. This suggested that people, irrespective of their social class, operate with a range of definitions of health that are not simply connected. Thus promoting health and preventing disease are not direct opposites, that is, positives and negatives, and while women had clear recipes about how to maintain health, they did not necessarily feel they were applicable to disease prevention.

While people consider that diet, exercise, rest and relaxation might contribute to maintaining health, it does not follow that such activities will prevent the onset of illness or disease. Ideas about disease causation tend to emphasize biological rather than behavioural factors.

There are diseases to which certain types of people are presumed to be more susceptible than others. Heart disease provides the classic example where people with certain temperaments, who are overweight and who are obsessively active are considered as being most likely to be susceptible. These ideas reflect medical epidemiology, which has identified type A and type B behaviours as being more or less prone to heart disease. Thus, people are able to identify heart disease 'candidates' based on information given by health educators (i.e. those who eat saturated fats, do not do any exercise and who are hyperactive). However, as Davison et al. (1991) point out, people collectively develop a 'lay epidemiology' which recognizes that not all candidates have heart attacks while some do, and this must therefore be due to chance. Health promoters, keen to present unequivocal, simplified and straightforward messages, fail to address these anomalies and so underestimate the sophistication of lay thinking. Davison goes on to point out that it 'is ironic that such evidently fatalistic cultural concepts should be given more rather than less explanatory power by the activities of modern health education, whose stated goals lie in the opposite direction'.

There appears to be a moral dimension to health. In Cornwell's (1984) study, people were keen to present themselves as being healthy, and initial statements on health status often bore no relation to their medical histories. For example, one woman described herself as healthy and lucky in that she had good health, and yet:

> Kathleen's medical history included having such bad eye sight as a child that she was expected to be blind by the age of twenty, lung disease including tuberculosis in her late teens, a miscarriage, a thyroid deficiency which requires permanent medication, and six years prior to interviews, a hysterectomy.

As well as an insistence on good health and a scorn of hypochondriacs and malingerers, the analysis of 'public accounts' revealed a necessity to be able to prove the 'otherness' of illness as a separate thing that happened to the person and was not something for which they could be held responsible.

## LAY VIEWS OF MEDICINES AND DRUGS

The rich and complex nature of people's views is evident in accounts of their use of medicines which have been either prescribed by general practitioners or bought over the counter. In those countries where Western bio-medicine is dominant, two contrasting images of drugs appear to prevail (Morgan 1996). On the one hand, medicines are seen positively as being cures, miracles, remedies and effective treatments. On the other hand, they are seen as being harmful, dangerous and may be ineffective or have bad side effects. Such images are evident in the media; for example, tales of wonder drugs and medical disasters are fairly commonplace in newspapers and on television. Research into people's ideas and use of drugs has found evidence of both of these positive and negative views of drugs, although they do appear to be more tempered and considered than those that appear in the media.

Based on an analysis of 30 qualitative interviews with men and women from a range of social backgrounds in London, Britten (1996) was able to classify her interview transcripts into what she termed orthodox and unorthodox accounts (Box 8.3). Aspects of these orthodox and unorthodox views can be discerned in Morgan's (1996) study of 'white' and African–Caribbean patients' use of anti-hypertensive drugs. From interviews carried out with 30 'white' and 30 African–Caribbean men and women who had being prescribed such drugs for at least a year, the researchers learned how different people managed and used their drugs in different ways. They identified three different types of responses to this drug regimen. There were what they labelled as 'stable' adherents (16 'white' and 8 African–Caribbean), who took the medicines as prescribed and who did not express any major worries or concerns about taking their tablets. Two further groups identified were the 'problematic' adherents (10 'white' and 4 African–Caribbean) and those who did not take the drugs as prescribed (2 'white' and 18 African–Caribbean). These people were concerned about the actual or possible adverse effects of the drugs. They expressed concerns such as not wanting to become dependent on drugs, and were anxious about the potential for long-term addiction. Some made use of alternative remedies such as herbal treatments. The extent to which these concerns led people to either reduce their dosage or to stop taking the drugs altogether was linked to their assessment as to the seriousness of their condition and to the benefits of taking the medicines. Among those African–Caribbean patients who had concerns about the drugs, the most common response was to take the drugs irregularly, taking them as and when they felt they needed them and in response to their blood pressure levels. Therefore, they were less likely than the white patients to stop altogether. Those groups who had concerns about the long-term use of these drugs mirrored the responses of the unorthodox group identified by Britten (1996). As with this unorthodox group, they were also more likely to use alternative, traditional remedies which were considered to be more 'natural'. These studies capture

## BOX 8.3   ORTHODOX AND UNORTHODOX ACCOUNTS OF MEDICINES

Britten classified 26 of her interview transcripts into what she termed orthodox and unorthodox accounts. The eight orthodox accounts were categorized as such because people articulated a faith in modern medicine, believed in its efficacy and tended to take medicines for granted. By contrast, 17 unorthodox accounts were attributed to those people who expressed not only concerns about the harmful effects of medicines, and especially their dangerous side effects, but they also had less faith in medicine in general. Furthermore, they were more favourably disposed to alternative and what they perceived to be more natural forms of treatments or remedies. While some of the views expressed in the orthodox accounts were found in the unorthodox accounts, the converse was not true.

Britten also identified four main themes in the orthodox accounts. First, 'correct behaviour', in that people presented themselves as taking medicines as prescribed by their doctors and that this was the right thing to do. Second, 'own use of medicines' referred to the fact that people would interpret and modify their use of prescribed drugs. For example, they might try and wean themselves off a drug or try and manage without medications such as antibiotics to give their body a chance to deal with the illness itself. Third, this group were happy with their doctor's prescribing habits. Finally, potential criticisms of doctors were either not evident or were 'diffused'.

Three issues were important in the accounts of the larger unorthodox group. First was their aversion to medicine. In particular, medicines were seen as being artificial, unsafe and unnatural. They highlighted the potential side effects of drugs and the possible long-term effects of introducing alien chemicals into the body. Medicines could, for example, lower the immune system. This is not to say that people did not acknowledge that medicines could do good, it was just that they were very conscious of the possible harmful effects. Second, because of their potential dangers, the people in this group preferred not to take drugs if at all possible. Finally, this group were more critical of doctors, with the most common criticism being about over-prescribing. This final view is an interesting one because it is at odds with the dominant medical view of patients, wherein patients are considered to make unrealistic demands for prescriptions when they are unnecessary.

Adapted from Britten, N. 1996. *Modern Medicine: Lay Perspectives and Experiences*. London: UCL Press, 48–73.

the views of some men and women living in London in the 1990s. It is important to remember that they will be shaped by their social and historical context. The African–Caribbean men and women in Morgan's (1996) study were born in the Caribbean. It is possible that their children's generation might hold different views. This is true of course for any social group.

The critical point here is that people's views and practices are shaped by their context – a finding that is replicated again and again in social research. For example, Murdoch et al.'s (2013) study into asthma patients' use of inhalers found that, when interviewed, their reasons for not using the inhalers was related to a multiplicity of factors that were weighed up in relation to pragmatic needs and benefits of use. There was a moral dimension to their accounts, however, with patients being aware that resisting medication use might implicate them as 'bad patients' in the eyes of care professionals. However, their own assessments of need and experiences of non-use confirmed that their health did not appear to be compromised. A systematic synthesis of research into qualitative studies (Pound et al. 2005) confirms these findings, revealing caution among patients when it comes to taking medicines, and the lay practice of testing medicines, mainly for adverse effects. The review concludes:

> Active accepters might modify their regimens by taking medicines symptomatically or strategically, or by adjusting doses to minimise unwanted consequences, or to make the regimen more acceptable. Many modifications appeared to reflect a desire to minimise the intake of medicines and this was echoed in some peoples' use of non-pharmacological treatments to either supplant or supplement their medicine.

The implication for practice is the need to take the patients' perspectives into account, the context of their lives and how they 'experience' their illness.

## THE EXPERIENCE OF ILLNESS

Biophysical changes have significant social consequences. Illness reminds us that the 'normal' functioning of our minds and bodies is central to social action and interaction. In this respect, the study of illness throws light on the nature of the interaction between the body, the individual and society. If we cannot rely on our bodies to function 'normally', then our interaction with the social world becomes perilous; our dependency on others may increase and, in turn, our sense of self may be challenged. To illustrate, the onset of rheumatoid arthritis can result in a severe restriction of bodily movements; this may mean that the sufferer becomes dependent upon others to perform tasks previously carried out by him or herself. As discussed above, there is a moral and cultural dimension to this. Within a culture which emphasizes independence and self-reliance, for example, a condition which limits that which previously had been presumed to be 'normal' functioning can be threatening to the sufferer's self-esteem. Essentially, then, chronic illness can impact on a person's daily living, their social relationships, their identity (the view that others hold of them) and their sense of self (their private view of themselves). It is on these experiences of illness that sociologists have focused their attention. Responses to illness, then, are not simply determined by either the nature of biophysical symptoms or individual motivations, but are shaped and imbued by the social, cultural and ideological context of an individual's biography. Thus, illness is at once both a very personal and a very public phenomenon.

## THE SICK ROLE

Illness is often related to one's capacity to work and/or fulfil one's social obligations. However, the presence of illness must be sanctioned by the medical profession. This forms the central premise of Parsons' (1951) concept of the sick role.
Parsons makes a distinction between the biological basis of illness and its social
basis and argues that to be sick is a socially as well as a biologically altered state.
Thus, the sick role delineates a set of rights and obligations; these are that a person
who is sick cannot be expected to fulfil normal social obligations and is not held
responsible for their illness. In turn, however, the sick role obliges that the sick
person should want to get well, and to this end, must seek and co-operate with
technically competent medical help. It appears that this 'role' is acknowledged
within the lay discourse of Western societies, as can be seen by the comments
made in interviews cited by Herzlich and Pierret (1987): 'When one is sick, one
obviously tries to get better as soon as possible. Personally, I do everything I can, I
try to do my utmost to be cured as quickly as possible...I would be a good patient
come to think of it'.

The sick role therefore indicates that the person who makes an effort to get well
will be granted a social status, as Herzlich and Pierret again explain:

> To be sick in today's society has ceased to designate a purely biological state and come
> to define a status, or even a group identity. It is becoming more and more evident that
> we perceive the reality of illness in these terms, for we tend to identify our neighbour
> as a 'diabetic,' almost in the same manner as we identify him [sic] as 'a professor,' or
> 'a mason.' To be 'sick' henceforth constitutes one of the central categories of social
> perception.

Thus, illness may become part of the identity of the sufferer and this is especially
significant, as we shall see, for those with long-term illnesses.

The concept of the sick role as described by Parsons is an ideal type and therefore does not necessarily correspond with empirical reality. Indeed, a moment's
reflection on our own experiences is likely to bring to mind circumstances where
the sick role did not apply. For example, we might have symptoms but refuse to seek
out professional help, or we might feel ill but carry on with activities which may
make our condition worse. Furthermore, as discussed above, the patient may not
rely solely on the advice and information given by the doctor, but may be effective
in seeking out his or her own information and developing his or her own expertise.
However, the sick role is a useful concept with which to assess actual illness behaviours and experiences. Let us take two examples of divergence from the ideal: first,
the issue of 'accessing' the sick role; and second, the issue of other people 'legiti-
mizing' the sick role.

### Access to the Sick Role

If a person adopts the sick role when they feel ill, they have an obligation to get well,
and this first requires that they seek medical advice. However, most people – most of
the time – do not go to the doctor when they are ill. Indeed, prevalence studies have

revealed that most symptoms are never seen by practitioners (Hannay 1980) – there is a 'symptom iceberg'. Certainly, most of the time, if people have a cold, bad back pain or a bout of hay fever, they probably would not want to bother their general practitioner. Conversely, if they did, general practitioners would get rather irritated, as one of the main sources of exasperation with their work is patients who present with trivial conditions. However, it is not only trivial symptoms that fail to reach health professionals: studies have also found that people suffering from extreme pain do not necessarily seek help.

People do not respond to the biophysical aspects of symptoms, but rather to the meaning of those symptoms. Many 'common' ailments (e.g. stomach pains, head-aches or a stiff neck) may be 'explained away' or be 'normalized'. They may be attributed to circumstances such as working late at night, eating too much strong cheese or sitting in a draft. If these ailments do turn out to be manifestations of a more serious illness, it may take some time for this to be recognized. Thus, accessing the sick role can take a long time.

## Lay Legitimization of the Sick Role

Legitimacy of access to the sick role can be compounded by moral evaluations. This may even occur when someone has received confirmation of sick role status from a health professional. For example, the credibility of a medical diagnosis may well be undermined for those who are only mildly affected by a disease or those who have remissions. As a respondent in Robinson's (1988) study of multiple sclerosis articulates:

> Some people can't understand why I'm in a wheelchair sometimes and not other times ... with some as long as I look cheerful and say I'm feeling fine they can cope with me but if I say I don't feel well they ignore the remark, or say I *look* well! I feel that some of them think I'm being lazy or giving up if I'm in a wheelchair, and they are inclined to talk right over my head to my pusher [emphasis in original].

Conditions such as chronic pain, which do not fit into any medical category and are idiopathic (i.e. they have no identifiable cause), are especially problematic for sufferers, as are diagnostic labels that are contested, such as chronic fatigue syndrome/myalgic encephalomyelitis (Dumit 2006) and fibromyalgia (Barker 2011).

We have seen that entering the sick role is more complex than the original concept suggests, as meanings and perceptions interfere with the process. Finally, there are also pragmatic constraints which prevent the straightforward acquisition of a sick status. For example, it may be impossible to be relieved of normal social duties if these involve caring for others and/or the general running of the household. Graham (1984) points out:

> While a mother is quick to identify and respond to symptoms of illness and disability in others, she appears less assiduous in monitoring her own health. Her role in caring for others appears to blunt her sensitivity to her own needs. Being ill makes it difficult for individuals to maintain their normal social roles and responsibilities: since the mother's roles and responsibilities are particularly indispensable, mothers are reluctant to be ill.

In recent decades, the scientific literature has tended to locate the causes of disease in features of people's personalities. If the personality is the source of illness (e.g. if the stressful or anxious person is more likely to get coronary heart disease or cancer), then this can have significant implications for the sufferer's sense of self, the reactions of others and the ability to overcome the illness.

The sick role, then, constitutes a culturally specific, ideal, typical response to illness. The reality of everyday life, however, is more complex than the concept itself suggests. The interpretation of symptoms, the decision to seek help and the conferring of rights and expectations to the sick person are mediated by the social and cultural environment. A key dimension of the sick role is that it is incumbent on the sick person to make every effort to get well. Clearly, this might be inappropriate for those people who are chronically ill. Help may come not just from professionals, but also friends, relatives and others who share common experiences.

## SELF-HELP GROUPS

It is evident that patients are not simply passive recipients of care; rather, they and their relatives and friends are also providers of that care – a fact that has long been recognized by sociologists of health and illness. Thus, lay people develop considerable amounts of expertise and knowledge which may even surpass that of the so-called 'experts' within the medical profession. This knowledge and experience may be shared among those people who suffer from the same illness. Self-help groups have been set up, sometimes at the instigation of, and sometimes in opposition to, the medical profession to provide informal support for those people with certain conditions, to educate people more generally about a particular disease, to support relevant research and to lobby for change. Self-help groups concerned with illness are arguably a relatively new phenomenon and form 'part of the larger protest movement' that is becoming evident in contemporary Western societies. These processes are likely to be accelerated within the context of the information society.

Self-help groups provide support on both individual and collective levels. For their individual members, they may offer emotional support and may be invaluable during the early stages of a person's illness career to overcome social isolation and loneliness. As many members have expertise in the provision of care, practical assistance may also be available. The ability to provide this level of support may contribute to the positive identity of people who are sick. This is also facilitated by a sense of solidarity which can be achieved among those who share a common problem. At the collective level, the establishment of solidarity among members of a self-help group may result in the pursuit of change at a political level. It can result in the mobilization of those concerned to become more active consumers of care and engage in activities which are aimed at overcoming prejudice and discrimination.

## PROFESSIONAL–PATIENT RELATIONSHIPS

Continuing the theme of change, it is argued here that the nature of relationships between lay people and experts has changed during the last few decades. Growth of lay knowledge, legitimacy of experience and declining faith in 'experts' are likely to impact on professional and patient or client interactions. The professional–patient relationship, once characterized as a meeting between the knowledgeable expert and the ignorant lay person, is now more appropriately, and more accurately, described as a 'meeting between experts' (Tuckett et al. 1985). The fact that people are encouraged to take responsibility for their own health and are more knowledgeable about factors which influence their health status adds to this view. Many illnesses today are associated with social and behavioural factors, and these are matters which are becoming 'common knowledge'. Consultations are increasingly likely to include discussions about lifestyle choices and not just focus on writing prescriptions for specific pathological conditions.

Research indicates that practitioners have often neglected to take the patient's view seriously, and this has been identified as a serious limitation of contemporary formal health care. This is important because, as we have seen, most people are able to develop sophisticated accounts about health and illness. The social science literature has revealed that lay people want to, can and do play an important part in interactions with trained health care workers, and the quality of interaction impacts upon the outcomes of health care. Such outcomes might include the extent to which a patient recovers from an illness for which he or she has been treated or the level of satisfaction with the health care provided.

Patients, then, may have more knowledge about their condition than health care professionals. People often accumulate expertise about their own bodies and come to have a special knowledge of their experience of health and illness. It is thus frustrating if the practitioner does not want to acknowledge the patient's view. One woman who was describing the difficulties she had in making the doctor listen to her put it thus: 'I've lived with this body for seventy odd years. If I don't know when it's not working properly I don't know who does' (Sidell 1992).

At a time when behavioural factors are increasingly being recognized as the antecedents of many illnesses, value judgements may be made as to the patient's culpability for their illness. This can result in patients' feeling guilty about their symptoms. Value judgements may also be made about the suitability of treatment. For example, in the summer of 1993, much controversy was generated in the UK media as a result of decisions taken by some medical consultants not to administer tests and carry out coronary bypass surgery on people who continued to smoke. They argued that the resources should not be spent on people if they smoke as they have little chance of recovery. Decisions such as these are considered by many to be value judgements rather than purely clinical decisions. The debate, which focused on the need to ration resources and direct them to those cases who will benefit most, highlights the extent to which responses to individual patients are likely to vary according to the economic and political context in which they are made.

Patients who are not satisfied with their interactions with health care professionals may deal with conflicts in a number of ways. For example, they may formally complain about a practitioner. In recent years, there has been a significant increase in complaints made within the National Health Service. It has been suggested, however, that there may still be an iceberg of dissatisfaction, because although many more people are complaining about health professionals, especially doctors, most people do not know how to complain.

For those people who do complain about primary health care practitioners, two concerns are particularly prevalent: first, the manner of practitioners; and second, difficulties in convincing them of the seriousness of a patient's condition for whom a visit is being requested. The ability to be supportive and empathetic to patients is also recognized by lay people to be an essential quality of health professionals. For example, one patient, in a letter of complaint, wrote: 'It would seem that Dr X lacks some of the qualities that will give his patients feelings of trust and understanding, qualities which I feel are essential for a good [general practitioner]' (Nettleton and Harding 1994). Furthermore, lay people do not always accept the clinical decisions of 'experts' uncritically. Indeed, another complainant cited in the same study reported how, after being prescribed a particular drug, looked it up in the British National Formulary, and finding no reference to her condition, did not collect the medication.

Patients, then, are not simply passive recipients of care, but are active participants in the processes of health care work. The relationship between professionals and patients is likely to be enhanced if practitioners are able to recognize and encourage patients to be involved. As patients and clients have access to ever more information, this point is likely to become especially salient.

## CONCLUSION

For most people, interactions with health professionals form their main encounters with health care services, and prescribed medicines are the most common form of treatment in Western medicine. People's knowledge and ideas about their treatments and how they actually experience health and illness will be contingent on the social context in which they live out their lives. This chapter has indicated that the social context is constantly changing, and the current pace of change is very rapid indeed. This is not least because of the growing proliferation of knowledge and information that people have available to them. Thus, lay people bring to their encounters with professionals considerable amounts of knowledge, information and expertise, which may be derived from a wide range of sources, be it their own personal experience or a specialist website on the Internet. During the last few decades, the contribution that lay people make to these interactions has been acknowledged, and it has been suggested that their participation has increased. This increasingly active role played by the clients, patients or lay people may be emblematic of wider social transformations, such as: a decline in faith in 'experts'; a questioning of modern scientific knowledge; the emergence of a consumer culture; and the formation of an information society.

## FURTHER READING

Albrecht, G.L., Fitzpatrick, R. and Scrimshaw, S. 1999. *The Handbook of Social Studies in Health and Medicine*. London: Sage.

Blaxter, M. 2010. *Health* (2nd Ed.). Cambridge: Polity Press.

Nettleton, S. 2013. *The Sociology of Health and Illness* (3rd Ed.). Cambridge: Polity Press.

Taylor, K.M.G., Nettleton, S.J. and Harding, G. 2003. *Sociology for Pharmacists: An Introduction* (2nd Ed.). London: Taylor & Francis.

## REFERENCES

Barker, K.K. 2011. Listening to Lyrica: Contested illnesses and pharmaceutical determinism. *Social Science and Medicine*, **73**(6), 833–842.

Blaxter, M. 2010. *Health* (2nd Ed.). Cambridge: Polity Press.

Britten, N. 1996. Lay views on drugs and medicines: Orthodox and unorthodox accounts. In: S. Williams and M. Calnan (Eds.), *Modern Medicine: Lay Perspectives and Experiences*. London: UCL Press, 48–73.

Calnan, M. 1987. *Health and Illness: The Lay Perspective*. London: Tavistock.

Cornwell, J. 1984. *Hard Earned Lives: Accounts of Health and Illness from East London*. London: Tavistock.

Currer, C. 1986. Concepts of mental well- and ill-being: The case of Pathan mothers in Britain. In: C. Currer and M. Stacey (Eds.), *Concepts of Health, Illness and Disease: A Comparative Perspective*. Lemington Spa: Berg, 183–200.

Davison, C., Davey Smith, G. and Frankel, S. 1991. Lay epidemiology and the prevention paradox: The implications of coronary candidacy for health education. *Sociology of Health and Illness*, **13**, 1–19.

Dumit, J. 2006. Illnesses you have to fight to get: Facts as forces in uncertain, emergent illnesses. *Social Science and Medicine*, **62**(3), 577–590.

Fox, N. and Ward, K. 2006. Health identities: From expert patient to resisting consumer. *Health*, **10**(4), 461–479.

Fox, N.J., Ward, K.J. and O'Rourke, A.J. 2005. The 'expert patient': Empowerment or medical dominance? The case of weight loss, pharmaceutical drugs and the Internet. *Social Science and Medicine*, **60**(6), 1299–1309.

Giddens, A. 2002. *Runaway World: How Globalisation Is Reshaping Our Lives*. London: Profile Books.

Giddens, A. 2013. *Modernity and Self-Identity: Self and Society in the Late Modern Age*. Oxford: John Wiley & Sons.

Graham, H. 1984. *Women, Health and the Family*. Brighton: Harvester Wheatsheaf.

Hannay, D.R. 1980. *The Symptom Iceberg: A Study of Community Health*, London: Routledge and Kegan Paul.

Herzlich, C. and Pierret, J. 1987. *Illness and Self in Society*. Baltimore: Johns Hopkins University Press.

Lupton, D. 2013. The digitally engaged patient: Self-monitoring and self-care in the digital health era. *Social Theory and Health*, **11**(3), 256–270.

Lupton, D. 2014. The commodification of patient opinion: The digital patient experience economy in the age of big data. *Sociology of Health and Illness*, **36**(6) 856–869.

Morgan, M. 1996. Perceptions and use of anti-hypertensive drugs amongst cultural groups. In: Williams, S. and Calnan, M. (Eds.), *Modern Medicine: Lay Perspectives and Experiences*. London: UCL Press, 95–116.

Murdoch, J., Salter, C., Cross, J., Smith, J. and Poland, F. 2013. Resisting medications: Moral discourses and performances in illness narratives. *Sociology of Health and Illness*, **35**(3), 449–464.

Nettleton, S. and Harding, G. 1994. Protesting patients: A study of complaints made to a family health service authority. *Sociology of Health and Illness*, **16**, 38–61.

Parsons, T. 1951. *The Social System*. London: Glencoe Free Press.

Pound, P., Britten, N., Morgan, M. et al. 2005. Resisting medicines: A synthesis of qualitative studies of medicine taking. *Social Science and Medicine*, **61**(1), 133–155.

Robinson, I. 1988. Reconstructing lives: Negotiating the meaning of multiple sclerosis. In: R. Anderson and M. Bury (Eds.), *Living with Chronic Illness: The Experiences of Patients and their Families*. London: Unwin Hyman, 43–66.

Sidell, M. 1992. The relationship of elderly women to their doctors, in J. George and S. Ebrahim (eds), *Health Care for Older Women*, Oxford: Oxford Medical Publications.

Tresidder, A. 2014. NICE should publish numbers needed to treat and harm for statins. *British Medical Journal*, 348, g3458.

Tuckett, D., Boutlon, M., Olson, C. and Williams, A. 1985. *Meetings Between Experts*. London: Tavistock.

Williams, R. 1983. Concepts of health: An analysis of lay logic. *Sociology*, **17**, 185–204.

# 9 Inequalities in Health and Health Care

*Mark Exworthy*

## CONTENTS

---

### KEY POINTS

- The social determinants of health refer to the range of interacting factors within the social structure of society that shape health and well-being.

- Health inequalities correlate with social class, with higher social classes enjoying increased health.
- The relationship between the need for health care and access to it is inversely proportionate, with those who need health care the most being the least likely to receive it.
- Health inequalities have been explained as a function of cultural and behavioural factors such as recklessness and irresponsibility, a function of belonging to a particular social class and a function of the way material living conditions are structured.
- Addressing health inequalities requires action at local, national and international levels.

## INTRODUCTION

This chapter provides an introduction to inequalities in health and health care. It examines the contrasting definitions of inequalities and the research evidence relating to them, and summarizes the key explanations for them. It then considers the strategies to tackle them in the UK. The chapter concludes by assessing the remaining challenges for reducing inequalities.

### WHAT ARE INEQUALITIES?

'Health inequality' is such a common term in everyday life (not least in health care organizations) that it seems strange to begin the chapter by clarifying the term itself. However, unless the term is clarified, then the way in which (research) evidence is interpreted and policies are implemented will be less than optimal. By clarifying what we mean by health inequalities, three key aspects are addressed.

### INEQUALITY AND EQUITY

Inequality and equity are related but different concepts. It is important to distinguish between (in-)equality and (in-)equity. The former divides units (of, say, resources or services) equally, while the latter may distribute them unequally depending on the characteristics of the users, recipients or clients. If we were using a cake as an analogy, equality would imply equal-sized slices for everyone, while equity would adjust those slices according to those who were hungry, those with a 'sweet tooth' or perhaps those who baked it (Stone 1998). For health care, equity is generally considered in terms of 'need'.

Definitions of equity focus attention on two questions: first, what is being distributed? This would include health (status) care or health itself, and the type of equity such as inputs (e.g. expenditure), access, use or outcome. The second question is: who is the 'target' (population or social group) of the distribution? This might include social class/socio-economic status, geography (urban/rural, etc.), gender and ethnicity (Powell and Exworthy 2003).

In practice, it is common for most health systems (including the National Health Service [NHS]) to focus on 'equal access to health care', applied universally to the whole population (rather than simply those insured). This approach, however, leads into philosophical questions about whether equal access should be sought even though groups in the population have unequal needs. Therefore, a more refined policy objective is to aim for 'equal access for equal need', recognizing that some may have better access than others (by virtues of their socio-economic position or where they live).

It should be noted that inequality is different to poverty or deprivation, although they are related concepts. In policy and practice, strategies to tackle poverty or deprivation often rely on binary approaches, such as classifying neighbourhoods as deprived or not deprived. Such strategies seek to remedy what has been termed as 'health gaps' between, say, the rich and the poor. This strategy does not always tackle the root causes of ill health and often neglects the structured nature of inequality.

> Health inequalities follow a social gradient ... health indicators show a stepwise relation to social position in a gradient which correlates higher social class with increased health throughout the different social groups ... health is related to an individual's position in society at every level (Department of Health 2002; quoted in Graham 2004).

This gradient is demonstrated in many examples; one such example is shown in Figure 9.1. The gradient has important implications for policy and practice, which are explored below.

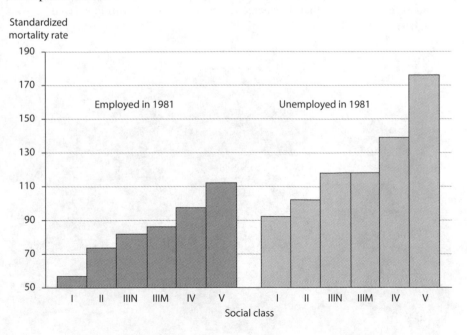

**FIGURE 9.1**   Mortality of men in England and Wales in 1981–1992, by social class and employment status at the time of the 1981 census. (Adapted from Marmot, M.G. 2010. *Fair Society, Healthy Lives. Strategic Review of Health Inequalities in England Post-2010.* London: UCL, p. 27; From Office of National Statistics Longitudinal Studies.)

## SOCIAL DETERMINANTS OF HEALTH

The social determinants of health are different from health inequalities, although they are often used in conjunction with each other. Health should be seen as the 'outcome of causal processes which originate in the social structure' of societies (Graham 2004). Social determinants of health refers to 'the range of interacting factors that shape health and well-being' (Marmot 2010). They include material circumstances, the social environment (such as housing), psychosocial factors, behaviour and biological factors. Each of these is, in turn, affected by factors such as level of education, income, employment and the societal context within which individuals live. This has been most commonly portrayed in the 'rainbow model' of Dahlgren and Whitehead (Figure 9.2), whereby layers of influence help to determine the level and quality of health for individuals and communities. The unequal distribution of these social determinants of health inevitably influences the nature of health inequalities.

A key theme in social determinants of health (and health inequalities) is the life-course perspective. This approach shows how influences early in life (including *in utero*) have long-term impacts later in life (Blane 2003). So, for example, the life chances of children are heavily shaped if they live in damp housing, have poor nutrition and/or do not receive a good education. For example, Poulton et al. (2002) found that 'low childhood socioeconomic circumstances have long-lasting negative influences on adult health, irrespective of what health cache one begins life with, or where one ends up in the socioeconomic hierarchy as an adult'. A conclusion of this and other studies is that the social gradient emerges in childhood and persists through to adulthood.

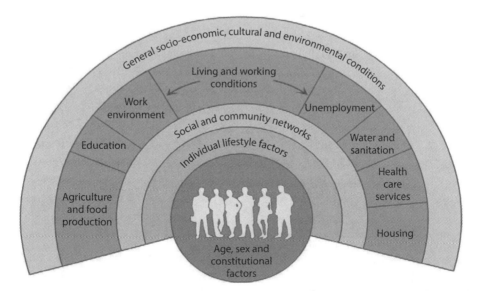

**FIGURE 9.2** General socio-economic, cultural and environmental conditions. (Adapted from Dahlgren, G. and Whitehead, M. 1991. *Policies and Strategies to Promote Social Equity in Health*. Stockholm: Institute of Futures Studies.)

## INEQUALITIES IN HEALTH CARE

'Health inequality' is a broad term that could also include inequalities in health status; that is, in terms of morbidity and/or mortality. However, the term could also refer to inequalities in health care; that is, in terms of access, provision or use. Given these caveats, a commonly accepted definition of health inequalities is 'The systematic disparities in health [status] (or in the major social determinants of health) between groups with different levels of underlying social advantage/disadvantage', including wealth, power, or prestige (Braveman and Gruskin 2003). By contrast, inequalities in health care have been defined as the 'differences in the quality of health care that are not due to access-related factors or clinical needs, preferences and appropriateness of intervention' (Smedley et al. 2002).

Health care inequalities are thus generated by the interaction of clinicians' interpretations of patients' needs and the interventions they prescribe.

### Inverse Care Law

A key theme in health care inequalities is the 'inverse care law', which proposes a relationship between the need for health care and its actual access and use. In short, those who need health care the most are least likely to receive it (Hart 1971). Examples of this 'law' can be found in most areas of health care, from NHS spending to the distribution of general practitioners to the use of hospital beds. Though written more than 40 years ago, Hart's paper has been influential in understanding and explaining patterns of health care inequalities. The fact that it still remains relevant shows the persistence of these inequalities despite action by clinicians, organizations and policy to remedy them.

### Clinical Practice Variations

The distinction between health inequalities and health care inequalities is evident in medical practice variations. Despite the image of modern health care as being based upon scientific knowledge, research has revealed variations in the ways in which health professionals practise (McPherson et al. 1982). However, it is axiomatic that the discretion inherent in professional work (such as in health care) is bound to generate differences in the ways in which practitioners act. Yet studies have shown that these variations persist when differences in health care need are taken into account. As such, 'medical practice variations' are often considered to be synonymous with health care inequalities.

Medical practice variations are evident at all levels – between countries, within countries and across small areas such as between different hospitals and practitioners. Explaining these 'variations' (or inequalities) is notoriously difficult and has generated a research sector of its own. As these variations focus on health care (rather than health *per se*), it is reasonable to look at the health care system for explanations. Andersen and Mooney (1990) highlight two possible explanations. One is what economists call 'supplier-induced demand'. In health care, the patient is heavily dependent upon the practitioner to undertake the course of action which is in their best interests. This dependence generates demands for more resources (such as interventions in the form of surgery or drugs), which would be unknown to the patient. These demands will vary according to the resources available to practitioners, thereby generating variations in rates of surgery or prescribing. A second explanation lies in the legacy of procedures being common without being sufficiently evaluated. However, this explanation raises a conundrum in the sense that the aims of some health care interventions are not always equivocal; for instance, some practitioners might disagree as to the best course of action for a patient.

Resulting from these two explanations is the notion that some variations may indeed be legitimate differences, but also medical practice variations are indicative of geographical inequities. While ensuring the equitable provision of health care resources, practitioners and managers need to promote the continuous evaluation of day-to-day practices, which should include an assessment of the impact on equity, inequality and variations.

## Medicines and Health Care Inequalities

By definition, examples of inequalities in terms of pharmacy focus on health care inequalities relating to service provision and fall into the area of medical practice variations. The pharmacy evidence selected for this chapter is orientated towards primary care, but many issues also apply to secondary care.

Majeed et al. (1996) considered factors which might affect the variations between general medical practices. Their unit of variation was the mean net ingredient cost of prescribed medicines per patient, and the study included 131 practices in southwest London. They found that about a third of the variation in prescribing costs could be explained using routine data, including age and other census characteristics, as well as practice characteristics. This means that two-thirds of the variation were due to other factors, such as general practitioners' knowledge and preferences. Healey and colleagues (1994) conducted a similar study. Their aim was to determine the implication of variations in general practitioner prescribing behaviour for the determination of prescribing budgets. They concluded that:

> ... 97% of the variation in practice prescribing costs can be explained by differences in practice list size, the proportion of patients aged 65 years and over, the proportion of patients living in 'deprived areas' and whether or not the practice qualifies for 'inducement payments'.

Weighted capitation formulae based on such factors are, in their view, justified. Linking prescribing behaviour to organizational factors was the purpose of a study by Houghton and Gilthorpe (1998) in 263 Birmingham practices. In particular, they focused on the impact of general practitioner fundholding. They found that fundholders spent less and prescribed fewer items than non-fundholders, even though prescribing activity was steadily increasing.

The conclusion of such evidence suggests that information on clinical effectiveness is not being used sufficiently. Although medical care is 'variable and uncertain' (Bunker 1990), health care inequalities persist. The positive responses to such evidence by practitioners have often been to establish a confidential and educational system of data feedback; negative responses have ignored or dismissed the evidence

(McColl et al. 1998). The positive responses have had some success (Keller et al. 1996; Centre for Reviews and Dissemination 1999). The suboptimal use of evidence has implications for resource allocation; practices not adopting the 'best evidence' may be at a financial disadvantage.

# EVIDENCE OF HEALTH INEQUALITIES

## SUMMARY OF EVIDENCE

Inequalities in health status and health care have been acknowledged for more than a hundred years (Klein 1996; Syme 1998), and research evidence has been accumulating for much of that time (Exworthy et al. 2006). Arguably, this phase of research evidence was first marked by the Whitehall studies of British civil servants (Marmot et al. 1978, 1991). These studies were significant because they included more than 10,000 civil servants working in a range of occupations with relatively stable employment. They found a steep inverse association between social class, as assessed by grade of employment, and mortality from a wide range of diseases (Marmot et al. 1991). Those in the highest employment grade had about a third the mortality rate of those in the lowest grade.

However, the growing volume of evidence has also been summarized by three significant reports which have had contrasting impacts upon policy. These reports are explored next.

## REPORTS OF EVIDENCE

In the past 35 years in the UK, three reports have been highly significant in the accumulation and synthesis of evidence about health inequalities. These are titled by the chairs of the committee or working parties which produced them: Sir Douglas Black, Sir Donald Acheson and Sir Michael Marmot.

### Black Report, 1980

A Labour government commissioned an inquiry in 1977, which delivered its report in 1980 when a Conservative government was in power. Famously, it was published on the August Bank Holiday and only 260 copies were made available (Townsend et al. 1988).

The Black Report (1980) described the pattern of health inequalities according to occupational class, sex, geography (by region), ethnicity and housing tenure in terms of mortality and morbidity (illness) by social class. It considered the trend of inequality patterns over time and made some international comparisons. It also addressed inequality in terms of the 'availability and use of health services'. A clear pattern emerged in which unskilled classes (social class V) had mortality rates 2.5-times those of professional classes (social class I) (Table 9.1). This pattern was consistent between men and women. The pattern is often called the social class gradient and is perhaps the most widely cited health inequality. This pattern is also replicated in geographical variations. The Black Report compared death rates (standardized mortality rates) by English and Welsh regions. There was a clear north–south division in

## TABLE 9.1
## Death Rates by Sex and Social Class (15–64 Years; Rates per 1,000 Population in England and Wales, 1971)

| Social Class Category | Occupational Type | Men | Women |
|---|---|---|---|
| I | Professional (e.g. lawyer, pharmacist) | 3.98 | 2.15 |
| II | Intermediate (e.g. teacher) | 5.54 | 2.85 |
| IIIN | Skilled non-manual (e.g. shop assistant) | 5.80 | 2.76 |
| IIIM | Skilled manual (e.g. bus driver) | 6.08 | 3.41 |
| IV | Partly skilled (e.g. farm labourer) | 7.96 | 4.27 |
| V | Unskilled (e.g. cleaner) | 9.88 | 5.31 |

*Source:* From Black, D. (Chair) 1980. *Inequalities in Health: Report of a Research Working Group.* London: Department of Health and Social Security.

these figures, with more southerly regions experiencing lower-than-expected mortality rates (Table 9.2).

## Acheson Report, 1998

This inquiry, commissioned by a Labour government in 1997 and chaired by Sir Donald Acheson, was charged with reviewing the latest information on health inequalities and identifying priority areas for future policy development. The report was divided into 'the current position' on inequalities and 11 priority areas for policy development; the focus here is on the former.

## TABLE 9.2
## Regional Variations in Mortality in England and Wales

| Standard Region | Standardized Mortality Rate by Age | Standardized Mortality Rate by Age and Class |
|---|---|---|
| Northern Yorkshire and Humberside | 113 | 113 |
| North West | 106 | 105 |
| East Midlands | 116 | 116 |
| West Midlands | 96 | 94 |
| East Anglia | 105 | 104 |
| South East | 90 | 90 |
| South West | 93 | 93 |
| Wales (south) | 114 | 117 |
| Wales (north) | 110 | 113 |
| *England and Wales* | *100* | *100* |

*Source:* From Black, D. (Chair) 1980. *Inequalities in Health: Report of a Research Working Group,* London: Department of Health and Social Security.

*Note:* As the England and Wales average is 100, standardized mortality rates above 100 imply a greater-than-expected mortality rate and vice versa.

## TABLE 9.3
## Mortality Rates (All Causes) for Men and Women (Aged 35–64) by Social Class over Time

| Social Class | 1976–1981 | | 1981–1985 | | 1986–1992 | |
|---|---|---|---|---|---|---|
| | Men | Women | Men | Women | Men | Women |
| I/II | 621 | 338 | 539 | 344 | 455 | 270 |
| III non-manual | 860 | 371 | 658 | 387 | 484 | 305 |
| III manual | 802 | 467 | 691 | 396 | 624 | 356 |
| IV/V | 951 | 508 | 824 | 445 | 764 | 418 |

*Source:* From Acheson, D. (Chair) 1998. *Independent Inquiry into Inequalities in Health*, London: The Stationery Office.

*Note:* Rates per 100,000 for England and Wales and age standardized.

The Acheson Report highlighted the trends over time which showed a decline in mortality rates for gender and social class groups, and yet the differentials between them had persisted or even increased. For example, the ratio of (male) mortality rates for social classes IV and V to classes I and II in 1976–1981 was 1.53, while the ratio in 1986–1992 had increased to 1.68 (Table 9.3). The Acheson Report examined five specific causes of death and made comparisons between different social classes. The broad social class gradient was persistent throughout these different causes and had remained despite a general decline in mortality rates. This is illustrated by deaths from lung cancer (Table 9.4). This summary of the evidence presented in the Black

## TABLE 9.4
## Standardized Mortality Rates for Lung Cancer in England and Wales by Social Class for Men Aged 20–64

| Social Class | 1970–1972 | 1979–1983 | 1991–1993 |
|---|---|---|---|
| I: professional | 41 | 26 | 17 |
| II: managerial and technical | 52 | 39 | 24 |
| IIIN: skilled, non-manual | 63 | 47 | 34 |
| IIIM: skilled manual | 90 | 72 | 54 |
| IV: partly skilled | 93 | 76 | 52 |
| V: unskilled | 109 | 108 | 82 |
| *England and Wales* | *73* | *60* | *39* |

*Source:* From Acheson, D. (Chair) 1998. *Independent Inquiry into Inequalities in Health*, London: The Stationery Office.

*Note:* Rates are per 100,000.

and Acheson reports is intended to provide an overview of the parameters of health inequalities generally. It would be difficult to do justice to the volume of evidence that currently exists. For example, there were 529 references in the Acheson Report. The reader is therefore directed to the reference list and contact list at the end of this chapter to explore these sources.

## Marmot Report, 2010

The World Health Organization (WHO) established a global Commission on the Social Determinants of Health, which was chaired by Professor Sir Michael Marmot and published in 2008. Following this report, in November 2008, the Department of Health commissioned a review (also chaired by Marmot) as 'a response to ... the government's commitment to reducing health inequalities in England'. The aim of the report was to influence policy beyond 2010 (when the national targets for reducing health inequalities [originally set in 2001] expired). For example, evidence suggests that these targets have not been met (Table 9.5).

The Marmot Review had four objectives:

1. To identify, for the health inequalities challenge facing England, the evidence most relevant to underpinning future policy and action.
2. To show how this evidence could be translated into practice.
3. To advise on possible objectives and measures, building on the experience of the current Public Service Agreement target on infant mortality and life expectancy.
4. To publish a report of the review's work that would contribute to the development of a post-2010 health inequalities strategy.

The collection, synthesis and interpretation of evidence were arguably more extensive than the Acheson Report from some 10 years earlier. Many more academics and other experts were involved in examining nine themes. While these themes

## TABLE 9.5
### National Health Inequality Targets: Evidence of Progress

|           | England                 | Spearhead Areas[a]      | Difference |
|-----------|-------------------------|-------------------------|------------|
| Men       | Life expectancy, years  | Life expectancy, years  | %          |
| 1994–1995 | 74.6                    | 72.7                    | 2.57%      |
| 2004–2006 | 77.3                    | 75.3                    | 2.63%      |
| Women     |                         |                         |            |
| 1994–1995 | 79.7                    | 78.3                    | 1.77%      |
| 2004–2006 | 81.6                    | 80.0                    | 1.96%      |

*Source:* From Department of Health. 2007. Health inequalities. Available from: http://webarchive. nationalarchives.gov.uk/ + /www.dh.gov.uk/en/Publichealth/Healthinequalities/index.htm.

[a] Spearhead areas were 88 of the most health-deprived areas in England that were the first to pilot various initiatives in the 2000s.

## TABLE 9.6
## Marmot Report: Policy Objectives and Recommendations

| Policy Objective | Recommendations |
|---|---|
| A: Give every child the best start in life | • Increased investment in early years<br>• Supporting families to develop children's skills<br>• Quality early-years education and childcare |
| B: Enable all children, young people and adults to maximize their capabilities and have control over their lives | • Reduce the social gradient in educational outcomes<br>• Reduce the social gradient in life skills<br>• Ongoing skills development through lifelong learning |
| C: Create fair employment and good work for all | • Active labour market programmes<br>• Development of good-quality work<br>• Reducing physical and chemical hazards and injuries at work<br>• Shift work and other work-time factors<br>• Improving the psychosocial work environment |
| D: Ensure healthy standard of living for all | • Implement a minimum income for healthy living<br>• Remove 'cliff edges' for those moving in and out of work and improve flexibility of employment<br>• Review and implement systems of taxation, benefits, pensions and tax credits |
| E: Create and develop healthy and sustainable places and communities | • Prioritize policies and interventions that reduce both health inequalities and mitigate climate change<br>• Integrate planning, transport, housing and health policies to address the social determinants of health<br>• Create and develop communities |
| F: Strengthen the role and impact of ill health prevention | • Increased investment in prevention<br>• Implement evidence-based ill health-preventative interventions<br>• Public health to focus interventions on reducing the social gradient |

*Source:* From Marmot, M.G. 2010. *Fair Society, Healthy Lives. Strategic Review of Health Inequalities in England Post-2010.* London: UCL.

are similar to the Acheson Report, there were also new ones, such as built environment, sustainable development and economics.

Recommendations were grouped into categories which did not always match the thematic approach taken during the process. The report made 20 recommendations across six main categories (Table 9.6).

## EXPLANATIONS FOR HEALTH INEQUALITIES

### Cultural and Behavioural Explanations

The focus in these explanations is mainly upon the individual's choice of lifestyle. Thus, individuals' 'reckless' or 'irresponsible' behaviour may have inimical consequences on their health. For instance, excessive amounts of drinking, smoking or eating may be detrimental to their health. While some point to the lack of education or understanding of these impacts upon an individual's lifestyle, others argue that it is an individual's free will to pursue such a lifestyle. However, the choice that individuals face is constrained by their circumstances, which are primarily shaped by their socio-economic situation. Thus, an unemployed person has much tighter constraints in terms of the options they have for pursuing a 'healthy' lifestyle. Access to shops selling cheap, good-quality foods may be limited by the lack of transport and income. Alternatively, the housing market may operate in such a way that only poor-quality, damp housing is available. The cultural norms of particular social groups or social classes influence the type of lifestyle that individuals pursue. Rates of smoking, for example, are higher among manual and unskilled occupational groups. Understanding behaviour in this cultural context makes a clear link between the structural explanations discussed later and individual lifestyles. As such, the two explanations are clearly inter-related, but the nature of that relationship is not yet fully understood.

## SOCIAL (OR NATURAL) SELECTION EXPLANATIONS

These explanations suggest that individuals with certain characteristics drift into lower social classes and thereby receive fewer economic rewards (such as lower salaries). As well as problems of identifying cause and effect, this thesis suffers from a lack of conclusive evidence to support it. It is unclear whether the bio-genetic composition of individuals alone would merit such a conclusion, although social processes, such as the job and housing markets, help generate a finely graded social system.

## STRUCTURED EXPLANATIONS

These explanations focus on the structure of society and material living conditions. They highlight the connection between socio-economic processes of employment, government expenditure and the impact upon health. At one level, this involves the link between hazardous occupations (such as coal-mining) and individual health, but it points more broadly to more endemic processes of an individual's chances to secure adequate housing, a balanced diet and gainful employment (among other things) so as to enable them to participate fully in society. Despite rising living standards and generally improving levels of health in the UK, there are areas of high deprivation and poverty that are clearly associated with income inequality. This form of inequality reflects not only the level of income earned, but also the net income taking into account benefits and taxation. The persistence of areas of deprivation points to the continuation of forces encouraging income inequality. Redistribution in the form of government taxation and expenditure is one way in which such inequality may be reduced, but its effects are moderated by the workings of a capitalist, market-based economy.

Although some social divisions are becoming less clear-cut than they once were (in part due to the changing nature of employment and the increased participation of women in the workforce) and living standards are rising, the general pattern of health inequalities remains. Several commentators, notably Wilkinson (1996), have sought to explain the persistent social class gradient in health inequalities. Wilkinson examined the degree of income inequality in various countries and concluded that the overall level of wealth (or poverty) was not a significant factor in explaining health inequalities, but rather the difference between the richest and poorest was such an explanatory factor (Wilkinson and Pickett 2010). Thus, income inequalities are related to health inequalities. Moreover, those societies with lower income inequalities had higher levels of 'social capital', which translated through unspecified mechanisms into the level of health. Others have sought to operationalize Wilkinson's thesis by examining the mechanisms of social capital within societies. Social capital refers to the social solidarity between citizens, promoting feelings of well-being and social cohesion or inclusion – the systems and processes by which individuals feel part of society. This may be manifest in terms of turnout at elections, participation in social groups (e.g. sports clubs), voluntary organizations or church attendance or donations to charity (Putnam 2001). One problem of the social capital thesis is establishing the precise connection between health and these multifarious types of social capital; the causal mechanisms are not very clear-cut.

## TACKLING HEALTH INEQUALITIES

Inequalities in health and health care are complex and deep-rooted phenomena that lie beyond the scope of health care systems alone, and thus are not simply amenable to remedy by government interventions or practitioners. Indeed, the social determinants of health lie well beyond any health care interventions. They involve interactions between age, sex and constitutional (genetic) factors and individual lifestyle factors, social and community networks and general socio-economic, cultural and environmental conditions (Dahlgren and Whitehead 1991). As such, health services can play only a small role in tackling health inequalities, but in certain ways, these roles may still be important (Benzeval et al. 1995). This sense of perspective is manifested, for example, by the Acheson Report, which devotes only nine pages to the role of the health service in reducing health inequalities, but 68 pages to factors such as taxation and benefits, education, housing, employment, environment, pollution and transport.

Broadly, action to tackle health inequalities takes places at local, national and international levels. Some strategies at one level may, of course, be negated by actions at another level. Any assessment of action at these three levels is partial, but a summary is offered below. Further sources of information can be found at the end of this chapter.

### LOCAL ACTION

The NHS makes a significant contribution to promoting equity and reducing health inequality and especially health care inequality. The existence of the NHS with a reasonable degree of (geographical and social) access and services that are (mostly) free at the point of delivery is, in itself, a major contribution to ensuring a reasonable degree of access to health services for the whole population. However, it can also perpetuate and even magnify some inequalities.

The NHS is often the single largest employer in most areas. It is in a unique position to promote diversity in the workforce and to foster good working practices (such as a sense of occupational control). It also procures goods and services from all sorts of suppliers (from catering to pharmaceuticals), but could do so in more equitable ways.

In 2013, Health and Well-being Boards (HWBs) were created in each area to coordinate public health activities (including action on health inequalities) between local government (where public health functions now reside) and Clinical Commissioning Groups (CCGs), which secure health services from the NHS and other providers. Humphries and Galea (2013) found that 'public health and health inequalities are the highest priorities in the [joint health and well-being strategies] of most boards, but they have not yet begun to grapple with the immediate and urgent strategic challenges facing local health and care systems'.

A common strategy to foster equity being used by many organizations (in the NHS and elsewhere) is equity impact assessments or audits. These are similar to health impact assessments. An equity audit is 'a decision support tool which walks users through the steps of identifying how a program, policy or similar initiative will impact population groups in different ways ... The end goal is to maximize positive impacts and reduce negative impacts that could potentially widen health disparities between population groups' (http://www.health.gov.on.ca/en/pro/programs/heia/). These audits can also identify unintended consequences of strategies and policies (see further information below). All of these local strategies need to 'compete' with equally pressing imperatives, such as finance (Exworthy et al. 2002).

## NATIONAL ACTION

Many argue that decisions by national governments have a more profound impact on health inequalities than other public (or even possibly private) organizations. In particular, their policies on taxation and public spending have significant impacts upon the life chances of the population. Their decisions have the potential for redistribution of resources, which shape the social determinants of health and health inequalities.

A key tension in national (health) policy rests on governments' roles in influencing the private sector. For example, the UK Coalition Government (elected in 2010) pursued a strategy of 'responsibility deals' with the private sector, in which voluntary agreements are reached for adopting health-promoting practices, rather than implementing mandatory regulation. One such deal includes public health. Food and drink (but not tobacco) companies are involved in a partnership with government to address issues such as food labelling and salt content, in pursuit of tackling obesity. Gilmore et al. (2011) argue that partnership with the private sector is not problematic *per se*, but that it should not be given such a prominent role in policy making. Bryden et al. (2013) echo this view, but also noted unexpected consequences:

> If properly implemented and monitored, voluntary agreements can be an effective policy approach, though there is little evidence on whether they are more effective than compulsory approaches. Some of the most effective voluntary agreements include substantial disincentives for non-participation and sanctions for non-compliance.

One illustration of the approach is in the government-sponsored campaign for healthy lifestyles called 'Change4Life'. Favouring solutions which focus on lifestyle and ignoring wider structural factors (Hunter et al. 2009), this campaign is poorly funded (£14 million per year) compared to the marketing budgets of the food industry (more than £1 billion per year) (Bosley 2014).

Governments have often sought to promote 'joined-up' solutions to tackle complex social problems like health inequalities. Joined-up government is a solution when 'responsibility for tackling the health gap does not reside within one policy sector or department but rather is a total or whole government issue' (Exworthy and Hunter 2011), Although joined-up government can help keep issues on the policy agenda, there remains a lack of integration across government ministries to have a sustained and significant impact on health inequalities.

## INTERNATIONAL ACTION

Until relatively recently, international action on tackling health inequalities has been weak. The WHO Commission on Social Determinants of Health was a watershed in encouraging governments across the world to tackle health inequalities seriously. The 'spread of life expectancy of 48 years among countries and 20 years or more within countries is not inevitable'. Marmot (2005) had prompted the initiative, which accumulated evidence, developed national case studies and fostered actions by civil society. The European Commission (among others) have also pursued strategies to tackle social determinants of health and health inequalities (see further information below). However, the action at an international level needs to be set against the countervailing forces of globalization and neo-liberal policies of organizations such as multinational corporations and the World Trade Organization (Pollock and Price 2000; Navarro 2007).

## CONCLUSION

Benzeval (1999) summarizes the evidence of health inequality thus:

> The weight of evidence seems to suggest that it is the cumulative effect of people's material and social circumstances that are the most important determinants of health inequalities.

The NHS seems to be in constant reorganization (whether as part of government policy or local organizational imperatives), and so it is speculative to assess the outcomes of current policy initiatives (such as CCGs or HWBs) on the future state of health inequalities. However, some factors can be identified which might affect their 'success'. A number of factors appear to be essential for strategies towards health inequalities and health care inequalities to be effective. A far from exhaustive list is shown in Box 9.1. If governments are serious about making significant and securing sustained progress in reducing inequality, these factors also need to be accompanied by a degree of income redistribution.

**BOX 9.1   ESSENTIAL FACTORS FOR EFFECTIVE POLICIES TO REDUCE HEALTH AND HEALTH CARE INEQUALITIES**

- Clarity of objectives in inequality policies; that is, clarity of 'who' and 'what'.
- Inclusion of equity and reducing inequality as governing principles in the day-to-day work of practitioners and agencies.
- Strong incentives for partnership to overcome traditional resistance at both government department and local agency levels.
- Wider structural reform, including equity considerations in education, employment, transport and nutrition.
- Measures to monitor and assess progress towards reducing inequality.

Inequalities are beyond the scope of health services alone. Partnerships are essential but extremely difficult to achieve. In addition, other policy pressures are likely to impinge and trade-offs are inevitable. In order to be serious about reducing inequalities, policy makers and practitioners need to be clear about the timescales (i.e. which strategies should be tackled first and when change might be evident) and the (social and financial) costs of their proposals (i.e. what the opportunity costs are of pursing this proposal). In short, it is not sufficient to simply present the evidence about inequalities; this must also be backed up by an understanding and commitment to change that recognizes the demands that practitioners and policy makers face.

## ACKNOWLEDGEMENT

The author is grateful to those agencies which have funded his research on health inequalities, including the ESRC (award no: L128251039), Joseph Rowntree Foundation and Commonwealth Fund of New York.

## FURTHER READING AND INFORMATION SOURCES

Equity audits
   http://www.health.gov.on.ca/en/pro/programs/heia/
   http://www.apho.org.uk/default.aspx?RID=40141
   http://www.pha.org.nz/documents/health-equity-assessment-tool-guide1.pdf

European Union: health inequalities
   http://www.health-inequalities.eu/

European Union: social determinants and health inequalities
   http://ec.europa.eu/health/social_determinants/policy/commission_
   communication/index_en.htm

Health Equity Network
'The Health Equity Network aims to encourage active and fruitful collaboration between specialists from different disciplines in addressing and debating issues of equity and inequality in health'
https://www.jiscmail.ac.uk/cgi-bin/webadmin?A0=health-equity-network

Health and well-being boards
http://www.kingsfund.org.uk/projects/new-nhs/health-and-wellbeing-boards

Institute of Health Equity, University College London
http://www.instituteofhealthequity.org/

National Institute for Health and Care Excellence: health inequalities—concepts, frameworks and policy
http://www.nice.org.uk/niceMedia/documents/health_inequalities_concepts.pdf

Royal College of Nursing: tackling health inequalities
http://www.rcn.org.uk/development/practice/public_health/topics/tackling_health_inequalities

Royal Pharmaceutical Society: map of evidence (keyword search: health inequalities)
http://www.rpharms.com/moe/moe

World Health Organization (Europe): health determinants
http://www.euro.who.int/en/health-topics/health-determinants

World Health Organization (Europe): social determinants of health
http://www.euro.who.int/__data/assets/pdf_file/0005/98438/e81384.pdf

World Health Organization: social determinants of health (including Commission on Social Determinants of Health)
http://www.who.int/social_determinants/en/

## REFERENCES

Acheson, D. (Chair) 1998. *Independent Inquiry into Inequalities in Health*. London: The Stationery Office.

Andersen, T. and Mooney, G. 1990. *The Challenges of Medical Practice Variations*. London: Macmillan.

Benzeval, M. 1999. Tackling inequalities in health: Public policy action. In: Griffiths, S. and Hunter, D.J. (Eds.), *Perspectives in Public Health*. Abingdon: Radcliffe Medical Press, 34–46.

Benzeval, M., Judge, K. and Whitehead, M. (Eds.) 1995. *Tackling Inequalities in Health: An Agenda for Action*. London: King's Fund.

Black, D. (Chair) 1980. *Inequalities in Health: Report of a Research Working Group*. London: Department of Health and Social Security.

Blane, D. 2003. The life-course, the social gradient and health. In: M.G. Marmot and R. Wilkinson (Eds.), *Social Determinants of Health*. Oxford: Oxford University Press, 54–77.

Bosley, S. 2014. The truth about obesity: 10 shocking things you need to know. *Guardian*, June 23, 2014. Available at: http://www.theguardian.com/lifeandstyle/2014/jun/23/truth-about-obesity-10-shocking-things-need-to-know.

Braveman, P. and Gruskin, S. 2003. Defining equity in health. *Journal of Epidemiology and Community Health*, **57**(4), 254–258.

Bryden, A., Petticrew, M., Mays, N. et al. 2013. Voluntary agreements between government and business—A scoping review of the literature with specific reference to the public health responsibility deal. *Health Policy*, **110**(2), 186–197.

Bunker, J. 1990. Variations in hospital admissions and the appropriateness of care: American pre-occupations? *British Medical Journal*, **301**, 531–532.

Centre for Reviews and Dissemination 1999. Getting evidence into practice. *Effective Health Care*, **5**, 1–16.

Dahlgren, G. and Whitehead, M. 1991. *Policies and Strategies to Promote Social Equity in Health*. Stockholm: Institute of Futures Studies.

Department of Health 2007. Health inequalities. Available at: http://webarchive.nationalarchives.gov.uk/ + /www.dh.gov.uk/en/Publichealth/Healthinequalities/index.htm.

Exworthy, M., Berney, L. and Powell, M. 2002. How great expectations in Westminster may be dashed locally: The local implementation of national policy on health inequalities. Policy and Politics, **30**(1), 79–96.

Exworthy, M., Bindman, A., Davies, H.T.O. and Washington, A.E. 2006. Evidence into policy and practice? Measuring the progress of policies to tackle health disparities and inequalities in the US and UK. *Milbank Quarterly*, **84**(1), 75–109.

Exworthy, M. and Hunter, D.J. 2011. The challenge of joined-up government in tackling health inequalities. *International Journal of Public Administration*, **34**(4), 201–212.

Gilmore, A.B., Savell, E. and Collin, J. 2011. Public health, corporations and the new responsibility deal: Promoting partnerships with vectors of disease? *Journal of Public Health*, **33**(1), 2–4.

Graham, H. 2004. Tackling health inequalities in England: Remedying health disadvantages, narrowing health gaps or reducing health gradients? *Journal of Social Policy*, **33**(1), 115–131.

Hart, J.T. 1971. Inverse care law. *Lancet*, **297**(7696), 405–412.

Healey, T., Yule, B. and Reid, J. 1994. Variations in general practice prescribing: Costs and implications for budget setting. *Health Economics*, **3**, 47–56.

Houghton, G. and Gilthorpe, M.S. 1998. Variations in general practice prescribing: A multilevel model approach to determine the impact of practice characteristics, including fundholding and training status. *Journal of Clinical Effectiveness*, **3**(2), 75–79.

Humphries, R. and Galea, A. 2013. Health and wellbeing boards: One year on. London: King's Fund. Available at: http://www.kingsfund.org.uk/sites/files/kf/field/field_publication_file/health-wellbeing-boards-one-year-on-oct13.pdf.

Hunter, D.J., Popay, J., Tannahill, C. et al. 2009. Learning lessons from the past: Shaping a different future. Marmot Review Working Committee 3; cross-cutting sub-group report. In: M.G. Marmot (Ed.), *Fair Society, Healthy Lives. Strategic Review of Health Inequalities in England post-2010*. London: UCL. Available at: http://www.ucl.ac.uk/marmotreview/documents.

Keller, R.B., Chapin, A.M. and Soule, D.N. 1996. Informed inquiry into practice variations: The Maine Medical Assessment Foundation. *Quality Assurance in Health Care*, **2**, 69–75.

Klein, R. 1996. Acceptable inequalities. In: Day, P. (Ed.), *Only Dissect: Rudolf Klein on Politics and Society*. Oxford: Blackwell, 389–406.

Majeed, A., Cook, D. and Evans, N. 1996. Variations in general practice prescribing costs: Implications for setting and monitoring prescribing budgets. *Health Trends*, **28**, 52–55.

Marmot, M.G. 2005. Social determinants of health inequalities. *Lancet*, 365(9464), 1001–1104.

Marmot, M.G. 2010. *Fair Society, Healthy Lives. Strategic Review of Health Inequalities in England post-2010.* London: UCL.

Marmot, M.G., Davey-Smith, G., Stansfield, S. et al. 1991. Health inequalities among British civil servants: The Whitehall II study. *Lancet*, **337**, 1387–1393.

Marmot, M.G., Rose, G., Shipley, M., and Hamilton, P.J.S. 1978. Employment grade and coronary heart disease in British civil servants. *Journal of Epidemiology and Community Health*, **32**, 244–249.

McColl, A., Roderick, P., Gabbay, J., Smith, H. and Moore, M. 1998. Performance indicators for primary care groups: An evidence based approach. *British Medical Journal*, **317**, 1354–1360.

McPherson, K., Wennberg, J.E., Hovind, O.B. and Clifford, P. 1982. Small-area variations in the use of common surgical procedures: An international comparison of New England, England, and Norway. *New England Journal of Medicine*, **307**(21), 1310–1314.

Navarro, V. (Ed.) 2007. *Neoliberalism, Globalization, and Inequalities: Consequences for Health and Quality of Life.* Amityville: Baywood Publishing.

Pollock, A. and Price, D. 2000. Re-writing the regulations: How the World Trade Organisation could accelerate privatisation in health-care systems. *Public Health*, **356**, 1995–2000.

Poulton, R., Caspi, A., Milne, B.J. et al. 2002. Association between children's experience of socioeconomic disadvantage and adult health: A life-course study. *Lancet*, **360**(9346), 1640–1645.

Powell, M. and Exworthy, M. 2003. Equal access to health-care and the British NHS. *Policy Studies*, **24**(1), 51–64.

Putnam, R. 2001. *Bowling Alone: The Collapse and Revival of American Community.* New York: Simon Schuster.

Smedley, B.D., Stith, A.Y., and Nelson, A.R. (Eds.) 2002. *Unequal Treatment: Confronting Racial and Ethnic Disparities in Health Care.* Washington, DC: National Institute of Medicine.

Stone, D. 1998. *Policy Paradox: The Art of Political Decision Making.* New York: W.W. Norton and Company.

Syme, S.L. 1998. Social and economic disparities in health: Thoughts about Intervention. *Milbank Quarterly*, **76**(3), 493–505.

Townsend, P., Davidson, N. and Whitehead, M. 1988. *Inequalities in Health.* London: Pelican.

Wilkinson, R.G. 1996. *Unhealthy Societies: From Inequality to Well-being*, London: Routledge.

Wilkinson, R. and Pickett, K. 2010. *The Spirit Level: Why Equality Is Better for Everyone.* London: Penguin.

# 10 Promoting Health

*Alison Blenkinsopp, Claire Anderson and Rhona Panton*

## CONTENTS

---

### KEY POINTS

- Health behaviours have wider determinants than the individual choices that people make.
- This wider context has to be recognized and understood by pharmacists in order for them to practice health promotion effectively.
- Information alone is unlikely to change behaviour.
- Pharmacists can use the body of evidence about behaviour change techniques to inform their practice.

---

## INTRODUCTION

Greater efforts to prevent ill health are recognized globally as crucial for the future, driven by the recognition of the contribution of individual health behaviours to major diseases. Interventions of various sorts are being made to encourage individuals to improve their diet and become more physically active, lose weight if they are overweight or obese, stop smoking, reduce their alcohol intake and practice safe sex to prevent unwanted pregnancies and a range of infectious diseases such as human immunodeficiency virus and chlamydia.

Community pharmacy teams are well placed to act as health promoters. The UK continues to be at the leading edge of health-promoting pharmacy practice, with the Healthy Living Pharmacy movement providing a focus for development in community pharmacy. Health promotion is commonly perceived as being about lifestyle change and personal choice, and the pharmacist's role tends to be discussed in that context. However, health promotion has a wider meaning, incorporating a range of actions with the potential to improve health. This chapter will present health promotion and the pharmacist's role in its wider context. It will begin by presenting definitions and models for health promotion and will then go on to consider three myths: the myth of individual control over health, the myth of the unenlightened public and the myth that information alone changes behaviour. Finally, we review health promotion in pharmacy practice and consider the evidence for pharmacists' contributions to health promotion.

## WHAT IS HEALTH PROMOTION?

Health promotion aims to maintain and enhance good health and prevent ill health. It has been argued that 'the overall goal of health promotion may be summed up as the balanced enhancement of physical, mental and social facets of positive health, coupled with the prevention of physical, mental and social ill-health' (Downie et al. 1992). The term encompasses a range of activities and issues, including both individual and societal aspects. At one end of this range are government policies and legislation affecting health. These include actions with a direct influence on health (e.g. legislation to ban tobacco smoking in public places), as well as those which affect the determinants of health (e.g. social welfare and benefits policies).

Pharmacists' undergraduate training in the UK is regulated by the General Pharmaceutical Council, whose required learning outcomes include: 'Identify inappropriate health behaviours and recommend suitable approaches to interventions'; 'Promote healthy lifestyles by facilitating access to and understanding of health promotion information'; and 'Play an active role with public and professional groups to promote improved health outcomes' (General Pharmaceutical Council 2011).

These learning outcomes broaden pharmacists' thinking beyond the traditional bio-medicalization of health, where health and illness are considered as exclusively biologically determined (see also Chapter 8). Pharmacists and other health professionals provide information to promote and maintain good health, to support people's actions and behaviours related to health and to contribute to improving quality of life. However, pharmacists may still feel more comfortable linking the offering of such advice to the use of medicines and other health-related goods, as the provision of medicines remains their core function.

Beattie's strategies of health promotion (Beattie 1990) are useful ways to explore the pharmacist's current and potential future contribution (Figure 10.1).

In Beattie's framework, pharmacists' involvement in health promotion to date has primarily fallen within quadrant 1 – providing expert information to individual clients. It is easy to see how health professionals, who well know the health consequences of certain behaviours, may be tempted to act in a 'telling' rather than a 'discussing' mode. However, the evidence shows that people tend not to respond positively to such approaches. Current thinking is that the pharmacist's most effective contribution would be through adopting a general style consistent with quadrant 3 – working with individuals to negotiate change.

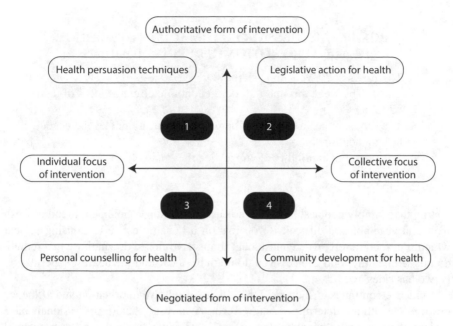

**FIGURE 10.1**   Strategies for health promotion. (Adapted from Beattie, A. 1990. *Sociology of the Health Service*. London: Routledge, Kegan and Paul.)

Health professionals engage in 'people-centred health promotion', which is:

> An enterprise involving the development over time, in individuals and communities of basic and positive states of and conditions for physical, mental and social and spiritual health. The control of and resources for this enterprise need to be primarily in the hands of the people themselves, but with the back up and support of health professionals, policy makers and the overall political system. At the heart of this enterprise are two key concepts: one of development (personal and community) and the other of empowerment. (Raeburn and Rootman 1998)

Thus, health promotion embraces the notions of community as well as individual development. Tannahill's model for health promotion includes health education, prevention and health protection (Downie et al. 1992). Pharmacists have an important role as an articulate and informed advocate for their community, in lobbying at local and national levels and in supporting local community groups working for health improvement. However, in order to engage effectively with the health promotion agenda, pharmacists need to understand their relationship with the social and economic context. In the next section, three myths which relate to health promotion are considered.

## MYTH 1: INDIVIDUALS EXERCISE CONTROL OVER THEIR HEALTH

Over the last decades, the evidence of inequalities in health has mounted (see Chapter 9 for a fuller discussion). Health chances are determined by a more complex set of

**BOX 10.1   ISSUES FOR PHARMACISTS OFFERING
HEALTH PROMOTION IN DEPRIVED AREAS**

- Their own socio-economic status
- The gap between this and the socio-economic circumstances of their customers
- The implications in terms of differences in educational level, vocabulary and culture
- The potential credibility of any advice they may offer

factors than simply peoples' lifestyle choices. Purchasing wholemeal bread or fresh fruit and vegetables is difficult if you live on a housing estate or housing project which is a 'food desert', where most local shops have closed down, those that remain do not sell healthy food choices, you do not have a car and the nearest supermarket is two bus rides away.

Evidence continues to show how the effects of relative deprivation and affluence on future health are determined before birth. As a result, health professionals have revised their assumptions about the extent to which individuals can exercise real choices about their health, and previous 'victim-blaming' approaches have been recognized for what they were – inappropriate and unrealistic. The concepts of 'social exclusion' and 'disadvantage' are used worldwide to describe those in societies who are most in need of support, financial and otherwise. For pharmacists working in deprived areas and providing services for people whose health chances most need to be improved, the challenges have to be recognized. Pharmacists should reflect on several issues (Box 10.1).

Pharmacists should work closely with client groups within local communities (e.g. drug users, mothers and toddlers). Playing a more active part in determining the needs of the communities is the basis for pharmacists to consider how they, acting as facilitators, can help empower individuals to meet their needs.

### THE ROLE OF LIFESTYLE

Pharmacists can offer information and advice about a range of issues, including those highlighted in Box 10.2.

It should be recognized that advice and information are not given in a vacuum and no individual is a 'blank sheet'. People bring with them their own beliefs and information systems about health to the pharmacy, and the pharmacist needs to be aware of the background against which further information might be offered (see also Chapter 8).

## MYTH 2: THE UNENLIGHTENED PUBLIC

In the past, it was believed that lack of information was the reason why people made less healthy lifestyle choices. With the proliferation of information, the public has

> **BOX 10.2   ISSUES ABOUT WHICH PHARMACISTS CAN OFFER INFORMATION AND ADVICE**
>
> - Smoking cessation
> - Baby and child health
> - Healthy eating
> - Physical activity
> - Drug misuse
> - Contraception and sexual health
> - Stress
> - Oral health
> - Concordance in medicine taking (e.g. for treatments to prevent heart disease and osteoporosis)
> - Prevention of accidents
> - Prevention and early diagnosis of cancer (e.g. skin cancer)
> - Promotion of screening and vaccination programmes

become increasingly better informed about the factors that affect health. The lay media is awash with stories and information on health, and the Internet enables access to detailed technical information which would once have been the sole province of health professionals. Smartphones have massively widened Internet usage and most people will have already looked for information about their disease state or condition before consulting a health professional (see also Chapter 8).

Research shows that the public is generally well aware of the health risks of smoking, yet people continue to smoke, and far from declining, smoking among women and children is increasing. Why is this? People make their own risk–benefit calculations in relation to behaviour (Butler et al. 1998). Smoking might be seen as the only way of coping with an otherwise unbearable life, and living longer by giving up smoking may not be an attractive prospect. Thus, 'concepts of future' play a key role. The underlying theme of many health-promotion messages has focused on extending life. As Pitts (1996) puts it, 'The aim of much preventive health therefore is to substitute an early death, say before the age of 60 years in the UK, for a later one'. Such an outcome may not be perceived as a benefit and thus an incentive to change by those who are poor. Consequently, pharmacists need to adapt the message to the circumstances of the recipient.

## MYTH 3: INFORMATION ALONE CHANGES BEHAVIOUR

It might be expected that the changes in the public's knowledge about health would lead to the adoption of healthier lifestyles. However, research shows that providing information does not in itself inevitably lead to the expected effect (Ley 1988). In particular, providing negative information about the consequences of behaviours that are likely to be harmful to health does not work.

Pharmacists have an important role to play in interpreting health information and in clarifying areas where the messages seem to be in conflict or information has been misunderstood. Pharmacists can interpret new findings and set them in the context of the bigger picture.

## Can Behaviour Be Changed?

Even though information in itself is unlikely to result in behaviour change, it is an important part of attempts to persuade people to adopt healthy choices. There is now a body of evidence upon which to base efforts to change behaviour (NICE 2014).

Research by behavioural psychologists has resulted in the development and testing of a model to explain why individuals change and why they sometimes revert to previous behaviour. The trans-theoretical model (TTM) of behaviour change drew on theories from several disciplines to develop a model which is both explanatory and the basis for tailoring intervention (Prochaska and DiClemente 1992). The TTM is commonly referred to as the 'stages of change' model and has been tested in a range of behaviours where change could enhance health. There are five stages: pre-contemplation, contemplation, preparation, action and maintenance. Table 10.1 describes each stage and sets out their implications for pharmacists.

The stages are not linear and the TTM should be regarded as a cycle which people may enter at any stage, leave and re-join (Figure 10.2). People who want to stop smoking or misusing drugs, for example, often make several attempts before they eventually quit. Failure at one attempt does not mean that a future attempt cannot be successful. An individual may re-enter the cycle at the planning or action stages, or may revert to pre-contemplation for a period.

---

**TABLE 10.1**

**Applying the Stages of Change Model in Pharmacy Health Promotion**

| Stage | Behaviour | Implications for Pharmacist Intervention |
|---|---|---|
| Pre-contemplation | The individual is content with current behaviour and has no intention of changing; is not considering change | Listen and respond to questions Attempts to persuade are unlikely to be successful |
| Contemplation | The person is thinking about the possibility of changing, but has made no plans to change | Listen and respond to questions Provide information |
| Preparation | The decision has been made to change and the person is getting ready to make the change | Help in planning and goal-setting |
| Action | The change is implemented | Encourage return to pharmacy to discuss progress Supportive approach |
| Maintenance | The person works to prevent relapse to the previous behaviour | Continue supportive approach |

*Source:*   Adapted from Berger, B. 1997. *Journal of the American Pharmaceutical Association*, **NS37**, 321–329.

---

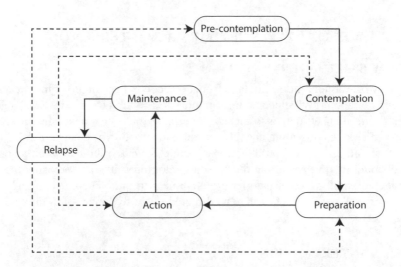

**FIGURE 10.2** The stages of change cycle.

**BOX 10.3   POSSIBLE QUESTIONS PHARMACISTS MIGHT ASK TO ESTABLISH THE POSITION OF AN INDIVIDUAL IN RELATION TO THE STATES OF CHANGE MODEL OF BEHAVIOUR**

- Have you ever thought about changing/stopping?
- Would you like to try to change?
- Would you like some information about…?
- If you could use some help, I am available here, just ask to speak to me.

Pharmacists can use the model in practice by using careful questioning to assess which stage the person is currently at and tailoring information, advice and questions appropriately (Ashworth 1997). Appropriate questions or approaches might include those shown in Box 10.3.

One of the key elements of this approach is that when an individual is in the pre-contemplation stage, health professionals should not attempt to push them to the next stage. Information might be offered, but the person is left to make their own decision. Pre-contemplation may continue for months or years.

There is evidence that even the shortest of interventions can be effective, providing they are delivered in a way that has been shown to work (Box 10.4).

## HEALTH PROMOTION IN PHARMACY PRACTICE

Pharmacists wishing to develop 'health-promoting' activities need to adopt a style of consulting which involves listening and negotiating rather than telling; crucially

## BOX 10.4   TYPES OF PHARMACY INTERVENTION

### VERY BRIEF INTERVENTION

A very brief intervention can take from 30 seconds to a couple of minutes. It is mainly about giving people information or directing them on where to go for further help. It may also include other activities, such as raising awareness of risks or providing encouragement and support for change. It follows an 'ask, advise, assist' structure. For example, very brief advice on smoking would involve recording the person's smoking status and advising them that stop-smoking services offer effective help to quit. Then, depending on the person's response, they may be directed to these services for additional support.

### BRIEF INTERVENTION

A brief intervention involves oral discussion, negotiation or encouragement, with or without written or other support or follow-up. It may also involve a referral for further interventions, directing people to other options or more intensive support. Brief interventions can be delivered by anyone who is trained in the necessary skills and knowledge. These interventions are often carried out when the opportunity arises, typically taking no more than a few minutes for basic advice.

### EXTENDED BRIEF INTERVENTION

An extended brief intervention is similar in content to a brief intervention but usually lasts more than 30 minutes and consists of an individually focused discussion. It can involve a single session or multiple brief sessions.

Adapted from National Institute for Health and Care Excellence 2014. *Behaviour Change: Individual Approaches.* NICE Public Health Guidance 49. London: NICE.

taking into account the individual's social circumstances. This may involve the role of family members, carers or friends in the management of therapy, while taking into consideration living conditions, health status and socio-economic resources. Any pharmacist may participate in health promotion and those working in community and hospital practice are well placed to do so. Their level of input can be classified as:

Level 1: displaying leaflets on health topics and responding to requests for advice and information about health.

Level 2: in addition to level 1 activities, offering information and advice opportunistically and proactively, working in a coordinated way with community-based health care workers.

## BOX 10.5   THE COMPONENTS OF PHARMACISTS' HEALTH PROMOTION ACTIVITIES

- Using the pharmacy premises effectively to promote health through the display of posters and leaflets on health topics.
- Providing an advice or counselling area.
- Using written information opportunistically to supplement verbal advice (e.g. using a leaflet on healthy eating, as well as selling a bulk laxative, as part of the response to a customer asking for advice on constipation).
- Offering one-to-one advice about individual behaviours (e.g. smoking cessation); this might often be linked with the sale of nicotine replacement therapy.
- Offering clinics (perhaps in conjunction with local medical practices) on specific topics such as the menopause.
- Targeting individuals known to be at risk (e.g. those receiving prescription medicines for angina or osteoporosis) and discussing management options, involving family, friends and carers in management if appropriate, considering with the individual the effect of the treatment on their quality of life and offering further information if required.
- Networking with other health professionals and health agencies to participate in activities and campaigns that address the local community's health needs.

The difference in these two levels is essentially that, in the first, the pharmacist is passive and working at an individual level, and in the second, they are active and using community networks effectively.

The components of health promotion input from pharmacists are summarized in Box 10.5. Pharmacists should adopt a holistic approach and think creatively about the opportunities to promote health. By 'holistic' we mean addressing issues not traditionally associated with pharmacy, but which may be linked to the sale or supply of medicines or health-related goods. Pharmacists may be uncomfortable when providing dietary advice or recommending physical activity programmes. This initial discomfort may be alleviated by targeting advice to particular groups of people, for instance:

- Targeting information about effective physical activity to those receiving prescriptions for medicines to prevent or treat osteoporosis. This might be the availability and timing of local sessions to promote strength and balance as part of a 'falls reduction programme'.
- Asking patients presenting prescriptions for medicines for heart problems whether they would like further information about diet and physical exercise.

Forward-looking health care organizations are experimenting with, for example, the prescription of exercise sessions by pharmacists, in which the patient receives vouchers for exercise sessions at local leisure facilities.

## THE EVIDENCE FOR PHARMACISTS' CONTRIBUTION TO HEALTH PROMOTION

In medicine, the randomized controlled trial (RCT) is considered the gold standard for the generation of evidence (see also Chapter 22). However, RCTs may not encompass the sorts of multi-component behavioural interventions that are utilized in health promotion programmes. There has been a vigorous debate about appropriate research methodologies to evaluate health promotion programmes. One of the major methodological difficulties is differentiating the effects of health promotion initiatives from other services and information which the public might obtain. Another issue is measuring the resultant health gain, since many health promotion initiatives are designed for long-term effects (e.g. preventing heart disease). Educational gain following a health promotion intervention may be more readily measured.

Reviews of published studies show that there is evidence to support community pharmacy involvement in health promotion (Brown et al. 2012; Fajemisin 2013; Anderson et al. 2004) and that this is strongest for smoking cessation, cardiovascular disease prevention, hypertension and diabetes.

Research suggests that while pharmacists themselves are committed to involvement in health promotion, the feasibility of spending time on a one-to-one basis in patient-centred health promotion with their customers depends on the staff skill mix and working arrangements. In particular, personal involvement in the dispensing process acts as a barrier to spending more time at the 'front of the shop' talking with customers.

## CONCLUSION

Community pharmacy teams have the potential to contribute to health promotion activities in the community. To achieve this potential, pharmacists will need to develop working styles that embrace the notions of negotiation and partnership with the public. Changes in working arrangements, particularly reducing the amount of time spent on the mechanical and technical aspects of dispensing, will be a prerequisite to the development of the health promotion role. As the public's access to information increases, the pharmacist's role in interpreting and contextualizing information will become more important.

## REFERENCES

Anderson, C., Blenkinsopp, A., Armstrong, M. 2004. Feedback from community pharmacy users on the contribution of community pharmacy to improving the public's health: A systematic review of the peer reviewed and non-peer reviewed literature 1990–2002. *Health Expectations* 7(3), 191–202.

Ashworth, P. 1997. Breakthrough or bandwagon? Are interventions tailored to stage of change more effective than non-staged interventions? *Health Education Journal*, **56**, 166–174.

Beattie, A. 1990. Knowledge and control in health promotion. In: J. Gabe, M. Calman and M. Bury (Eds.), *Sociology of the Health Service*, p. 162. London: Routledge, Kegan and Paul.

Berger, B. 1997. Readiness to change – Implications for pharmacy practice. *Journal of the American Pharmaceutical Association*, **NS37**, 321–329.

Brown, D., Portlock, J. and Rutter, P. 2012. Review of services provided by pharmacies that promote healthy living. *International Journal of Clinical Pharmacy*, **34**(3), 399–409.

Butler, C.C., Pill, R. and Stott, N.C.H. 1998. Qualitative study of patients' perceptions of doctors' advice to quit smoking: Implications for opportunistic health promotion. *British Medical Journal*, **316**, 1878–1881.

Downie, R.S., Fyfe, C. and Tannahill, A. 1992. *Health Promotion: Models and Values*, Oxford: Oxford University Press.

Fajemisin, F. 2013. Community pharmacy and public health. Solutions for Public Health. Available at: http://www.sph.nhs.uk/sph-documents/community-pharmacy-and-public-health-final-report.

General Pharmaceutical Council 2011. *Future Pharmacists: Standards for the Initial Education and Training of Pharmacists*. London: General Pharmaceutical Council.

Ley, P. 1988. *Communicating with Patients*. London: Chapman and Hall.

National Institute for Health and Care Excellence 2014. *Behaviour Change: Individual Approaches*. NICE Public Health Guidance 49. London: NICE.

Pitts, M. 1996. *The Psychology of Preventive Health*. London: Routledge.

Prochaska, J.O. and DiClemente, C.C. 1992. Stages of change in the modification of problem behaviours. In M. Hersen., R.M., Eisler and P.M. Miller (Eds.), *Progress in Behaviour Modification*, p. 183. New York: Sycamore Press.

Raeburn, J. and Rootman, I. 1998. *People-Centred Health Promotion*. Chichester: Wiley.

# 11 Compliance, Adherence and Concordance

*Robert Horne*

## CONTENTS

**KEY POINTS**

- It is thought that approximately half of all medicines prescribed for long-term conditions are not taken as directed.
- Non-adherence has costs in relation to the missed opportunity for health gain for the patient and the financial burden on health care providers.
- Good prescribing requires an understanding and knowledge of psychology as well as pharmacology.
- Non-adherence to prescribed medications may be intentional or unintentional.
- Four terms are commonly used in relation to medication taking: compliance, adherence, persistence and concordance. These may be used interchangeably, which can be confusing. 'Adherence' is the term of choice to describe patients' medicine-taking behaviour.
- The consequences of non-adherence will depend on several factors, including whether the prescription was appropriate for the patient and the type of illness and treatment.
- Defining and measuring adherence for clinical and research purposes is notoriously difficult.
- The choice of adherence measures represents a compromise in which the accuracy and comprehensiveness of the measure are balanced against reactivity and the practical, ethical and cost limitations. Valid and reliable self-report scales are often used to measure adherence.
- Four common myths surround non-adherence, which should be dispelled, namely that: (a) adherence rates are higher in severe diseases; (b) patients are non-adherent based on socio-demographic factors; (c) 'once-a-day' treatments solve the problem; and (d) providing clear instruction will resolve the problem.
- Non-adherence may be linked to a patient's beliefs about the illness and the necessity of medication, as well as to concerns about potential adverse effects.
- Helping patients to manage their medication requires a no-blame, patient-centred approach that takes account of their perceptions of their illness and treatment and the degree to which they wish to be involved in treatment decisions.
- To get the most from prescribed medicines, pharmacists and other health care professionals should address patients' beliefs about their treatments, as well as their abilities to use them.

## INTRODUCTION

Pharmacy practice serves to facilitate the appropriate use of medicines. In traditional approaches to clinical pharmacy, it was thought that this could be achieved by helping to ensure that individual patients received the 'correct medicine in the correct dose at the correct time'. However, providing a patient with the appropriate medication is only the first stage in the therapeutic process. The patient then has to use the medicine in a way that ensures optimum benefit. If one assumes that the prescription was evidence-based and appropriate, then presumably this will be achieved by following the prescriber's instructions. However, it is thought that approximately half of all medicines prescribed for long-term conditions are not taken as directed.

The fact that many patients do not use medication as advised has generated much research and debate over the last three decades, and it has become a major issue in medical care. The topic identifies some of the limitations of modern medicine and highlights the vital role of self-care in the treatment of illness. It shows that good prescribing requires an understanding and knowledge of psychology as well as pharmacology. Non-adherence to prescribed medication may be intentional as well as unintentional. Many patients actively decide to take their medication in a way that differs from the instructions. At first glance, it may seem odd that someone would go to the trouble of consulting a physician and then not follow the prescribed treatment. Understanding why patients might do this has been a key target for recent research into adherence.

This chapter will examine the causes of non-adherence, dispelling four common myths about non-adherence and presenting the perceptions and practicalities approach (PAPA), a simple framework for understanding non-adherence and how to address it. The chapter will pay particular attention to the psychology of adherence and will illustrate how research into patients' perceptions of their illnesses and treatments has led to new thinking about adherence, informing new models of care that support patients to get the best from medicines, with implications for practice in pharmacy and medicine.

## COMPLIANCE, ADHERENCE, PERSISTENCE AND CONCORDANCE: EXPLAINING TERMINOLOGY

The subject of medication taking has generated an extensive literature and some controversy. The complexity of the topic is illustrated by the fact that four terms are commonly used in relation to medication taking: compliance, adherence, persistence and concordance. It is therefore worth taking some time here to explain the definitions and why I have chosen to adopt the term 'adherence' in this chapter.

### COMPLIANCE

Until relatively recently, the most common term for following treatment instructions was 'compliance'. Compliance may be simply defined as 'the extent to which the patient's behaviour matches the prescriber's recommendations'.

Although the term 'compliance' is commonly used in the medical and pharmaceutical literature, it has been criticized because it has negative connotations in terms of the clinician–patient relationship. It seems to denote a relationship in which the role of the clinician is to decide on the appropriate treatment and issue the relevant instructions, whereas the role of the patient is to passively follow 'the doctor's orders'. Within this connotation, noncompliance may be interpreted as patient incompetence in being unable to follow the instructions, or worse, as deviant behaviour.

## ADHERENCE

The term 'adherence' has been adopted by many as an alternative to compliance in an attempt to emphasize that the patient is free to decide whether to follow the prescriber's recommendations and that failure to do so should not be a reason to blame the patient. Adherence develops the definition of compliance by emphasizing the need for agreement and may be defined as 'the extent to which the patient's behaviour matches agreed recommendations from the prescriber'.

## PERSISTENCE

Persistence is the act of continuing a treatment for the prescribed duration and does not give an indication as to whether a patient adheres to the recommended timing, dose or frequency. It may be defined as 'the duration of time from initiation to discontinuation of therapy'.

## CONCORDANCE

Concordance is a relatively recent term, predominantly used in the UK. Its definition has changed over time from one that focused on the consultation process in which doctor and patient agree therapeutic decisions that incorporate their respective views, to a wider concept that stretches from prescribing communication to patient support in medicine taking. Concordance is sometimes used incorrectly as a synonym for adherence.

It can be seen that these terms are related but different. Two issues underpin this. First, whether patients should take their medicines or not depends on whether the prescribing was appropriate – we do not want to promote patients taking inappropriate medicines. Hence, all terms refer back in varying degrees to the act of prescribing. Second, all of these terms involve varying normative agendas in terms of understandings of what is good and right about prescribing and medicine taking (see Horne et al. [2005] for a more detailed discussion).

## RECOMMENDATION ON TERMINOLOGY: LET US STICK WITH *ADHERENCE*

These four terms are sometimes used interchangeably, which can be confusing. For this reason, a National Institute of Health Research-commissioned review recommended 'adherence' as the term of choice to describe patients' medicine-taking behaviour (Horne et al. 2005), and this was subsequently endorsed by the National Institute for Health and Care Excellence (NICE) Medicines Adherence Guideline (Nunes et al. 2009).

It is important to recognize that adherence may not always be a good outcome, as a prescription may be inappropriate or not reflect the patients' changing needs. Adherence is appropriate and beneficial if it follows a process that allows patients to influence the decision making if they wish and an appropriate choice of medicine is made by the prescriber.

More recently, a collaboration funded by the EU Commission (the Ascertaining Barriers to Compliance or ABC project) endorsed the term 'adherence' as the most appropriate overarching descriptor of the 'process by which patients take their medication as prescribed', but further divided the process of 'adherence' into three quantifiable phases: initiation, implementation and discontinuation. Vrijens and colleagues (2012) define these terms as follows: initiation occurs when the patient takes the first dose of the prescribed medication; discontinuation occurs when the patient stops taking the prescribed medicine (for whatever reason); and implementation is the extent to which the patient's actual dosing corresponds to the prescribed dosing regimen, from initiation until the last dose. Persistence is the time between initiation and the last dose before discontinuation.

## CONSEQUENCES OF NON-ADHERENCE

The consequences of non-adherence will depend on several factors such as those outlined below.

### WHETHER THE PRESCRIPTION WAS APPROPRIATE FOR THE PATIENT

Concern about non-adherence seems to be fuelled by an implicit assumption that high adherence is good for patients and low adherence is bad. This will only be true if the prescription represents the best treatment option for the individual patient. Individualizing the prescription to the needs of the patient is a complex process, wherein the clinician needs to apply principles of therapeutics, knowledge of current evidence (usually obtained from data of large-scale clinical trials and therefore requiring extrapolation to the individual) and prescribing policies to the needs of the individual, while taking into account the patient's preferences (Barber 1995). The practice of clinical pharmacy may have a useful input into this process, if accepting the assumption that the role of the health care professional is to help the patient make an informed decision about adherence rather than to 'improve compliance' *per se*. If we take a leap of faith and imagine that each prescription represents the best possible intervention for each particular patient, then non-adherence represents a significant loss to patients, the health care system and the pharmaceutical industry. For the patient, it is a lost opportunity for health gain; for the health care system, it is a potential waste of resources (medicines are purchased but not used) and there is a possible increase in future demands for health care related to the lack of treatment effect. The pharmaceutical industry also loses, as patients whose adherence is low may redeem their prescriptions less frequently. For many illnesses and their treatments, the relationship between adherence and outcome is unclear. However, for most licensed medicines, we assume that the evidence from the clinical trials necessary for approval of the drug implies that low rates of adherence to medication will be associated with less favourable outcomes (as the medicine has to be taken to have an effect!).

### THE TYPE OF ILLNESS AND TREATMENT

The impact of adherence varies across conditions, ranging from minor effects on outcomes in some conditions to making the difference between life and death in

**BOX 11.1   A CLASSIC STUDY ILLUSTRATING THE IMPORTANCE OF ADHERENCE TO HEALTH OUTCOMES**

- A review of 21 studies of medication adherence found the odds of dying among those with high adherence to medication were almost half those of the group with low adherence (Simpson et al. 2006). Interestingly, while those who adhered to medication were significantly less likely to die than those who adhered to placebo, there was also an 'adherence effect' in the placebo group, with the odds of dying among high adherers to placebo being approximately half those of low adherers to placebo. The explanation for the observed 'healthy adherer' effect is not clear. It may be due to the fact that patients who are highly adherent to medication are more likely to engage in other health behaviours. It may also reflect the fact that high adherence is a behavioural marker of the placebo effect (Horne and Clatworthy 2010).
- See Pressman et al. (2012) for a more recent examination of the mechanism behind this remarkable effect. The authors conclude that 'the underlying explanation for the association (between adherence to placebo and mortality) remains a mystery'.

others. For some diseases, treatments and situations, there is more supporting evidence for the concept of adherence as 'good' than in others. A priority for adherence research and the development of adherence interventions is therefore to focus on the conditions where adherence matters most (i.e. in conditions where there is strong evidence supporting the benefits of medication and where high levels of adherence to treatment are essential to ensure efficacy or prevent problems such as treatment resistance). Although more work needs to be done to develop a framework for adherence priorities, we can immediately identify examples that fit the criteria; for example, highly active anti-retroviral therapy for human immunodeficiency virus infection, pharmacological treatment of diabetes, immunosuppressant medication following transplantation, preventer medication in asthma, medicines for severe mental illness, anti-tuberculosis treatment and anti-cancer agents (Horne and Clatworthy 2010; Horne et al. 2005).

These examples do not constitute a comprehensive list but are mentioned to illustrate the type and range of conditions for which we might consider adherence to be particularly important. However, there is also evidence that even adherence to placebos may be beneficial, as illustrated in Box 11.1.

## How We Define and Measure Non-Adherence

Defining and measuring adherence for clinical and research purposes is notoriously difficult. There are numerous ways in which patients' behaviour can differ from recommendations, with varying implications for clinical outcomes. For example, a patient could take all the required doses of a medication, but not at the correct time, miss occasional doses, take 'drug holidays' (i.e. miss three or more days' doses), take lower or fewer doses than prescribed, never take the medication or take larger or more frequent doses than prescribed.

A detailed discussion of definitions and measurement is beyond the scope of this chapter, but is dealt with elsewhere (Clatworthy et al. 2009; Horne and Clatworthy 2010). There is currently no 'gold standard' measure of adherence which can be used within the resource restraints of studies outside the controlled conditions of clinical trials. Interpreting studies comparing the performance of various adherence measures is therefore difficult. Each of the available methods has certain flaws which limit the accuracy, reliability or practical application of the technique. With the possible exception of electronic measurement devices, most of the available techniques function as indicators of adherence rather than exact, quantitative measures of behaviour. An interesting recent development is the inclusion of a microchip in the medicine formulation that sends a signal when the medicine comes into contact with stomach acid. This offers the potential to record whether and when a specific dose of medicine was taken (http://www.proteus.com). However, this new technology has yet to be widely applied in clinical studies or practice.

The easiest and cheapest way of assessing non-adherence might be to simply ask the patient. However, patient self-report measures of adherence are often criticized for being subjective and prone to response bias. People might overestimate their adherence because of poor recall or because they are reluctant to admit to non-adherence (Box 11.2).

Despite its limitations, patient report is the only method that might tell us why the person was non-adherent (e.g. was it intentional or unintentional?). For example, a self-report measure of adherence revealed that after 10 days of taking a new medication prescribed for a chronic illness, 30% of patients were non-adherent, 55%

---

**BOX 11.2   THE PRESSING NEED FOR HONEST DISCLOSURE OF NON-ADHERENCE**

In 2005, the National Institute of Health Research-commissioned review of compliance adherence and concordance found that:

One of the main problems with adherence assessment in clinical practice is that most non-adherence remains undisclosed. Patients rarely volunteer reports of non-adherence and professionals rarely ask. If they do, then many patients are reluctant to give truthful reports of non-adherence because they fear that this will offend the prescriber. One of the urgent requirements, therefore, is to develop methods and techniques for facilitating honest disclosure of medication-taking behaviour, and open, non-judgemental discussions about adherence within medication-related consultations.

of whom reported that their non-adherence was unintentional and 45% reported it being intentional (Barber et al. 2004). The accuracy of self-report may be improved by taking steps to reduce self-presentational bias by 'normalizing' non-adherence and by limiting questions to behaviours rather than reasons for behaviours (see the Medication Adherence Report Scale of Cohen et al. [2009] as an example).

The choice of adherence measures represents a compromise in which the accuracy and comprehensiveness of the measure are balanced against reactivity and the practical, ethical and cost limitations. Valid and reliable self-report scales are often used to measure adherence in 'naturalistic' studies (e.g. following up a group of chronically ill patients who are treated in the community) and may have the potential for more widespread application in clinical practice. However, they are much more accurate for reports of non-adherence than adherence. They might be used to order respondents on an adherence continuum, but do not give an accurate assessment of how much medication was consumed.

## COST OF NON-ADHERENCE

If we assume the recommended treatment was appropriate, non-adherence can have numerous costs in addition to the missed opportunity for health gain for the patient. Non-adherence to medication places a substantial financial burden on health care providers. A report published by the UK NICE estimates that hospital admissions resulting from medication non-adherence cost the UK National Health Service up to £196 million annually (NICE 2009). In addition, the report suggests that up to £4 billion per year is wasted on prescribed medications that are not taken as directed. Lack of therapeutic benefit due to undisclosed non-adherence could also lead to escalating treatment costs (increased dose/switch to more expensive regimen) or further costly diagnostic tests (Hughes et al. 2001). The wider economic costs of non-adherence have not been fully evaluated and further health economics modeling studies are needed to improve our understanding of the effects of non-adherence on health utilities (Horne and Clatworthy 2010).

## UNDERSTANDING THE CAUSES OF NON-ADHERENCE: TOWARDS MORE EFFECTIVE SOLUTIONS

Improving adherence seems to be easier said than done. A series of systematic reviews for the Cochrane Collaboration have examined the efficacy of the most comprehensively tested adherence interventions across illnesses. The good news that adherence can be improved is tempered by the disappointing news that even the best-quality interventions do not seem to have major or sustained effects (Kripalani et al. 2007).

The NICE Medicines Adherence Guidelines (Nunes et al. 2009) concluded that although no single 'off-the-shelf' intervention could be recommended, several principles could be applied to develop more effective solutions. This can be achieved by understanding the causes of non-adherence. To do this, we need to dispel some common myths about adherence (Box 11.3) and view non-adherence from the patients' perspectives.

> ## BOX 11.3   FOUR MYTHS OF NON-ADHERENCE
>
> Myth 1 – the more severe the disease, the higher the level of adherence.
> Myth 2 – non-adherence can be understood in terms of socio-demographic variables.
> Myth 3 – simpler dosage regimens guarantee adherence.
> Myth 4 – providing more information about a therapy improves adherence.

## THE CAUSES OF NON-ADHERENCE: DISPELLING FOUR COMMON MYTHS

### Myth 1: Adherence Rates Are Higher in More Severe Diseases

There is circumstantial evidence that general levels of adherence may be higher in some conditions than others. Similarly, adherence rates in acute conditions are often higher than in chronic diseases, especially where treatment of the latter seems to produce little symptomatic benefit. However, the fact that considerable variation in adherence is noted among patients with the same disease suggests that variations in adherence arise from the effect of the disease on the individual, rather than from a property of the disease which has a generalizable effect on adherence in all patients. In order to understand non-adherence, we should therefore focus on patients and how they interpret or manage the challenges imposed by the disease. This principle is illustrated by a classic review in which non-adherence was not predicted by the type or severity of the disease, with rates of 25%–30% noted across 17 studies (DiMatteo 2004).

### Myth 2: The Non-Adherent Patient

No clear relationship has emerged between race, gender, educational experience, intelligence, marital status, occupational status, income and ethnic or cultural background and adherence behaviours. Similarly, the relationship between age and adherence appears to be complex and inconsistent. Some studies find younger people are more adherent and others find the opposite, and other studies find no effect of age at all.

There is little evidence that adherence behaviours can be explained purely in terms of trait personality characteristics. Even if stable associations existed, they would serve to identify certain 'at-risk' groups to facilitate the targeting of interventions, but could do little to inform the type or content of interventions. Furthermore, socio-demographic characteristics and personality traits are not generally amenable to change and therefore present few opportunities for interventions. Establishing a link between socio-demographic or personality variables does little to explain why such factors are associated with high or low adherence. We are therefore none the wiser about what to do to facilitate adherence, since we cannot change a person's age, gender or personality. Moreover, the idea that stable socio-demographic factors (e.g. age, gender or intelligence) or dispositional characteristics (i.e. personality) are the main determinants of adherence is discredited by evidence that adherence rates do not just vary between patients, but also within the same patient over time and between different aspects of the treatment. This is not to say that socio-demographic or dispositional characteristics are irrelevant. Rather, it would seem that associations with adherence may be indirect and best explained by the influence of socio-demographic and dispositional characteristics on other relevant parameters, such as motivation or capability to adhere.

In summary then, the typical 'non-adherent patient' is something of a myth: most of us are non-adherent some of the time. Stable characteristics, such as the nature of the disease and treatment, or socio-demographic variables influence the adherence behaviour of some patients more than others. This has led to a greater emphasis on understanding the interaction of the individual with the disease and treatment, rather than identifying the characteristics of a mythical 'non-adherent patient'.

## Myth 3: 'Once-a-Day' Treatments Solve the Problem

The formulation or packaging of the medication may act as a barrier to adherence. Some patients may have difficulty in swallowing large capsules or may lack the manual dexterity to use complex dosage forms such as pressurized metered-dose inhalers or to open blister packs or child-resistant containers. Patients with arthritic conditions may be particularly prone to these problems.

There is evidence to support the common-sense notion that the more complex the treatment demands, the lower the adherence. There are several sources of complexity: the prescription of a large number of individual medications, the need to take medication at frequent intervals or medications which are difficult to use, such as inhaler devices. Complex regimens carry the risk of information overload and related problems of poor understanding or poor recall of instructions. Additionally, a complex regimen may be so disruptive to the patient's daily routine that they become de-motivated and may avoid or delay doses. The observed relationship between regimen complexity and non-adherence seems to have led to the assumption in some quarters that simply reducing the frequency of dosing is enough to prevent non-adherence. This is evidenced by the marketing of 'once-daily' pharmaceuticals. However, there is little evidence to suggest that this strategy alone is sufficient to prevent non-adherence. Complexity *per se* is not the key issue, but instead it involves how well the treatment fits in with the individual patient's routine, expectations and preferences.

Simplifying the regimen can be helpful for many patients, but non-adherence also occurs with once-daily treatments. We need to think beyond formulation and dosage regimens.

## Myth 4: Providing Clear Instruction Is Not Enough

Providing clear instructions, although essential, is not enough to guarantee adherence. Patients do not always understand prescription instructions and may forget considerable portions of what clinicians tell them. It is well recognized that many patients have a poor understanding of the terminology that is often used by doctors in communicating details about their illness, and many patients have little or no understanding of the details of their medication regimen. However, the relationship between a patient's knowledge of their medication regimen and their adherence to it is by no means simple or clear-cut. Improving knowledge does not necessarily improve adherence.

Often in medicine we tell patients what we want them to hear. This can create an information–action gap. People don't blindly follow health advice, even if it comes from trusted clinicians. Rather, we evaluate the advice and make a 'common-sense' decision about whether to follow it. This will be covered in more detail later, but here it is sufficient to note three things:

1. In order to change behaviour, information has to either concur with our beliefs about the behaviour or change those beliefs: information needs to persuade as well as inform (Karamanidou et al. 2008).
2. Many patients are dissatisfied with the type and amount of medicines information they receive (Bowskill et al. 2007).
3. Information should be targeted to the needs of the individual, both in terms of content (what it says) and complexity, so that it addresses outstanding questions and conveys recommendations (Raynor et al. 2007). It should match patients' own levels of health literacy and their ability to obtain, process and understand basic health information needed to make appropriate health decisions (Ngoh 2009).

## The PAPA

The PAPA provides a conceptual framework for moving beyond the myths of adherence to developing effective, patient-centred solutions. The PAPA is represented by Figure 11.1 and the main principles are given below.

The many reasons why an individual might not follow treatment recommendations can be summarized under two categories: they cannot or they do not want to. The causes of non-adherence are often complex and related to both intentional and unintentional processes. For example, non-adherence may be unintentional when the

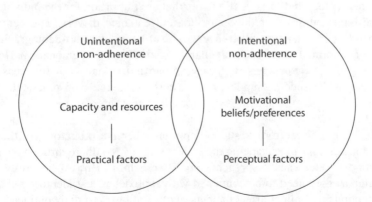

**FIGURE 11.1** The perceptions and practicalities model of adherence. The figure does not represent a comprehensive model of non-adherence but rather serves to illustrate that interventions to support adherence need to address motivation as well as capacity (i.e. both perceptions and practicalities).

patient wants to follow the treatment recommendations but is prevented from doing so by barriers beyond their control, such as poor recall or comprehension of instructions, difficulties in administering the treatment, simply forgetting or because they cannot afford to pay for it. Unintentional non-adherence results from limitations in capacity and resources that reduce the person's ability to adhere. Non-adherence is considered to be intentional if it results from a decision on the part of the patient to avoid taking the treatment or to use it in a way that is at odds with the recommendations of the prescriber. In reality, these categories overlap and are not mutually exclusive. There is a degree of overlap between intentional and unintentional non-adherence. Motivation may overcome resource barriers, and resource barriers may reduce motivation. However, it is clear that adherence is a product of two things: motivation and ability. Both are influenced by an interaction between internal factors (such as beliefs and capabilities) and external or environmental factors (such as communication and prompts to action). These are discussed in more detail below and are illustrated in Figure 11.2.

## THE PAPA MODEL

The PAPA reminds us to take account of these factors when trying to help patients to adhere to appropriately prescribed medicines. It emphasizes the need to move beyond the 'practical support' designed to improve the patient's ability to adhere to also address the perceptual factors affecting their motivation to start and continue with the treatment. Enhancing motivation and ability requires different types of interventions (Michie et al. 2011). For example, motivation might be addressed by cognitive behavioural techniques or motivational interviewing, whereas ability might be enhanced by interventions that increase capacity to adhere (e.g. help with the costs of unaffordable treatments) or improve capability (e.g. reminder systems to reduce forgetting).

Support should be tailored to meet the needs of individuals by assessing the specific perceptual and 'practical' factors that are important for the individual and tailoring interventions to reduce barriers and enhance drivers. The perceptions and capabilities influencing adherence will be affected by socio-demographic, cultural and economic factors and trait characteristics (such as personality). However, the effects of these variables will vary among individuals. For this reason, the assessment of the specific support needs (both perceptual and practical) of each individual should be the starting point for adherence interventions. One size does not fit all.

In clinical practice, efforts to support optimal adherence often focus on the practicalities; for example, by enhancing the patient's ability to adhere through instruction and reminders, etc. These approaches are often helpful. However, to fully impact on adherence, they need to be combined with approaches that identify and address the perceptions that might affect patients' motivation to start and continue with the treatment.

Perceptions are less frequently addressed in practice, but have recently become a focus for research into non-adherence, with studies identifying the importance of patients' beliefs about medication.

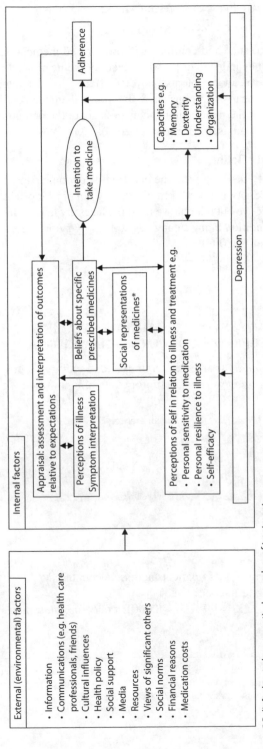

* Beliefs about pharmaceuticals as a class of treatment

**FIGURE 11.2**  Conceptual map of determinants of adherence.

## How Patients Evaluate Prescribed Medication: The Necessity Concerns Framework

Patients' motivation to start and continue with prescribed medication is influenced by the way in which they judge their personal need for medication (necessity beliefs) relative to their concerns about potential adverse effects. As illustrated in Box 11.4, studies spanning long-term conditions show that non-adherence is related to doubts about personal need for the treatment and concerns about the potential adverse consequences of using it as advised (Horne et al. 2013).

### Medication Necessity Beliefs

To arrive at a necessity belief, we ask the question, 'How much do I need this treatment?' Perceived necessity is not a form of efficacy belief. We might believe that a treatment will be effective but not that we need it. Necessity beliefs are influenced by perceptions of the condition being treated, as well as by symptom expectations and experiences (Cooper et al. 2004).

---

### BOX 11.4   SYSTEMATIC META-ANALYSIS OF THE NECESSITY-CONCERNS FRAMEWORK

Studies across a range of illnesses, countries and cultures indicate that the necessity-concerns framework is useful for explaining low adherence.

Low adherence

| Doubts about personal necessity of medication | Concerns about *potential* adverse effects |

**Meta-analysis**[*]

94 studies covering 24,864 patients across 18 countries

23 different long-term conditions

Necessity odds ratio = 1.918, p < 0.0001; concerns odds ratio = 0.476, p < 0.0001

---

[*] Horne, R., Chapman, S.C.E., Parham, R. et al. 2013. Understanding patients' adherence-related beliefs about medicines prescribed for long-term conditions: A meta-analytic review of the Necessity-Concerns Framework. *PLoS ONE*, **8**, e80633.

## Medication Concerns

One obvious source of concern is the experience of symptoms as medication 'side effects' and the disruptive effects of medication on daily living, but this is not the whole picture. Many patients receiving regular medication who have not experienced adverse effects are still worried about possible problems in the future. In a survey of over 1,800 patients in the UK, 35% reported that their maintenance treatment caused unpleasant side effects. However, more patients were concerned about long-term effects (73%) or that taking medication regularly would make it less effective (57%) or cause dependence (52%) (Horne et al. 2009).

## PERCEPTIONS OF ILLNESS: THE COMMON-SENSE MODEL

Howard and Elaine Leventhal (an American psychologist and doctor, respectively) and their colleagues have developed a theory of illness and treatment-related behaviour, called the common-sense model (CSM) (Leventhal et al. 2012; Leventhal 2014). This places the patients' perceptions of their illness and treatment as key to understanding illness-related behaviours such as adherence.

The CSM suggests that when we are faced with a 'health threat' (e.g. experiencing symptoms or being told by a physician that we have a particular disease), our first response is to form a 'mental map' or 'model' of the condition. This helps us to 'make sense' of the condition and guides the action we take to remedy the perceived problem. Patients' models of illness are referred to using several terms: illness beliefs, illness perceptions and illness representations. For the purposes of this discussion, these terms are considered interchangeable as they essentially mean the same thing: the patient's personal ideas about their illness. Leventhal and colleagues suggest that illness perceptions have several important attributes, as shown in Box 11.5.

## COMMON-SENSE ORIGINS OF MEDICATION NECESSITY BELIEFS AND CONCERNS

### Necessity Beliefs

Two factors appear to have a particularly strong link to patients' perceptions of the necessity for prescribed medication: their beliefs about the illness and their experience of symptoms. Patients will be more likely to agree with the necessity for prescribed medication if this accords with their perceptions of the illness. For example, an asthma patient who perceives their asthma to be a fairly short-lived problem with few personal consequences (i.e. 'I am ill when I suffer from an asthma attack but otherwise feel normal') may not have strong beliefs in the necessity of regular prophylactic medication and may be more inclined to manage their condition using medication for symptomatic relief alone. The effect of symptom experiences on views about medication necessity may be complex. At one level, symptoms may stimulate medication use by acting as a reminder or by reinforcing beliefs about its necessity. However, patients' expectations of symptom relief are also likely to have an important effect. This could be problematic if the expectations are unrealistic. For example, a patient who expects their newly prescribed anti-depressant medication to

## BOX 11.5   IMPORTANT ATTRIBUTES
## OF ILLNESS PERCEPTIONS

- Patients' personal ideas about their illness are often organized around five components: identity, timeline, cause, consequences and control/ cure. These can be thought of as the answers to five basic questions about the illness or health threat: What is it? How long will it last? What caused it? How will it/has it affected me? Can it be controlled or cured? People form a mental model or representation of the illness, which is made up of their answers to these questions.
- Perception of symptoms has a strong influence on patients' ideas about their illness and upon subsequent behaviour. Patients are more likely to perceive their condition as a problem and try to rectify it if they associate it with unpleasant symptoms. This is illustrated by the example of asthma in Box 11.6. In other words, the experience of symptoms is fundamental to our thinking about illness. Taking a treatment for a condition which does not appear to have any symptoms may appear to go against 'common sense' unless the patient is provided with a clear rationale for why the treatment is being recommended (e.g. for prophylaxis).
- Illness perceptions influence behaviour and outcomes. Patients' own ideas about the illness may have a stronger influence on their behaviour than the advice of health care practitioners.

relieve their symptoms of depression after a few doses is likely to be disappointed when they find that the medication takes several days or weeks to have any effect. This might cause them to believe that the medicine is ineffective and that continued use is not worthwhile. Symptom experience may also influence medication concerns if they are interpreted by the patient as medication side effects.

Until we experience a chronic condition, most of our experience of illness is symptomatic and acute. However, for many long-term conditions, the medical rationale for maintenance treatment is based on a prophylaxis model. The benefits of treatment are often silent and long term. This may be in stark contrast to our intuitive CSM of 'no symptoms, no problem' (Halm et al. 2006). Moreover, missing doses may not lead to an immediate deterioration in symptoms, thereby reinforcing the (erroneous) perception that high adherence to the medication may not be necessary. Related to this is the fact that people often stop taking treatments when they judge that the condition has improved (Box 11.6). These judgements are often based on potentially misleading symptom perceptions rather than on objective clinical indicators of disease severity (Horne et al. 2007).

People do not blindly follow treatment advice even from respected clinicians. Rather, we evaluate the advice and decide whether it is a good idea for us, based on our understanding of the illness and treatment. This is where an adherence problem often begins. In order to be convinced of a personal need for ongoing medication, we

**BOX 11.6  ILLUSTRATING THE IMPORTANCE OF THE FIT BETWEEN PERCEPTIONS OF ILLNESS AND TREATMENT: THE CASE OF ASTHMA**

For many long-term conditions, including asthma, the medical rationale for maintenance treatment is based on a prophylaxis model. The benefits of treatment are often silent and long term. This may be in stark contrast to our intuitive common-sense model of 'no symptoms, no problem'[*]. The importance of illness representation in adherence to inhaled corticosteroids is illustrated by studies in the UK[†] and US[*]. Many patients considered themselves to be well when asthma symptoms were absent and took inhaled corticosteroids sporadically in response to symptoms. They doubted their personal need for preventer medication because the notion of asthma as a chronic condition needing continuous treatment was at odds with their experience of it as an episodic problem. Moreover, missing doses did not lead to an immediate deterioration in symptoms, thereby reinforcing the (potentially erroneous) perception that high adherence to the medication may not be necessary.

---

[*] Halm, E.A., Mora, P. and Leventhal, H. 2006. No symptoms, no asthma: The acute episodic disease belief is associated with poor self-management among inner-city adults with persistent asthma. *Chest*, **129**(3), 573–580.

[†] Horne, R. and Weinman, J. 2002. Self-regulation and self-management in asthma: Exploring the role of illness perceptions and treatment beliefs in explaining non-adherence to preventer medication. *Psychology and Health*, **17**(1), 17–32.

must first perceive a good fit between the problem (the illness or condition) and the solution (the medication) (Horne et al. 2009).

Medication concerns are often related to suspicions of pharmaceuticals as a class of treatments (Horne et al. 2009). Studies of peoples' beliefs about medicines show that some people have more negative attitudes towards pharmaceuticals as a class of treatment. They may be suspicious of pharmaceuticals and the pharmaceutical industry, seeing medicines as intrinsically harmful, addictive poisons that are overused by physicians and the health care system (Horne et al. 1999). This means they may be more reluctant to accept that the prescribed medication offers the best treatment for their illness and are likely to have stronger concerns about the potential adverse effects of medicines prescribed for them.

## IMPLICATIONS FOR PHARMACY PRACTICE

The PAPA has informed NICE adherence guidelines in the UK (Nunes et al. 2009), which were developed to help health professionals support patients in making informed choices about and adhering to prescribed medication. A simple three-step approach would be a good start.

1. Communicate a 'common-sense' rationale for why the treatment is needed. Patients need to perceive a close fit between the problem and the proposed

solution (e.g. regular use of maintenance treatment) and to be provided with a convincing 'story' for why medication is still necessary, even when symptoms are not present or when symptom resolution is delayed.

2. Elicit and address patient concerns about the medication and help the patient to make treatment choices that are informed by an understanding of the likely risks and benefits, rather than by potentially erroneous beliefs or misconceptions about the condition and treatment. It is important to understand this from the patient's perspective. For example, the patient may be worried about subjective side effects that clinicians may perceive to be clinically insignificant.

3. Identify and address potential practical barriers and make the regimen as convenient and easy to take as possible.

Pharmacists are in a good position to help patients get the best from medication by adopting a 'partnership model' which takes account of patients' perceptions of their medications (see Box 11.7). The decision to take or not to take a medicine should, in almost all cases, be taken by the patient. However, this is problematic if the decision is based on mistaken perceptions about the relative benefits and risks of treatment. Clinicians could help patients by ensuring that their decision is informed by the best available evidence, rather than by mistaken beliefs about the necessity of the medication or misplaced concerns about adverse effects. This entails eliciting patients' views about their medication and addressing doubts and concerns in a frank and open discussion. It is important to take a 'no-blame approach' that facilitates honest disclosure of non-adherence and encourages patients to express doubts and concerns. Many are reluctant to do this because they believe that clinicians will perceive doubts about treatment as doubts about themselves.

---

### BOX 11.7   PATIENT PARTNERSHIP IN PRACTICE

How might it look in practice?

Patients differ in:

1. Desire to be involved in treatment decisions
2. Perceptions of medicines
3. Information needs
4. Capacity and resources to adhere to treatment

We need to:

1. Identify individual needs and preferences
2. Tailor intervention to:
   a. Address misconceptions, concerns and information needs
   b. Address practical problems reducing patients' ability to adhere to medicines

Communicating medication necessity beliefs and addressing concerns does not need to be resource intensive. Studies have shown that simple interventions such as text messaging (Petrie et al. 2012) and discussions with a pharmacist by telephone can effectively communicate treatment necessity and address concerns (Clifford et al. 2006). Supporting patients with a telephone call from a community pharmacy within 10 days of a new prescription was found to be a cost-effective way of providing adherence support (Elliott et al. 2008). Patients who received a call were significantly more likely to report higher adherence, more positive views about their medicines (stronger necessity beliefs and fewer concerns) and fewer medication-related problems relative to controls who received standard care (Clifford et al. 2006). This proof-of-principle study informed the UK Department of Health New Medicines Service (http://www.rpharms.com/health-campaigns/new-medicines-service.asp).

The challenge is to tailor support to meet individual needs (see Box 11.7). This may seem ambitious based on today's typical pharmacy services. However, medicines typically account for the single biggest source of expenditure in developed health economies, and the current high rates of non-adherence represent a startling inefficiency within the system. Improving the situation is likely to benefit the individual and society.

Adherence support begins at the point of prescribing and dispensing, but it may also be necessary during treatment review, as perceptions, capabilities and adherence can change over time. Over the course of a chronic illness, patients may need more than one opportunity to discuss their treatment with a health care practitioner. A single discussion at the start of treatment may not be enough. Patients should also be able to feed back their experiences of their medication and raise any concerns or questions which arise over the course of their treatment. In collaboration with other health care professionals, pharmacists have an important role in this. Box 11.8 identifies a number of opportunities for pharmaceutical care which focus on adherence issues.

## CONCLUSION

Non-adherence to medication is perceived to be a significant barrier to treatment efficacy and, if the prescription was appropriate, it is detrimental to patients and the health care system. Research shows that non-adherence may have many causes, but these may be simplified into perceptions and practicalities. Non-adherence may be linked to beliefs about the illness and the necessity of medication, as well as to concerns about potential adverse effects. When viewed from the patient's perspective, non-adherence is often seen to be a common-sense response to the illness and treatment as they see it. For example, it may be a logical – albeit mistaken – attempt to moderate the perceived risk of treatment by taking less medication.

Helping patients to manage their medication requires a no-blame, patient-centred approach which takes account of their perceptions of their illness and treatment and the degree to which they wish to be involved in treatment decisions. To get the most from prescribed medicines, pharmacists and other health care professionals should address patients' beliefs about their treatments, as well as their ability to use them. Patients frequently want to know 'why' as well as 'how'. They should be provided with a rationale for why their medication is necessary, and given an opportunity to

## BOX 11.8   SOME EXAMPLES OF HOW PHARMACISTS MIGHT SUPPORT ADHERENCE TO ESSENTIAL TREATMENTS

- Many general practitioners issue repeat prescriptions without conducting a full review of treatment. Not surprisingly, this is associated with low adherence rates and wastage of medication. This highlights the need for regular review of medication. Pharmacists could contribute to this by working closely with physicians to stimulate regular reviews of the treatment regimen.
- Once an appropriate treatment has been selected, the pharmacist could facilitate patient acceptability by ensuring that containers and labels are appropriate.
- The transfer of the patient between hospital and community often disrupts the continuity of care, and changes to the components or appearance of the medication regimen may lead to dissatisfaction or confusion about the medication. Continuity of care is dependent on adequate communication between patients, their carers and health practitioners in community and hospital settings. By liaising with these parties, hospital and community pharmacists might help prevent medication-related problems and facilitate the smooth transfer of care.
- An 'adherence-related drug history' could be used to elicit the patient's representations of their illness and treatment. A frank and open discussion between pharmacist and patient may afford an opportunity for the patient to 'feed back' their experience of the treatment and allow the pharmacist to identify requirements for explanation and information. This could provide the basis for the design of individual information/counselling, which builds on the patients' representations of the treatment. Additionally, it may form the basis of a contribution to subsequent prescribing decisions and the design of the patient's medication regimen.
- Within the UK National Health Service, the Medicines Usage Review* service and New Medicines Service[†] provide pharmacists with a vehicle to deliver more advanced services to help patients get the best from their medicines through optimal adherence.

---

* http://www.rpharms.com/health-campaigns/medicines-use-review.asp
† http://www.rpharms.com/nhs-community-pharmacy-contract-england/new-medicine-service.asp

discuss their concerns about its use. These approaches should be coupled with initiatives to overcome the practical difficulties of using the medication; for example, by making the regimen as convenient to use as possible and by tailoring it to fit the person's capabilities and lifestyle. These approaches should occur over the course of a chronic illness, providing patients with an opportunity for feedback.

## ACKNOWLEDGEMENTS

Professor Horne is supported by a National institute of Health Research Senior Investigator Award. Penny Reed helped in the production of the manuscript.

## FURTHER READING

Chater, A. and Cook, E. 2014. *Psychology Express: Health Psychology*. Harlow: Pearson.

French, D., Vedhara, K., Kaptein, A.A. et al. 2010. *Health Psychology* (2nd Ed.). Chichester: Wiley-Blackwell.

Ogden, J. 2012. *Health Psychology: A Textbook* (5th Ed.). Buckingham: Open Univ Press.

## REFERENCES

Barber, N. 1995. What constitutes good prescribing? *British Medical Journal*, **310**, 923–925.

Barber, N., Parsons, J., Clifford, S. et al. 2004. Patients' problems with new medication for chronic conditions. *Quality and Safety in Health Care*, **13**, 172–175.

Bowskill, R., Clatworthy, J., Parham, R. et al. 2007. Patients' perceptions of information received about medication prescribed for bipolar disorder: Implications for informed choice. *Journal of Affective Disorders*, **100**, 253–257.

Clatworthy, J., Price, D., Ryan, D. et al. 2009. The value of self-report assessment of adherence, rhinitis and smoking in relation to asthma control. *Primary Care Respiratory Journal*, **18**, 300–305.

Clifford, S., Barber, N., Elliott, R.A. et al. 2006. Patient-centred advice is effective in improving adherence to medicines. *Pharmacy World and Science*, **28**, 165–170.

Cohen, J., Mann, D., Wisnivesky, J. et al. 2009. Assessing the validity of self-reported medication adherence among inner-city asthmatic adults: The Medication Adherence Reporting Scale for Asthma. *Annals of Allergy, Asthma and Immunology* **103**, 325–331.

Cooper, V., Gellaitry, G. and Horne, R. 2004. Treatment perceptions and self-regulation in adherence to HAART. *International Journal of Behavioral Medicine*, **11**(Supplement 2004), 81.

DiMatteo, M.R. 2004. Variations in patients' adherence to medical recommendations: A quantitative review of 50 years of research. *Medical Care*, **42**, 200–209.

Elliott, R.A., Barber, N., Clifford, S. et al. 2008. The cost effectiveness of a telephone-based pharmacy advisory service to improve adherence to newly prescribed medicines. *Pharmacy World and Science*, **30**, 17–23.

Halm, E.A., Mora, P. and Leventhal, H. 2006. No symptoms, no asthma: The acute episodic disease belief is associated with poor self-management among inner-city adults with persistent asthma. *Chest*, **129**, 573–580.

Horne, R., Chapman, S.C.E., Parham, R. et al. 2013. Understanding patients' adherence-related beliefs about medicines prescribed for long-term conditions: A meta-analytic review of the Necessity-Concerns Framework. *PLoS ONE*, **8**, e80633.

Horne, R. and Clatworthy, J. 2010. Adherence to advice and treatment. In: D. French, K. Vedhara, A.A. Keptein and J. Weinman (Eds.), *Health Psychology*. Chichester: British Psychological Society and Blackwell Publishing Ltd., 175–188.

Horne, R., Cooper, V., Gellaitry, G. et al. 2007. Patients' perceptions of highly active antiretroviral therapy in relation to treatment uptake and adherence: The utility of the necessity-concerns framework. *Journal of Acquired Immune Deficiency Syndromes*, **45**, 334–341.

Horne, R., Parham, R., Driscoll, R. et al. 2009. Patients' attitudes to medicines and adherence to maintenance treatment in inflammatory bowel disease. *Inflammatory Bowel Diseases*, **15**, 837–844.

Horne, R. and Weinman, J. 2002. Self-regulation and self-management in asthma: Exploring the role of illness perceptions and treatment beliefs in explaining non-adherence to preventer medication. *Psychology and Health*, **17**(1), 17–32.

Horne, R., Weinman, J., Barber, N. et al. 2005. *Concordance, Adherence and Compliance in Medicine Taking: A Conceptual Map and Research Priorities*, London, National Institute for Health Research (NIHR) Service Delivery and Organisation (SDO) Programme. Available from: http://www.netscc.ac.uk/hsdr/files/project/SDO_FR_08-1412-076_V01.pdf (accessed 15 May 2015).

Horne, R., Weinman, J. and Hankins, M. 1999. The Beliefs about Medicines Questionnaire: The development and evaluation of a new method for assessing the cognitive representation of medication. *Psychology and Health*, **14**, 1–24.

Hughes, D.A., Bagust, A., Haycox, A. et al. 2001. The impact of non-compliance on the cost-effectiveness of pharmaceuticals: A review of the literature. *Health Economics*, **10**, 601–615.

Karamanidou, C., Weinman, J. and Horne, R. 2008. Improving haemodialysis patients' understanding of phosphate-binding medication: A pilot study of a psycho-educational intervention designed to change patients' perceptions of the problem and treatment. *British Journal of Health Psychology*, **13**, 205–214.

Kripalani, S., Yao, X. and Haynes, R. 2007. Interventions to enhance medication adherence in chronic medical conditions: A systematic review. *Archives of Internal Medicine*, **167**, 540–549.

Leventhal, H. 2014. The integration of emotion and cognition: A view from the perceptual–motor theory of emotion. In: *Affect and Cognition: The 17th Annual Carnegie Symposium on Cognition*. Hillsdale, NJ: Erlbaum, 121–156.

Leventhal, H., Bodnar-Deren, S., Breland, J. et al. 2012. Modeling health and illness behavior: The approach of the commonsense model. In: A. Baum, T.A. Revenson and J. Singe (Eds.), *Handbook of Health Psychology* (2nd Ed.). New York: Taylor and Francis, 3–36.

Michie, S., Van Stralen, M. and West, R. 2011. The behavior change wheel: A new method for characterising and designing behavior change interventions. *Implementation Science*, **6**, 42.

National Institute for Health and Care Excellence 2009. *Costing Statement: Medicines Adherence: Involving Patients in Decisions about Prescribed Medicines and Supporting Adherence*. London: National Institute for Health and Care Excellence.

Ngoh, L.N. 2009. Health literacy: A barrier to pharmacist-patient communication and medication adherence. *Journal of the American Pharmacists Association*, **49**, e132–e146.

Nunes, V., Neilson, J., O'Flynn, N. et al. 2009. *Clinical Guidelines and Evidence Review for Medicines Adherence: Involving Patients in Decisions about Prescribed Medicines and Supporting Adherence*. London: National Collaborating Centre for Primary Care and Royal College of General Practitioners, 364.

Petrie, K.J., Perry, K., Broadbent, E. et al. 2012. A text message programme designed to modify patients' illness and treatment beliefs improves self-reported adherence to asthma preventer medication. *British Journal of Health Psychology*, **17**, 74–84.

Pressman, A., Avins, A.L., Neuhans, J. et al. 2012. Adherence to placebo and mortality in the Beta Blocker Evaluation of Survival Trial (BEST). *Contemporary Clinical Trials*, **33**, 492–498.

Raynor, D.K., Blenkinsopp, A., Knapp, P. et al. 2007. A systematic review of quantitative and qualitative research on the role and effectiveness of written information available to patients about individual medicines. *Health Technology Assessment*, **11**, iii, 1–160.

Simpson, S.H., Eurich, D T, Majumdar, S.R. et al. 2006. A meta-analysis of the association between adherence to drug therapy and mortality. *British Medical Journal*, **333**, 15.

Vrijens, B., De Geest, S., Hughes, D.A. et al. 2012. A new taxonomy for describing and defining adherence to medications. *British Journal of Clinical Pharmacology*, **73**, 691–705.

# Section III

---

*Professional Practice*

# 12 Occupational Status of Pharmacy

*Geoffrey Harding and Kevin Taylor*

## CONTENTS

**KEY POINTS**

- Commentators differ as to what defines professional status.
- Occupations achieving professional status benefit in terms of privileges such as monopoly of practice, autonomy of practice and enhanced remuneration.
- Professional status may be considered the result of a social process, rather than just the acquisition of a number of specific attributes.
- The professional status of pharmacy has been both constrained and facilitated by recent development in health care and pharmaceutical service delivery.

## INTRODUCTION

Before addressing the occupational status of pharmacists as professionals, we shall first consider what is meant by the term 'profession'. We often talk about the 'pharmacy profession', but what does the term mean? Opinions vary as to what distinguishes an occupation as a profession. Some occupations, such as law and medicine, have acquired a pre-eminent status in society and have historically been endowed with power and prestige, commensurately attracting social and economic rewards. For these occupations, the term 'profession' has a specific meaning distinct from its more colloquial sense (i.e. the opposite of amateur). Thus, 'professional' sports people, though skilled and paid to play their chosen sport, do not possess the key characteristics of a profession. Occupations aspiring to professional status do so in order to gain and protect certain privileges such as a monopoly of practice, autonomy of action and enhanced remuneration. This chapter is divided into two sections in which we shall deal first with definitional issues of professions and professionalism, and second with an analysis of pharmacy as a profession.

## PROFESSIONS AND PROFESSIONALIZATION

### DEFINING PROFESSIONAL STATUS

There has been much debate over what defines a profession. The development of this debate is summarized in Box 12.1.

Until the 1970s, professions were conceptualized as privileged occupations within capitalist societies, uniquely characterized by a commitment to a universal standard of service which was delivered in a neutral and non-profit-motivated way. At this time, analyses of professions centred on identifying and listing attributes specific to professions (Goode 1960). This has been referred to as the 'attribute' or the 'trait' theory of professions. The most frequently cited traits of a profession are outlined in Box 12.2.

**BOX 12.1   LANDMARKS IN THEORETICAL
ANALYSES OF PROFESSIONS**

- Professions are essential to the maintenance of the social order; an important stabilizing force (Parsons 1939).
- Professions possess a statutory licence to perform certain actions (Hughes 1953).
- Professions possess characteristic traits (Goode 1960).
- Professions are self-regulating (Freidson 1970a).
- Professions need to promote an esoteric or indeterminate knowledge base in order to attract social and economic rewards within a free market (Jamous and Peloille 1970; Johnson 1972; Larson 1977).
- Professions have particular relations with both the State and the public (Ritzer 1975; Weber 1978).
- Occupations aspiring to be a profession undergo a 'professional project' (MacDonald 1995).

## CORE FEATURES OF A PROFESSION

The traits identified by Goode and others can be further distilled down to what might be considered the core features of professions. These are summarized in Figure 12.1.

To be granted entry into a profession, an individual must acquire specialized knowledge and undergo lengthy training. Extensive training is necessary, because the professional must possess a specialized knowledge, unavailable to the public, which in turn ensures the public's reliance on their service. During training, aspiring professionals also acquire the attitudes, values and belief systems specific to that profession (i.e. they undergo professional socialization). Another characteristic of a profession is that of service-orientation (i.e. a professional acts in the public's

**BOX 12.2   ATTRIBUTES OF PROFESSIONS**

- A profession determines its own standards of education and training.
- The student professional undergoes an extensive training and socialization process.
- Professional practice is legally recognized by some form of licensure.
- Licensing and admission boards are run by members of the profession.
- Most legislation which affects a profession is shaped by that profession.
- A profession commands high income, power and status and can demand high-calibre students.
- The professional is relatively free from lay evaluation.
- The norms of practice enforced by the profession are often more stringent than legal controls.
- A profession is likely to remain a lifetime occupation.

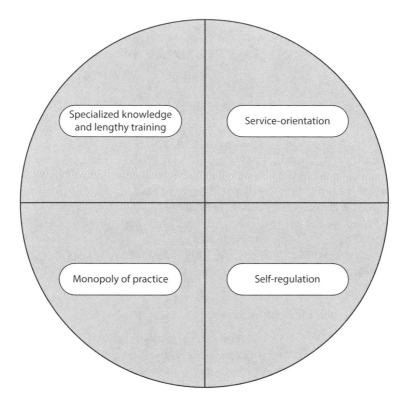

**FIGURE 12.1**    Core features of a profession.

best interests, rather than pursuing their own self-interest). This is very important because professions have a monopoly of practice granted and secured by the State, which also sanctions their right to monitor and control their activities. For example, in most countries, pharmacists have an exclusive legal right to sell certain categories of medicines, but are bound by their own code of professional practice not to exploit this monopoly for personal financial gain. Professions also determine the content and scope of training, arbitrate over eligibility of membership and assess competency to practice (i.e. they 'self-regulate'). This is necessary, it is argued, because the specialized skill and knowledge of the professional precludes non-professionals from evaluating or regulating their activities.

## A FUNCTIONALIST ANALYSIS OF PROFESSIONS

Some commentators have suggested that professions achieve their high status because they perform functions vital to the workings of modern industrialized society, rather than simply because they possess particular attributes. Within sociology, this has been referred to as a 'functionalist' analysis. A functionalist perspective regards society as analogous to a living organism. All social institutions function to ensure the cohesion of the social order, rather like the various physiological systems which function to ensure our body's healthy state. Complex industrial societies depend on expert knowledge and informed judgement, and the function of professions is to supply this for the benefit of the community.

While both the trait and the functionalist approaches have been supplemented by more critical analyses, it is apparent that professions do: (a) possess certain important characteristics; and (b) fulfil an important social function.

## PROFESSIONAL JUDGEMENTS

Professionals claim to make 'professional judgements' (see also Chapter 13) based on particular forms of knowledge and skill that are esoteric and frequently cannot be fully articulated in written form (codified). Jamous and Peloille (1970) have described how a professional judgement is informed by a greater proportion of indeterminate knowledge than technical knowledge (i.e. professional judgements are characterized by a high indeterminate/technical knowledge ratio). Indeterminate knowledge is personal knowledge acquired through professional experience, while technical knowledge is rational and codified (i.e. available from texts). The centrality of a professional judgement for professions has been identified in the case of medicine by Elliot Freidson (1970b), who describes the 'clinical mentality'. The professional, Freidson argues, 'believes what he is doing' (i.e. is likely to display personal commitment to a chosen course of action and is essentially pragmatic, relying on results rather than theory, and trusting personal rather than book knowledge). Similarly, pharmacists might be argued to exercise their professional judgements when deciding on the appropriate response to patients' symptoms.

Professional judgements do not in themselves demarcate a professional. To obtain, sustain and justify its status, it is not sufficient for an occupation to claim its judgements to be 'professional'. The State and public must also place sufficient value on an occupation's knowledge (esoteric or otherwise) for professional status to be conferred.

## THE PROCESS OF BECOMING A PROFESSION

So far, it has been assumed that what constitutes a profession is dependent on something special or exceptional about a particular occupation. However, while the length of training, service-orientation, ethical practice and expertise are all significant in convincing the State and the public of its importance, they are not 'causes' of an occupation achieving professional status. The success of medicine, for instance, in establishing and promoting itself as a profession has been argued not to be attributable to the quality of medical knowledge or doctors' expertise (Wright 1979). When doctors first organized themselves as an occupational group, there was no evidence that they were any more effective than astrologers in influencing health. Historically, doctors rather than astrologers were successful in establishing their claim to professional status because of the high social standing of doctors and their patrons.

How an occupation both achieves and maintains professional status is termed the process of 'professionalization'. This process involves the profession in successfully controlling its relationship with those who fund and use its services. Professionalization is a dynamic process founded on complex social relations between the public, the occupational group and the State. In this sense, it may be considered an accomplishment achieved through negotiation: it is not given by right, but is subject to continual validation by the State and public. Thus, the professions must be sensitive to the social, political and technological change which may undermine their claims to privileged status. For example, the emergence of a consumer culture has led to more open accountability in professional practice and challenges to the traditional basis of professional authority and self-regulation.

## THE PROFESSIONAL PROJECT

What can an occupational group do to legitimize its claim to professional status? The professionalization process involves the deployment of a strategy which has been termed a 'professional project' (Larson 1977). The success of this project does not rely on attaining a list of attributes, but rather on an occupational group: (a) persuading the State that its work is reliable and valuable; and (b) the public's willingness to accept – or their inability to successfully challenge – the group's area of expertise.

## MYSTIFICATION AND SOCIAL DISTANCE

A 'professional project' depends in part on the power relationship between the occupation's members and the public. An important element of this relationship is that of 'mystification' (Johnson 1972). An occupation that aspires to professional status may only achieve this objective if it succeeds in promoting its knowledge and services as mystical or esoteric. By creating a dependence on their knowledge and skills, members of such occupations effectively reduce the areas of knowledge and experience they share with those they serve. This increase in the 'social distance' between themselves and their clients provides professionals with an opportunity for autonomous control over their practices by warding off potential challenges to their status from the lay public.

A successful claim to professional status is an outcome of ongoing political struggles and power conflicts, not just with the public and the State, but also with rival occupational groups. An occupation becomes a profession not so much because of improvements in its skills and knowledge, but rather because the profession's leaders are successful in convincing the State and public that autonomy and self-regulation best serve the interests of all concerned. Thus, it may not be the characteristics of professionals *per se* that determine their status so much as their relationships with the public, the State and other occupations. Instead of pondering the question of whether or not an occupation is a profession, it may therefore be more appropriate to consider the circumstances in which occupations attempt to establish and maintain themselves as professions.

## PHARMACY AS A PROFESSION: HOW DOES IT MEASURE UP?

Pharmacy's status as a profession has been the subject of numerous analyses, as summarized in Box 12.3.

> **BOX 12.3   KEY ANALYSES OF PHARMACY'S OCCUPATIONAL STATUS**
>
> - Pharmacy is an incomplete profession (Denzin and Mettlin 1968).
> - Changes in their activities have resulted in the deprofessionalization of pharmacists (Birenbaum 1982; Holloway et al. 1986).
> - Professional boundaries in pharmacy are potentially problematic (Eaton and Webb 1979; Messier 1991).
> - Pharmacy lacks autonomy and mystique (Turner 1987).
> - Pharmacy has a symbolic function (Dingwall and Wilson 1995; Harding and Taylor 1997).

## APPLYING THE CRITERIA OF THE 'TRAIT THEORY' TO PHARMACY

Pharmacists exhibit a number of professional 'traits'. They have a virtual monopoly of practice in dispensing prescribed medication and in the sale of certain over-the-counter (OTC) medicines. They possess specialized knowledge and undergo lengthy training; pharmacy is service-orientated. While historically health professions have been self-regulating, following the notorious 'Shipman case' and the Bristol Heart scandal, which revealed inadequate self-regulation of professional practice, health professions' practice is now subject to scrutiny by external agencies. For pharmacy, this role has been assumed in Great Britain by the General Pharmaceutical Council, while the Royal Pharmaceutical Society, which was formerly responsible for the self-regulation of pharmacists and pharmacy premises, is now the representative body for its members. Overall, pharmacy exhibits a majority of professional traits.

However, pharmacy has been described by Denzin and Mettlin (1968) as an example of 'incomplete professionalization'. This, they claim, is due to pharmacy's failure to recruit altruistic people; to exercise control of the supply and manufacture of drugs; to develop a unique body of scientific knowledge; and to maintain occupational unity. This analysis has, however, been challenged by Dingwall and Wilson (1995), who argue that when these features are considered in the context of the professions of medicine and the law, doctors and lawyers are no more 'professional' than pharmacists.

Notwithstanding this, we have seen that professionalization is a dynamic process. If pharmacy is to establish and sustain its status as a profession, the concept of a professional project has to be embraced. However, several factors, outlined in Table 12.1, might hinder its future claim to privileged occupational status.

## CONSTRAINTS TO PHARMACY'S OCCUPATIONAL DEVELOPMENT

### Social Closure

For an occupation to aspire to professional status, its members must be licensed for practice by the State (Hughes 1953). In the case of community pharmacy, this correlates with their legal entitlement to dispense prescribed drugs and medical appliances. Clearly, some form of formal qualification to practise is required to protect the public

**TABLE 12.1**

**Factors Undermining Pharmacy's Professional Status**

| Factors | Consequences |
| --- | --- |
| Consumerism | Public's willingness to challenge professional knowledge and authority |
| Technology | Automation, routinization and loss of mystique |
| Mercantilism | Juxtaposition of market forces and service-orientation |
| Corporatization of pharmacy | Bureaucracy in pharmacy and diminished professional autonomy |
| Failure to achieve social closure | Non-exclusivity of pharmacists' functions |
| Incomplete control over medicines | Dependence on physicians and diminishing responsibility for over-the-counter medicines |

from unlicensed practitioners, but the credentials required to practise the core function of pharmacy – dispensing or supplying prescribed medications – are not exclusive to pharmacy. Currently, in the UK at least, physicians, dentists and nurses may all, in certain limited circumstances, supply medication to patients. Thus, credentialism as a means of excluding competitors from supplying prescribed medication, or 'social closure', is not effective in distinguishing the occupation of pharmacy as a profession. Pharmacists, however, do have an exclusive legal entitlement to sell certain categories of medicines (pharmacy medicines), establishing an element of 'social closure'. This may become key to pharmacy's future professional project, as highly effective medicines are increasingly reclassified from 'prescription only' to 'pharmacy medicines'.

## Controlling the Use of Medicines

Denzin and Mettlin (1968) claim that while possessing a licence and mandate to supply prescribed drugs, pharmacists have:

> ... failed to engage in long term activities which ensure their control over the social object around which their activities are organised ... the drug. ... The major problem which prevents pharmacy from stepping across the line of marginality is its failure to gain control over the social object which justifies existence of its professional qualities in the first place.

That is to say that, historically, pharmacists have not been legally entitled to prescribe potent medications, requiring to supply them in accordance with prescribers' instructions. However, in recent years, patient group directions and the ability of pharmacists to be supplementary and independent prescribers (within the limits of their professional competence) have meant they do have a limited but growing control over the social object. However, it remains the case that in the large majority of cases, who uses which prescribed drug, for which ailment and how remain largely beyond the controlling power of pharmacists.

The prescribing and dispensing functions of physicians and pharmacists continue to emphasize the differences in control each has over medications. However, it should be noted that doctors' access to prescribable medicines may be constrained by legislation, National Institute for Health and Care Excellence guidelines and formularies.

Pharmacists, on the other hand, may have 'control' in terms of their contribution to formularies, input on ward rounds, the choice of product for a generically prescribed drug, refusal to dispense prescriptions on legal or therapeutic grounds and simply through pharmacy opening hours and stock holding.

## Drug Information

An occupation's professional status is founded on the promotion of its advice and services as indispensable and esoteric in nature. Claims to the indispensable nature of pharmacists' advice and information are undermined by the fact that pre-packaged medicines contain written inserts giving detailed instructions for their use. Moreover, pharmacists compete with other sources of advice and information, such as doctors, the media, the Internet and the lay community (see also Chapter 8). The open and wide availability of alternative sources of advice and information on minor illnesses and medication thus challenges pharmacy's claim to privileged occupational status on the basis of the esoteric, indeterminate and indispensable nature of its knowledge base. However, professional judgement can be argued to be necessary when pharmacists ensure the individual patient's informational requirements are met, tailoring written information and, in so doing, drawing on their indeterminate knowledge and professional experience.

## Commodification of Medicines

The wide availability of medicines from non-pharmacy outlets, together with the increasing deregulation of medicines once obtained exclusively from pharmacies, means that medicines are increasingly perceived by the public and promoted by the manufacturers and suppliers as commodities, qualitatively indistinguishable from other retail goods. If medicines can be purchased from supermarkets, petrol filling stations, etc., it follows that no accompanying 'expert' supervision or advice is necessary when they are purchased, essentially making the pharmacist's contribution in this area redundant.

## Mercantilism

Community pharmacists practice in an economic environment where commercial viability is of primary importance. Commercial interests would appear to be at odds with the ethos of impartial service-orientation and professional altruism (see also Chapters 1 and 2). Consequently, pharmacists may experience 'role strain' or 'role ambiguity', as they balance the conflicting demands of professional and retail practice. For instance, evidence suggests that pharmacy proprietors are more likely than employee pharmacists to recommend customers to purchase a product. Even when the provision of goods or services would be beneficial to customers, these may only be offered when pharmacists perceive there to be sufficient demand and that it is commercially advantageous to do so. That said, there is also evidence suggesting that conflict between professional altruism and commercial interests is not inevitable.

## Pharmacy Ownership

In recent years, there has been an increasing proliferation of multiple and supermarket-based pharmacies (see also Chapters 1, 2 and 4). Successful large organizations such as these require complex bureaucratic procedures for maximizing their efficiency and profitability. This results in rationalized, standardized pharmaceutical services as dictated by corporate policies. This has implications for the professionalization of pharmacy, since it has been claimed that the intrinsic knowledge and skill of an occupation claiming professional status '... is asserted to be so esoteric as to warrant no interference by laymen, and so complex, requiring so much judgment, from case to case as to preclude governing it by an elaborate system of detailed work rules or by supervision exercised by a superior official' (Freidson 1994).

The increasing corporatization of community pharmacy thus raises questions as to whether the professional autonomy of pharmacists is susceptible to compromise by commercial interests, with their activities constrained, controlled and regulated by routinized bureaucratic procedures.

## Technology

The increased availability of pre-formulated medicines and the emergence of original-pack and patient-pack dispensing clearly diminish the utilization of pharmacists' compounding and formulating skills, and the time taken to dispense medicines is less than in the past, particularly with the introduction of dispensing robots (see also Chapters 2 and 3). Consequently, the 'mystique' traditionally associated with the compounding aspects of their role has largely disappeared. Likewise, pharmacists' intellectual input into the dispensing process has been largely usurped and rationalized by computer software which identifies potential drug interactions and inappropriately prescribed doses, and produces medicine labels with appropriate directions and warnings. Pharmacy's exposure to such occupational and technological change has been described as an example of 'deprofessionalization', wherein the increasing automation of tasks has undermined the traditional basis for its claim to professional status (Birenbaum 1982; Holloway et al. 1986). Thus, pharmacists' expertise and practice becomes routinized and the public may perceive them as merely suppliers of pre-packaged medicines. Correspondingly, there is limited scope for pharmacists to bring their own unique knowledge and skills to their day-to-day tasks. That is to say, they are too highly trained for the jobs they do, hence the proliferation of articles and statements from commentators in recent years claiming that pharmacists' skills are 'underutilized'.

When a profession's specialized knowledge becomes codified and rationalized, its very existence is threatened. As Turner (1989) suggests, 'Objective changes in tasks, brought about for example, by technological advance, inevitably threaten to transform or possibly obliterate, a particular profession'.

## OPPORTUNITIES FOR OCCUPATIONAL DEVELOPMENT

Health care is continually developing. As pharmacists take on new responsibilities, this will necessarily impact on their occupational status. Table 12.2 illustrates the impact that developmental changes may have on their claims to professional status based on the application of theoretical analyses of professionalization.

## TABLE 12.2
### Evaluation of Pharmacy's Professionalizing Strategies

| Strategy | Advantages | Disadvantages |
|---|---|---|
| Promoting open access | Platform for indeterminate knowledge | Diminishes value of experts' time |
| Devolving dispensing duties | Reduction in time spent on technical activities | Distances pharmacists from their traditional role |
| Promoting advisory function (e.g. Healthy Living Pharmacies) | Opportunities for professional judgement<br>Responsibility for health, not just medicines | May eclipse 'core supply functions' |
| Pharmaceutical care | Defines boundaries of pharmaceutical responsibility | Possible boundary encroachment |
| Enhancing service delivery (e.g. Medicines Use Reviews, New Medicines Service) | Opportunities for professional judgement<br>Delivers best practice | Constrains professional autonomy |
| Promoting a symbolic function | Exclusive function of pharmacy | Ethereal and unevaluated |

## Promotion of Pharmacists as the First Port of Call for Health Issues

Pharmacists are increasingly being promoted as 'first port of call' health profession-als, available to the public without appointments, providing advisory and health care services. This development reflects the changing nature of primary care delivery, optimizing the use of services other than general practice or hospital accident and emergency services (which are increasingly under strain) and not least constraints on the health care budget. The rationale for pharmacists acting as 'gatekeepers' to primary health care rests on their ability to make a professional judgement regarding the appropriate action in response to patients' symptoms, including self-treatment or referral to other services. However, in adopting such a strategy, it is important for pharmacists and pharmacy leaders to recognize the symbolic importance of ration-ing the public's claims on professionals' time. This demarcates a social distance between professional and public by reinforcing the concept that because a profes-sional's time is highly valued, it must be rationed.

## Devolution of Dispensing Activities

In recent years, the de-skilling associated with dispensing prescribed medication has reduced pharmacists' input in the dispensing process. Concomitant with this has been the professionalization and, more recently, registration and regulation of pharmacy technicians as credentialed members of the pharmacy workforce with particular responsibility for the technical aspects of dispensing. This has provided an opportu-nity for pharmacists to increase their other activities in, for example, the provision of health care advice and diagnostic testing, with the manipulative aspects of dispens-ing being largely devolved to pharmacy technicians, with pharmacists' involvement restricted to checks for accuracy. These developments form part of a professionalizing strategy, as pharmacists take on new roles and responsibilities in health care.

## Pharmacists as Health Care Advisors

Assuming an advisory role on medication and other health issues and offering diagnostic tests such as blood cholesterol and blood pressure measurement provides pharmacists with an opportunity to shed their image of over-educated and underutilized health workers. This has led to the recent concept of the Healthy Living Pharmacy (see also Chapter 2) in which pharmacists help reduce inequalities in health by delivering health and well-being services and offering proactive health advice. This development has the effect of increasing pharmacists' indeterminate/technical knowledge ratio (i.e. as pharmacists become increasingly involved in providing health care advice and education and interpreting test results, there is a commensurate rise in the use and promotion of their indeterminate knowledge, enhancing claims to professional status).

## Pharmaceutical Care

The various activities pharmacists currently perform have, in recent years, been encompassed by the concept of 'pharmaceutical care', defined as 'the responsible provision of drug therapy for the purpose of achieving definite outcomes that improve a patients quality of life' (Hepler and Strand 1990). What actually comprises pharmaceutical care remains open to interpretation. To some, it is indistinguishable from clinical pharmacy, while in the community it might be argued to encompass pharmaceutical services additional to dispensing, such as the provision of advice to patients, residential homes and other primary care workers. The practice of pharmaceutical care, with its emphasis on the patient and, in particular, its outcome-orientation, will, it has been argued, serve as a professionalizing strategy by imparting to pharmacy the key elements of other health care professionals, namely a practice philosophy, a process of care and a practice management system (Cipolle et al. 1998). Pharmaceutical care requires pharmacists to be directly responsible and accountable to patients for the outcomes of drug therapy, and as such represents an opportunity for pharmacists to exercise control over medicines use. Recent developments in this area for which community pharmacists in the UK are remunerated include Medicines Use Reviews (a consultation between patient and pharmacist reviewing prescribed medication, resolving any issues and feeding back to the prescriber) and the New Medicines Service (provide support for people with long-term conditions receiving a new medicine with the aim of 'medicines optimization', improving medicines adherence). Putting pharmaceutical care into practice, however, will necessarily involve pharmacists in negotiating with other health professionals where this impinges on their areas of professional responsibilities (see also Chapters 2 and 15). This has been referred to in the context of the development of clinical pharmacy as 'boundary encroachment' (Eaton and Webb 1979).

## Advanced Practice

Since 2005, in the UK, the establishment of consultant pharmacists (senior professionals with advanced roles in patient care, professional education, research in a specific area of practice and professional leadership) has afforded pharmacists the opportunity to enhance their occupational standing within the health care team. Moreover, since 2003 and 2006, supplementary and independent prescribing by pharmacists have been legally permitted. An independent pharmacist prescriber is entitled to prescribe any medication autonomously, for any condition, within their clinical competence, with some exclusions, including controlled drugs for the treatment of addictions.

## The Symbolic Transformation of Drugs into Medicines

Historically, the physical transformation from drug to medicine was almost the sole province of pharmacists, as they compounded medicines from their constituent ingredients. While this physical transformation function is now undertaken predominantly within the pharmaceutical industry, the symbolic meaning and value attributed to a medicine is still acquired within the pharmacy.

Pharmacists are authorized by the State and the public to transform potent pharmacological entities into medicines (i.e. they inscribe prescribed or purchased drugs with a particular meaning for the user [e.g. to alleviate or control a biological dysfunction]). For example, warfarin, a rodenticide, is transformed into a medicine with specific meaning for a patient when supplied by a pharmacist for a specific medical purpose. Similarly, aspirin can be considered a drug because of its ability to inhibit a particular enzyme. However, aspirin can also be considered a commodity, widely available to the public to relieve mild-to-moderate pain. In such circumstances, aspirin is loaded with no more symbolic significance than any other product available from retail outlets, because it is supplied beyond the surveillance of drug 'experts'. However, when aspirin is selected (from a range of alternative drugs) by a pharmacist sanctioned to interpret its appropriateness for a specific individual, this commonly available drug has the potential to be symbolically transformed into a medicine.

This benefits the public by investing a prescribed or purchased product with 'added value', in that a drug becomes a medicine for an individual's specific condition. Moreover, opportunities for pharmacists' input into such transformations may increase in the future due to the accelerating rate of reclassification of prescription to OTC medicines. This important social function is taken for granted by both pharmacists and the public and has not been exploited, yet it is a function which pharmacists alone are able to perform.

## CONCLUSION

Increasingly, questions are being raised as to whether the privileged status of professions can be justified. Professions have historically wielded disproportionate power and influence, with minimal accountability for their activities. Increasingly, the State and public are questioning professional practice, and traditional 'restrictive practices' are being eroded. Pharmacy is no exception. Currently, there are important questions concerning pharmacists' activities and their contributions to the provision of health care. This will have implications for their relationships with other health professionals, as well as their relationships with the public. If pharmacy is to maintain and sustain a privileged occupational status in the future with its effective monopoly of practice, it must respond strategically to social, political and technological changes. This response should be in the form of a 'professional project' which capitalizes on pharmacists' unique knowledge and skills. Privileged occupational status is not bestowed. It is an outcome of continual negotiation of social relationships between the public, the State and the occupation.

## FURTHER READING

Cipolle, R.J., Strand, L.M. and Morley, P.C. 2012. *Pharmaceutical Care Practice: The Patient Centered Approach to Medication Management* (3rd Ed.). New York: McGraw-Hill.

Petrakaki, D., Barber, N. and Waring, J. 2012. The possibilities of technology in shaping healthcare professionals: (re/de-) professionalisation of pharmacists in England. *Social Science and Medicine*, **75**, 429–437.

Turner, B.S. 1995. *Medical Power and Social Knowledge* (2nd Ed.). London: Sage Publications, Chapter 7, 129–152.

## REFERENCES

Birenbaum, A. 1982. Reprofessionalisation in pharmacy. *Social Science and Medicine*, **16**, 871–878.

Cipolle, R.J., Strand, L.M. and Morley, P.C. 1998. *Pharmaceutical Care Practice*. New York: McGraw-Hill.

Denzin, N.K. and Mettlin, C.J. 1968. Incomplete professionalisation: The case of pharmacy. *Social Forces*, **46**, 375–381.

Dingwall, R. and Wilson, E. 1995. Is pharmacy really an "incomplete profession"? *Perspectives on Social Problems*, **7**, 111–128.

Eaton, G. and Webb, B. 1979. Boundary encroachment: Pharmacists in the clinical setting. *Sociology of Health and Illness*, **1**, 69–89.

Freidson, E. 1970a. *Profession of Medicine: A Study in the Sociology of Applied Knowledge.* New York: Dodd, Mead and Co.

Freidson, E. 1970b. *Professional Dominance*. Chicago: Atherton Press.

Freidson, E. 1994. *Professionalism Reborn: Theory, Prophecy and Policy*. Cambridge: Polity Press.

Goode, W.J. 1960. Encroachment, charlatanism and the emerging professions: Psychiatry, sociology and medicine. *American Sociological Review*, **25**, 902–914.

Harding, G. and Taylor, K.M.G. 1997. Responding to change: The case of community pharmacy in Great Britain. *Sociology of Health and Illness*, **19**, 547–560.

Hepler, C.D. and Strand, L.M. 1990. Opportunities and responsibilities in pharmaceutical care. *American Journal of Hospital Pharmacy*, **47**, 533–543.

Holloway, S.W.F., Jewson, N.D. and Mason, D.J. 1986. "Reprofessionalisation" or "occupational imperialism"?: Some reflections of pharmacy in Britain. *Social Science and Medicine*, **23**, 323–332.

Hughes, E.C. 1953. *Men and Their Work*. Glencoe: The Free Press.

Jamous, H. and Peloille, B. 1970. Changes in the French university hospital system. In: J.A. Jackson (Ed.), *Professions and Professionalisation*. Cambridge: Cambridge University Press, 109–152.

Johnson, T. 1972. *Professions and Power*. London: Macmillian Education Ltd.

Larson, M.S. 1977. *The Rise of Professionalism: A Sociological Analysis*. London: University of California Press.

Macdonald, K.M. 1995. *The Sociology of the Professions*. London: Sage Publications.

Messier, M.A. 1991. Boundary encroachment and task delegation: Clinical pharmacists on the medical team. *Sociology of Health and Illness*, **12**, 310–331.

Parsons, T. 1939. The professions and the social structure. *Social Forces*, **17**, 457–467.

Ritzer, G. 1975. Professionalisation, bureaucratization and rationality: The views of Max Weber. *Social Forces*, **53**, 627–634.

Turner, B. 1987. *Medical Power and Social Knowledge*. London: Sage Publications.

Turner, B. 1989. Review of Abbott, A. *Sociology*, **23**, 472–473.

Weber, M. 1978. *Economy and Society*. Berkeley: University of California Press.

Wright, P. 1979. A study of the legitimisation of knowledge: The success of medicine, the failure of Astrology. In: R. Walls (Ed.), *On the Margins of Science*. Keele: Sociological Review Monograph 17.

# 13 Duty of Care, Professionalism, Ethics and Ethical Dilemmas

*Dai N. John and Richard O'Neill*

## CONTENTS

**KEY POINTS**

- Pharmacists' competencies include evidence-based decision making while also considering the ethical implications of these decisions.
- All pharmacists require a knowledge of their statutory legal obligations.
- Pharmacists are required to make complex ethical choices on matters which are not clearly designated in law.
- Maintaining competence and effectiveness as a practitioner requires pharmacists to participate in continuing professional development.
- The pharmacist's extended role involves a close involvement with patients, which in turn increases the opportunities to deal with ethical problems.

## INTRODUCTION

Pharmacy education has traditionally emphasized the acquisition of specialized knowledge and the development of selected skills required in the preparation and distribution of medicines. Over recent years, a greater involvement in the selection and supply of medicines has come about, necessitating a much wider range of skills in which competence must be achieved. Central to these changes is a greater emphasis on the provision of advice and information to patients, carers and other health and social care professionals.

The aim of pharmacists' early education is to provide a durable foundation for a lifetime of practice. As well as an understanding of theory and its application to practice (knowledge and skills), the development of personal effectiveness, together with a sense of appropriate behaviours, attitudes and values within a framework of professional behaviour, is a necessary requirement of preparation for practice. This is addressed and developed during supervised experience in practice and, thereafter, by ongoing self-development and learning. Competence in problem-solving and communication are essential elements in pharmacy practice. As problem-solvers, pharmacists need to be able to think clearly and logically and to make, and take responsibility for, decisions based on sound analysis and appropriate evidence. This requires a recognition of personal limitations, an ability to self-appraise, a commitment to continuing competence and due regard to the legal, professional and ethical implications that accompany decisions and action taken.

## THE REGULATION OF PHARMACY

Pharmacists in the UK are expected to provide a wide range of services within or outside the National Health Service, from the supply of medicines to the provision of cognitive services (see Chapter 10). Advising on the management of minor ailments and ensuring patients can make informed choices about over-the-counter (OTC) medicines requires competence in symptom recognition and a detailed knowledge of non-prescription medicines. These are areas of everyday practice where pharmacists are expected to take decisions and make professional judgements.

Increased responsibility implies a potential for increased liability and an increased basis for misconduct or malpractice. Health care and health care professionals are regulated not by a single body or group, but in a number of ways. The most direct form of regulation involves legislation and judicial precedents concerned with the standard and delivery of health care and enforced through the courts. Another form of regulation is entrusted to regulatory bodies established by law and given jurisdiction to enforce standards of conduct by controlling entry to the profession and through fitness-to-practise procedures (see Chapter 12). Pharmacists work in environments governed by ethics, with their primary focus being to serve the interests of the patient and the community. It is fundamental that both the legal controls on pharmacy and the ethical framework within which pharmacists operate allow them to exercise their professional discretion as independent health care professionals. In Great Britain, the pharmacy regulator is the General Pharmaceutical Council (GPhC). (For further information, see GPhC website [Reissner 2013].)

## LEGAL DIMENSION

There is a plethora of laws, regulations and standards with which the pharmacist is expected to comply, and liability may arise from a variety of different situations (see John 2013a,b; John 2013). The law may operate in a number of ways to maintain standards of pharmacists' practice (Box 13.1).

Liabilities that derive from the professional practice of pharmacy typically concern one of the following categories: pharmacy and medicine laws, including controlled drugs (criminal liability); standards of care (civil and criminal liability); or ethical/professional considerations (professional misconduct).

---

**BOX 13.1 WAYS IN WHICH THE LAW OPERATES TO MAINTAIN STANDARDS**

- The criminal law can be involved where harm was deliberately or recklessly caused.
- Health care regulatory law provides the registering bodies with the ultimate sanction: power to remove pharmacists from the register if their fitness to practise is currently impaired.
- Employers may, under the contracts of employment, discipline and dismiss.
- Administrative law (e.g. National Health Service [NHS]) can result in withholding payment from NHS contractors and can, under certain circumstances, withdraw the provision (and remuneration) of NHS services.
- The law of negligence (civil law) allows patients to sue pharmacists and their employers for compensation, should they suffer loss through a pharmacist's carelessness.

Pharmacists are expected to be familiar with the responsibilities and duties imposed upon them, and this necessitates a thorough knowledge and understanding of the law as it relates to pharmacy practice. Statutory obligations are, of course, wider than pharmacy legislation itself; they include many other areas, such as health and safety, consumer and environmental protection and employment legislation (see Appelbe and Wingfield 2013).

## NEGLIGENCE

In civil law, an individual who fails to take the care a reasonable person would exercise in any given situation is described as negligent. Clearly, there are degrees of negligence. Negligence which is so severe as to warrant punishment under the criminal law is described as gross negligence.

Liability in negligence arises when the breach of a duty owed by the defendant to the claimant (formerly referred to as the plaintiff) results in harm/damage that should have been foreseeable and reasonably avoidable (Box 13.2). It follows that the first step in establishing such liability is to show that such a duty exists. It is well established in law that pharmacists, in common with other health care professionals, owe a duty of care to their patients to act with a reasonable level of skill and care. Patients depend upon health care professionals and their standards of professional conduct, and rely on the special skills and knowledge of the pharmacist when she or he sells, dispenses or prescribes medicines, or provides advice. If a pharmacist makes a mistake or falls below the proper level of care, then harm may be caused to patients and to the public reputation of pharmacy. With regard to the dispensing process, a pharmacist's duty of care will relate to all aspects of checking the prescription, dispensing the medicine and providing advice and counselling. A cause of legal action may, therefore, relate to incorrect interpretation, failure to supply the correct medicine, mislabelling or from inappropriate (counter)-prescribing. A person has a duty of care to all those people whom he or she can reasonably foresee might be harmed by their actions or inactions. While it is reasonably foreseeable that forgetting or failing to check the correct dosage of a drug could cause harm, this may also apply to such actions as giving advice or failing to pass on critical information to patients or other health care professionals. There is a professional requirement for appropriate professional indemnity insurance cover to be in place so that, for example, any damages awarded to the claimant resulting from negligence can be met by the defendant.

---

### BOX 13.2   ELEMENTS OF THE TORT OF NEGLIGENCE

- The defendant owed a duty of care to claimant.
- There was a breach of that duty of care.
- The claimant suffered harm (loss).
- The harm was caused by the breach (causation).
- The resultant harm was reasonably foreseeable.

## STANDARD OF CARE

To be liable for negligence, there must also have been a breach of the duty of care by failing to provide the required standard of care. A pharmacist is not negligent when he or she acts in the way that reasonably competent members of the profession would act. The question is: what is the appropriate standard of care? Pharmacists are required to practise to a minimal common standard that takes into account evolving standards. This necessitates that pharmacists keep up to date and give due consideration to professional guidelines and changes in practice. The degree of skill demonstrated by pharmacists should be appropriate to the task undertaken and the standard of care should be related not to the individual, but to the position they hold. Otherwise, a subjective standard of care would mean that a patient's expectations would depend upon the experience of the particular professional. A single standard of care for patients can only be achieved by relating the reasonableness of a professional's conduct to the task that is undertaken and, therefore, what is objectively reasonable does not change with the experience of the professional. Thus, the minimum standard of care to be expected from a newly qualified pharmacist is no lower than that to be expected from an experienced one.

The courts have accepted that responsible practitioners recognize their own limitations. One way of meeting the appropriate standard of care is to seek help and advice when appropriate. As a matter of practice and common sense, inexperienced practitioners will normally undertake fewer complex tasks than their experienced colleagues and seek their assistance to check their work. In a retail pharmacy business, importantly, a pharmacist's responsibility for the supply of OTC medicines cannot be delegated, so even if the functions are performed by a medicines counter assistant, the pharmacist is ultimately responsible for them.

When a judge decides a case, details describing the rationale under which the case was decided (the *ratio decidendi*, or reasons) are published and may act as a precedent for subsequent cases. A body of law (case law) is thereby created which supplements statutes and regulations. The normal outcome of a successful action in negligence is damages, the amount being based upon the principle that the plaintiff should, as far as possible, be put into a position that he or she would have been in but for the injury to him or her. The primary purpose of law of negligence is to compensate the injured party and, as a secondary purpose, to deter negligent conduct.

Negligence involves some form of careless conduct and is usually the result of some inadvertence. Errors of judgement may not themselves amount to negligence; some errors may be consistent with the due exercise of professional skills, while others are so glaringly below proper standards as to make a finding of negligence inevitable. A single dispensing error can, if sufficiently serious, constitute misconduct on the part of the pharmacist.

## A PHARMACIST'S CIVIL LIABILITY

A pharmacist cannot act as a mere conduit in the supply of medicines. A pharmacist who knows (or should reasonably have known) of a potential problem with medicines and who can foresee (or should reasonably have foreseen) harm to the patient may be

> **BOX 13.3   EXAMPLES OF THE TYPES OF NEGLIGENCE CASES INVOLVING PHARMACISTS**
>
> - Pharmacist failed to inform the patient of the maximum dose to be taken of a prescribed medicine (the Migril® case).
> - Pharmacist misinterpreted the handwriting of the prescriber and supplied the wrong drug (the Daonil® case).
> - Pharmacist dispensed the wrong strength of a medicine (the Eplilm® case).
> - Pharmacist dispensed a higher dose of a medicine that had been incorrectly prescribed without checking an eight-fold increase in dose from that previously supplied medication (the dexamethasone case).

held accountable for failing to protect the patient's interests. While there remains the requirement to be error-free in the technical act of prescription processing, pharmacists are also required to recognize potential problems in a prescription and to take corrective action if a potential problem exists. See Box 13.3 for examples of the types of negligence cases involving pharmacists.

Damages were awarded against the pharmacist in each of these cases as their breach of their duty of care resulted in harm. For further information on each of these negligence decisions, see John and Reissner (2013).

## ETHICAL DIMENSION

Health care law governs professional practice and is an important regulator of professional standards and conduct. However, the law does not, and cannot, answer all questions about what constitutes ethically correct behaviour. There are many instances when professionals are confronted with choices that are significantly different in ethical terms, but on which the law is uncommitted. Ethical obligations are normally seen as going beyond the legal obligations. The law, by its nature, cannot enforce an ideal standard of care, but aims to prevent care falling below an acceptable minimum standard. Hence, the law of negligence is concerned with guaranteeing that a satisfactory level of competence is achieved. Unlike simple, reactive decisions made rapidly, professional judgements are complex and often demand the unravelling of ethical (moral) issues. They are questions of value beliefs and assumptions at personal and professional levels.

### MORALITY AND ETHICS

Morality concerns itself with relations between people and is made up of values and duties based on beliefs shared by society or a section of society; they tell those who share them what is right and wrong. Ethics is the application of values and moral rules to human activities; it centres around interpersonal relationships and how best to manage them. It is also concerned with the process of making moral judgements. There are three main approaches to resolving moral issues and health care dilemmas: virtue ethics, deontological (rule-based approach) and utilitarian (a form of consequentialism).

## VIRTUE ETHICS

Virtue ethics has its roots in the writings of Aristole and Socrates. Virtues are character traits and the decision is based on what a virtuous (or morally right) person would do. It is the character of the individual that determines a course of action. Examples include compassion, integrity and conscientiousness. That is, virtue ethics are not determined by the consequences of one's actions or conformity to a moral rule (see deontological and utilitarian theories below). There is a concern from some whether with a diverse population there can be agreement on what characteristics a good person possesses.

## DEONTOLOGICAL THEORY

Deontologists contend that morality is grounded in pure reason and objectivity. Decisions are ethically valid if they conform with a proper moral rule, and wrong if they violate such a rule. The person most closely associated with the deontological approach was Emmanuel Kant, who held that every person has an inherent dignity and as such is entitled to respect. This respect is shown by never using people to achieve goals or consequences; people are ends in themselves. The morally correct thing is always to be guided by moral duties, rights and responsibilities, and some actions are intrinsically immoral, irrespective of how positive or beneficial the consequences might be, while others are intrinsically moral, irrespective of how negative the consequences. Among the commonly accepted types of rules are telling the truth, keeping promises, respecting privacy, helping others and protecting the right to life. However, deontologists do not always agree on the same precepts, the importance they ascribe to different rules or how flexible they are in making exceptions to the rules. Adherence to moral rules, whatever the consequences, governs the deontologist's approach to ethical dilemmas. However, such a process is not self-evident. There is no obvious way to give order, or varying weight, to various duties, rights and responsibilities when the moral rules they have adopted come into conflict.

## UTILITARIAN THEORY

Utilitarianism places the focus on the consequences of actions. This approach was developed by Jeremy Bentham and John Stuart Mill. The attraction of the utilitarian theory is that it offers a simple explanation of what makes actions right or wrong: the right act being that which results in the best available outcome. A utilitarian approach to a dilemma would be to consider alternative courses of action, then predict the probable consequences of each of them and then evaluate the likely implications for everyone affected. Having weighed each value factor, the action that produces the best balance of benefits over burdens is the one that must be implemented. Conflicting moral rules can be disregarded: the best solution is that which leads to the best consequences overall. Duties, rights and responsibilities can be ignored with such an approach; people may be used as 'means to an end'.

## PRINCIPLISM (PRINCIPLES-BASED ETHICS)

Principlism is based on a set of four principles proposed by Beauchamp and Childress (2009) and has been widely accepted in health care (Table 13.1).

### Non-Maleficence

This is considered to be at the confluence of medical ethics and pharmacy and is the most compelling moral element driving decision making. Harm may be caused in many ways: by some deliberate action; by incorrect action perhaps through neglect or ignorance; or through omission, such as by failing to prevent others doing harm.

### Beneficence

This is closely allied with non-maleficence, in that it also concerns preventing harm or removing harm as well as bringing about positive good. According to Beauchamp and Childress (2009), a health professional would have a positive duty of beneficence towards a person when that professional has the capacity to promote the person's well-being.

### Respect for Autonomy

This involves individuals being able to formulate and carry out their own plans, desires, wishes and policies, thereby determining the course of their own life. Paternalism is often used to legitimize infringements of another's autonomy, supported as it is by the principle of beneficence. Paternalistic behaviour usually means acting on behalf of another person in that person's best interest. Competence in decision making is closely related to autonomous decision making and to questions about the validity of consent. The increasing emphasis on a more patient-centred approach to health care and patient involvement in decision making necessitates that patients receive adequate information in order to make informed choices about their health care. Patient preferences and values need to guide decisions about choices of treatment in addition to professional knowledge.

---

**TABLE 13.1**
**Ethical Principles**

| Principle | Application |
|---|---|
| Non-maleficence | Avoid harm |
| Beneficence | Act to benefit |
| Respect for autonomy | Respect choice |
| Justice | Treat fairly |

*Source:* Beauchamp, T.L. and Childress, J.F. 2009.
*Principles of Biomedical Ethics* (6th Ed.).
Oxford: Oxford University Press.

---

## Justice

This requires that the interests of those concerned are considered and the decisions made are based on what is fair, equitable and reasonable. That is, 'all equals should be treated equally'. Note how this differs from the statement 'all should be treated equally'. Distributive justice requires that benefits and burdens be distributed equitably, in accordance with the level of need or merit, not on other factors including, but not restricted to, gender, race, socio-economic status, profession and education.

## Other Factors

Other factors (referred to as focal virtues) have been highlighted by Beauchamp and Childress (2009), namely compassion, discernment, trustworthiness and integrity. Their view is that each one of these would be manifest in professionals following the four guiding principles.

For further information on ethics and ethical theory in a health context, see Herring (2014) (Chapter 1); Mason and Laurie (2013) (Chapter 1) and Wingfield and Badcott (2007) (Chapters 1–6).

## PROFESSIONAL/HEALTH CARE REGULATION DIMENSION

The role of a regulatory body is to set standards of professional practice and to safeguard the best interests of the public and the profession. Regulation is an important element of a profession and in contemporary society; with rising expectations of the professions, this cannot be taken for granted (see Chapter 12). The pharmacy regulators in Great Britain, Northern Ireland and Ireland are the GPhC, the Pharmaceutical Society of Northern Ireland and the Pharmaceutical Society of Ireland, respectively. The stringent level of professional care to be exercised by, and expected of, a pharmacist is evidenced, among other things, by the onerous obligations placed on them by the regulators' codes of ethics or standards. Pharmacists have a responsibility to remain up-to-date and to maintain competence and effectiveness as a practitioner, and to base the starting point of their practice on a 'best evidence' approach, but being mindful of principlism and individual patient characteristics. In order to fulfil this responsibility, it is necessary for them to engage with continuing professional development.

Pharmacists need to perfect a process of continual development in order to deal with the constant changes with which they are confronted and will continue to be confronted. Sources of medicines information are numerous, ranging from guidance of regulators, professional leadership bodies, pharmaceutical companies, medicines information centres, professional and scientific journals, formularies and bulletins and national (and/or local) guidelines. It is essential to appreciate the nature and source of the material, the date published/updated, whether it is independent (and to what extent) and whether it has been subject to external validation/peer review in order to determine the reliance that can be placed upon it. Individual pharmacists must decide how best to keep their knowledge and skills up-to-date and have access to the best evidence on which to base their practice.

ETHICS AND PHARMACY: CODES AND STANDARDS

All rules, whether legal, moral or customary, lay down standards of behaviour. They specify what ought to be done and aim to mark the boundaries between acceptable and unacceptable conduct. While the law requires that a basic standard of practice is maintained, codes of professional practice express a higher expectation and ethics requires that this standard be at the highest possible level.

A common feature of all professions is an ethical code, although terminology varies between countries and over time within the same jurisdiction; for example, a Code of Ethics, Code of Practice, Code of Conduct or Standards or Code of Conduct, Ethics and Performance. Such codes encompass those beliefs and behaviours with which members of the profession are expected to comply. They embody guiding principles by which a member of that profession (a registrant with a regulatory body) can judge their own conduct and by which this conduct can be viewed by others within and outside the profession. Codes may range from those which are extremely detailed, covering a wide spectrum of activities, to those which are shorter and more idealistic.

Codes typically comprise principles. Principles are rules that should always be obeyed unless an exception is available. Codes/standards and their principles may be supplemented with guidance to assist the professional in their decision-making process. A code, however detailed, cannot cover every situation.

The current codes of ethics/standards for the pharmacy regulators in Great Britain, Northern Ireland and Ireland are shown below in Box 13.4, Box 13.5 and Box 13.6, respectively. Although the wording differs, a review of the principles identifies that each is aligned with general ethical principles. Please check the regulators' websites for any updates.

---

**BOX 13.4   GENERAL PHARMACEUTICAL COUNCIL STANDARDS OF CONDUCT, ETHICS AND PERFORMANCE, JULY 2012**

The seven principles: as a pharmacy professional, you must:

1. Make patients your first concern.
2. Use your professional judgement in the interests of patients and the public.
3. Show respect for others.
4. Encourage patients and the public to participate in decisions about their care.
5. Develop your professional knowledge and competence.
6. Be honest and trustworthy.
7. Take responsibility for your working practices.

http://www.pharmacyregulation.org/sites/default/files/standards_of_conduct_ethics_and_performance_july_2014.pdf

## BOX 13.5   PHARMACEUTICAL SOCIETY OF NORTHERN IRELAND CODE OF ETHICS

As a pharmacist registered with the Pharmaceutical Society of Northern Ireland, you must:

- Make patients your first concern.
- Make the safety and welfare of patients your prime concern.
- The practice by a pharmacist of his/her profession must be directed to maintaining and improving the health, well-being, care and safety of the patient. This is the primary principle and the following principles must be read in light of this principle.
- Respect and protect confidential information.
- Show respect for others.
- Exercise professional judgement in the interests of patients and public.
- Encourage patients (and/or their carers as appropriate) to participate in decisions about their care.
- Maintain and develop professional knowledge and competence.
- Act with honesty and integrity.
- Provide a high standard of practice and care at all times.

http://www.psni.org.uk/documents/312/Code+of+Ethics+
for+Pharmacists+in+Northern+Ireland.pdf

## BOX 13.6   PHARMACEUTICAL SOCIETY OF IRELAND PRINCIPLES OF THE CODE OF CONDUCT

The Code of Conduct comprises and is contained in the six principles as follows:

1. The practice by a pharmacist of his/her profession must be directed to maintaining and improving the health, well-being, care and safety of the patient. This is the primary principle and the following principles must be read in light of this principle.
2. A pharmacist must employ his/her professional competence, skills and standing in a manner that brings health gain and value to the community and the society in which he/she lives and works.
3. A pharmacist must never abuse the position of trust which they hold in relation to a patient, and in particular, they must respect a patient's rights, including their dignity, autonomy and entitlements to confidentiality and information.
4. A pharmacist must conduct himself/herself in a manner which enhances the service which their profession as a whole provides to

society and should not act in a way which might damage the good name of their profession.

5. A pharmacist must maintain a level of competence sufficient to provide his/her professional services effectively and efficiently.

6. A pharmacist must be aware of his/her obligations under this Code and should not do anything in the course of practising as a pharmacist, or permit another person to do anything on his/her behalf, which constitutes a breach of this Code or impairs or compromises his/her ability to observe this Code.

> http://www.thepsi.ie/Libraries/Publications/Code_
> of_Conduct_for_pharmacists.sflb.ashx

## PROFESSIONALISM

Professionalism is often referred to as patient-centred professionalism, aligned with the principle of making the patient one's primary concern. It has been defined by many organizations and individuals in the USA (e.g. Popovich et al. 2011), the UK and elsewhere. Box 13.7 outlines the characteristics, traits or principles of or themes associated within the term patient-centred professionalism. (The principles are not in

---

### BOX 13.7  PRINCIPLES OF PATIENT-CENTRED PROFESSIONALISM

- Altruism and putting patients first
- Candour, honesty, integrity and trustworthiness
- Confidentiality
- Commitment to self-improvement and lifelong learning
- Empathy
- Decision making (ethically sound)
- Excellence in communication
- Expert knowledge and skills (competence and performance)
- Involving patients in decisions about their care
- Leadership skills
- Partnership working (with patients and professional colleagues)
- Patient safety
- Pride in one's profession
- Privacy, dignity and compassion
- Respect for others
- Supporting others to help themselves and helping patients make informed decisions
- Working within one's limitations and knowing when to seek help

any particular order, nor are all terms mutually exclusive.) A related term is person-centred care, a term preferred by many to patient-centred care; its starting point is valuing the patient as a 'whole person' and respecting their autonomy through the sharing of power and responsibility.

A number of qualitative studies have explored and described what is meant by patient-centred professionalism to patients, pharmacists and others in Great Britain (Elvey et al. 2012; Rapport et al. 2010a,b; Schafheutle et al. 2012). These empirical studies are helpful to pharmacy students and those involved in their professional socialization in that they provide context and explanation. Although patient-centred professionalism is a recognized term that has been used for several years, awareness of the term and its significance have increased following recent independent reports into the care that patients received within National Health Service organizations in Great Britain, namely the Francis Report (http://www.midstaffspublicinquiry.com/report) and the Andrews Report (http://wales.gov.uk/topics/health/publications/health/reports/care).

Both reports concluded that some patients were let down by individual health professionals and/or by management systems while in hospital and that this was unacceptable. In summary, patients needed to be put first. A joint statement from the Chief Executives of Statutory Regulators of Health Care Professionals in the UK was issued, stressing the essential duty for all professionals working with patients. The statement is provided in Box 13.8.

---

**BOX 13.8   JOINT STATEMENT FROM THE CHIEF EXECUTIVES OF STATUTORY REGULATORS OF HEALTH CARE PROFESSIONALS ON THE DUTY OF CANDOUR**

**Openness and Honesty – The Professional Duty of Candour**

Health professionals must be open and honest with patients when things go wrong. This is also known as 'the duty of candour'. As the Chief Executives and Registrars of statutory regulators of health care professionals, we believe that this is an essential duty for all professionals working with patients. Although it may be expressed in different ways within our statutory guidance, this common professional duty clarifies what we require of all the professionals registered with us, wherever they work across the public, private and voluntary sectors. We will promote this joint statement on 'the duty of candour' to our registrants, our students and to patients, ensuring our registrants know what we expect of them. We will review our standards and strengthen references, where necessary, to being open and honest, as appropriate to the professions we regulate. We will encourage all registrants to reflect on their own learning and continuing professional development needs regarding the duty of candour. We will also work with other regulators, employers and commissioners of services to help develop a culture in which openness and honesty are shared and acted on.

**The Professional Duty of Candour (*Continued*)**

Every health care professional must be open and honest with patients when something goes wrong with their treatment or care which causes, or has the potential to cause, harm or distress.

This means that health care professionals must:

- Tell the patient (or, where appropriate, the patient's advocate, carer or family) when something has gone wrong.
- Apologize to the patient (or, where appropriate, the patient's advocate, carer or family).
- Offer an appropriate remedy or support to put matters right (if possible) and explain fully to the patient (or, where appropriate, the patient's advocate, carer or family) the short- and long-term effects of what has happened.
- Health care professionals must also be open and honest with their colleagues, employers and relevant organizations, and take part in reviews and investigations when requested. Health and care professionals must also be open and honest with their regulators, raising concerns where appropriate. They must support and encourage each other to be open and honest and not stop someone from raising concerns.

http://www.pharmacyregulation.org/sites/default/files/joint_
statement_on_the_professional_duty_of_candour.pdf

## DECISION MAKING AND PROFESSIONAL JUDGEMENT

Ethics seeks to answer the questions 'what should we do?' and 'what should we not do?'. Ethics is concerned not only with making the right decisions, but also with justifying those decisions. When there are conflicting moral responsibilities – when in following one guiding principle we desert another – the situation becomes an ethical dilemma. Situations which involve some ethical decisions include those where there is more than one solution, no obvious correct solution and where ethical principles such as beneficence, non-maleficence, autonomy and justice conflict. In deciding how to act, health care professionals ought to consider certain principles for ethical decision making (Box 13.9).

These principles may act as guides in ethical decision making: a broad framework for organizing deliberations and debate. They should not be considered as a simple formula or an easy method for solving ethical dilemmas, but rather as a reminder of the key elements of ethical thinking. Ethical judgement depends crucially on questions of fact as well as questions of principles.

---

### BOX 13.9   PRINCIPLES FOR ETHICAL DECISION MAKING

- Avoid harm.
- Where possible, achieve benefit.
- Respect the autonomy of the individual.
- Consider fairly the interests of all those affected.

---

## ETHICAL DILEMMAS

Pharmacy ethics involves the application of ethical rules and principles to the practice of pharmacy. When faced with an ethical dilemma, a pharmacist is expected to use his or her professional judgement in deciding on the most appropriate course of action. An expanded professional role and a closer involvement with the patient will increase the opportunities for ethical problems to arise. Every encounter with a patient may potentially raise ethical issues, although such issues do not necessarily present ethical dilemmas. Many issues confronting the pharmacist are unambiguous and straightforward to resolve. Ethical dilemmas arise from fundamental conflicts among beliefs, duties and principles. Pharmacists can be faced with an ethical dilemma in diverse areas (e.g. see Box 13.10).

## RESOLVING DILEMMAS USING PRINCIPLISM

The application of ethical principles and decision making is needed to try to resolve such dilemmas, and this requires pharmacists to develop a working knowledge of formal and systematic ethical analysis, as well as learning to distinguish ethical issues from, for example, social or legal issues.

A multi-step process requiring judgement, reasoning and analysis has been adopted in pharmacy (Royal Pharmaceutical Society 2015; Wingfield and Badcott 2007). It involves evaluating facts and values, as well as duties, in order to arrive at

---

### BOX 13.10   ETHICAL DILEMMAS FACING PHARMACISTS

- When asked by a carer what a medicine is used for.
- When asked to supply a medicine that contravenes one's religious or moral beliefs.
- When asked to supply a medicine where there is no valid prescription.
- When considering whether or not to use a medicine for an unlicensed indication or at a dose or via a route not in accordance with the medicine's licence.
- When considering whether or not to disclose information to another health professional when the patient has explicitly stated their wish for you not to communicate this.

**BOX 13.11    STEPS IN THE PROCESS OF
ETHICAL DECISION MAKING**

1. Gather as much relevant information as possible in order to get the facts clear (these may include, but are not restricted to, clinical, legal, ethical and social information).
2. Identify the nature of ethical problem(s) being faced (if indeed there is one) and the values that are in conflict.
3. Analyse the problem by considering the various ethical approaches best suited to deal with it.
4. Explore the range of options or possible solutions that will best deal with the problem.
5. Choose the best solution for the particular problem, and be prepared to justify it, and document/record as appropriate.
6. Reflect on and evaluate the process and outcome.

a reasoned and justifiable solution to resolve the conflict. It is a process of problem solving which requires critical thinking, in which the cause, alternative actions and potential effects of each action must be considered. The steps in decision making are shown in Box 13.11.

This approach to dealing with dilemmas is used in many schools of pharmacy to help students develop the necessary skills.

### CONFLICTS BETWEEN THE FOUR BIOETHICAL PRINCIPLES

When dealing with an ethical dilemma, the four ethical principles (i.e. respect for autonomy, non-maleficence, beneficence and justice) may appear to be in conflict, and each needs to be balanced in determining the optimal resolution to that dilemma when considering all of the relevant facts. If we think about medicines, for example, many have side effects and certainly some of those will cause harm. However, pharmacological interventions may also provide benefit and so one considers the overarching effect of treatment (or choice of treatments). Patients need to be informed of the options and to be involved in decisions about their care. Considering respect for autonomy as a principle, a competent patient (with capacity) could refuse a specific treatment, or indeed any treatment. The health professionals could reach the conclusion that non-treatment would cause harm to the patient and also not provide benefit, but even so, the view is that respect for autonomy is the principle which prevails.

The question of what is right is not just decided within an ethical framework, but also within legal and professional obligations. The law establishes the ultimate standard for evaluating conduct and the pharmacy profession sets out those things that a pharmacist is obliged to do. Ethical analysis therefore requires that all of these elements are considered. For examples of such dilemmas, see Wingfield and Badcott (2007). The authors acknowledge themselves the important caveat that laws and codes change over time, but notwithstanding this caveat, Wingfield and

Badcott (2007) do talk through a number of pharmacy dilemmas that use the decision-making framework.

A review of the empirical ethics literature in pharmacy (Cooper et al. 2007) concluded that this was an under-researched area and was worthy of investigation, particularly as pharmacists now make significantly greater and more varied contributions to patient care and do so as members of multi-professional teams.

## CONCLUSION

One of the principal concepts of a professional is the ability to make personal professional decisions. Decision making is an expression of professional knowledge and responsibility. Pharmacists work with others, including patients themselves, to help patients gain maximum benefit from their medication, while having due regard for safety and the avoidance of unnecessary harm. Like other health care professionals, pharmacists are under a duty to exercise reasonable care and skill in all the disparate tasks they undertake, requiring a commitment to maintaining good standards of conduct, up-to-date knowledge and continuing competence. When faced with dilemmas, pharmacists need to make decisions and judgements. Sometimes, these are difficult, but being a member of a profession means pharmacists have responsibilities as well as rights. It does not mean that a pharmacist always makes a decision in isolation; in fact, often this would be inappropriate. When pharmacists make decisions, they must be adept at making sound decisions and judgements; patients, society and other members of the pharmacy profession expect nothing less.

## FURTHER READING AND SOURCES OF INFORMATION

### Useful Websites

General Pharmaceutical Council: www.pharmacyregulation.org
Pharmaceutical Society of Northern Ireland: www.psni.org.uk
Pharmaceutical Society of Ireland: www.thepsi.ie
Royal Pharmaceutical Society: www.rpharms.com
http://www.midstaffspublicinquiry.com/report
http://wales.gov.uk/topics/health/publications/health/reports/care
http://www.pharmacyregulation.org/sites/default/files/joint_statement_on_the_professional_
    duty_of_candour.pdf

## GENERAL TEXTBOOKS AND RESOURCES

Appelbe, G.E. and Wingfield, J. 2013. *Dale and Appelbe's Pharmacy Law and Ethics* (10th Ed.). London: Pharmaceutical Press.
Dickenson, D., Huxtable, R. and Parker, M. 2010. *The Cambridge Medical Ethics Workbook* (2nd Ed.). Cambridge: Cambridge University Press.
Herring, J. 2014. *Medical Law and Ethics* (5th Ed.). Oxford: Oxford University Press.
Mason, J.K and Laurie, G.T. 2013. *Mason and McCall Smith's Law and Medical Ethics* (9th Ed.). Oxford: Oxford University Press.
Merrills, J. and Fisher, J. 2013. *Pharmacy Law and Practice* (5th Ed.). London: Elsevier.

Royal Pharmaceutical Society 2015. *Medicines, Ethics and Practice: A Guide for Pharmacists* (39th Ed.). London: Royal Pharmaceutical Society of Great Britain.

## REFERENCES

Beauchamp, T.L. and Childress, J.F. 2009. *Principles of Biomedical Ethics* (6th Ed.). Oxford: Oxford University Press.

Cooper, R.J., Bissell, P. and Wingfield, J. 2007. A new prescription for empirical ethics research in pharmacy: A critical review of the literature. *Journal of Medical Ethics*, **33**, 82–86.

Elvey, R., Lewis, P., Schafheutle E., Willis S., Harrison S. and Hassell, K. 2012. *Patient-Centred Professionalism among Newly Registered Pharmacists*. Manchester: University of Manchester. Available at: http://www.pharmacyresearchuk.org/waterway/wp-content/uploads/2012/11/Patient_centred_professionalism_in_newly_registered_pharmacists.pdf.

Herring, J. (Ed.) 2014. Ethics and medical law. In: *Medical Law and Ethics* (5th Ed.). Oxford: Oxford University Press, 11–38.

John, D.N. 2013a. Pharmacy. In: G.E. Appelbe and J. Wingfield (Eds.), *Dale and Appelbe's Pharmacy and Medicines Law* (10th Ed.). London: Pharmaceutical Press, 303–323.

John, D.N. 2013b. Legal and ethical matters. In: J. Hall (Ed.), *Pharmacy Practice 'Integrated Foundations of Pharmacy'*. Oxford: Oxford University Press, 35–55.

John, D.N. and Reissner, D.H. 2013. Professional conduct. In: G.E. Appelbe and J. Wingfield (Eds.), *Dale and Appelbe's Pharmacy and Medicines Law* (10th Ed.). London: Pharmaceutical Press, 325–343.

John, T. 2013. Sources of law. In: G.E. Appelbe and J. Wingfield (Eds.), *Dale and Appelbe's Pharmacy and Medicines Law* (10th Ed.). London: Pharmaceutical Press, 1–20.

Mason, J.K. and Laurie, G.T. 2013. Medical ethics and medical practice. In: *Mason and McCall Smith's Law and Medical Ethics* (9th Ed.). Oxford: Oxford University Press.

Popovich, N.G., Hammer, D.P., Hansen, D.J. et al. 2011. Report of the AACP (American Association of Colleges of Pharmacy) Professionalism Task Force. *American Journal of Pharmaceutical Education*, **75**(10), S4.

Rapport, F., Doel, M.A., Hutchings, H.A. et al. 2010a. Through the looking glass: Public and professional perspectives on patient-centred professionalism in modern-day community pharmacy. *Forum Qualitative Social Research*, **11**(1), 7. Available at: http://www.qualitative-research.net/index.php/fqs/article/view/1301/2892.

Rapport, F., Doel, M.A., Hutchings, H.A. et al. 2010b. Eleven themes of patient-centred professionalism in community pharmacy: Innovative approaches to consultation about the concept 'patient-centred professionalism' in community pharmacy. *International Journal of Pharmacy Practice*, **18**, 260–268.

Reissner, D.H. 2013. Fitness to practise. In: G.E. Appelbe and J. Wingfield (Eds.), *Dale and Appelbe's Pharmacy and Medicines Law* (10th Ed.). London: Pharmaceutical Press, 345–368.

Royal Pharmaceutical Society 2015. Professionalism and professional judgement. In *Medicines, Ethics and Practice: A Guide for Pharmacists* (39th Ed.). London: Royal Pharmaceutical Society of Great Britain.

Schafheutle, E.I., Hassell, K., Ashcroft, D.M., Hall J. and Harrison, S. 2012. How do pharmacy students learn professionalism? *International Journal of Pharmacy Practice*, **20**, 118–128.

Wingfield, J. and Badcott, D. 2007. *Pharmacy Ethics and Decision Making*. London: Pharmaceutical Press.

# 14 The Pharmacy Workforce

*Karen Hassell and Sue Symonds*

## CONTENTS

---

### KEY POINTS

- More than half of pharmacists working in the community sector are employed by large multiples.
- In Great Britain, a large proportion (32%) of pharmacists work part-time.
- There is a demonstrable relationship between part-time work, gender and age.
- Black and ethnic minority groups constitute a significant proportion of pharmacy students and the qualified pharmacy workforce.
- Women comprise nearly half of the pharmacy workforce in most countries, and in Great Britain they represent the majority of registered pharmacists and pharmacy technicians.

---

## INTRODUCTION

The contribution of pharmacists to health care and health gain has been the subject of considerable debate. Notable, too, is the amount of attention that has been given in the last decade to the impact that the changing demographics and employment patterns in pharmacy have had on the supply and demand for pharmacists and other pharmacy support workers. The aim of this chapter is to outline the features which characterize the current pharmacy workforce, to explore what changes have taken

**TABLE 14.1**

**Pharmacy Workforce Data in Ten Countries**

| Country | Number of Pharmacists | % Female |
|---|---|---|
| Finland | 3,125 | 77 |
| Germany | 78,322 | 67 |
| France | 73,259 | 67 |
| Italy | 81,856 | 66 |
| Portugal | 13,379 | 79 |
| Saudi Arabia | 14,528 | 13 |
| South Africa | 12,813 | 59 |
| Great Britain | 44,751 | 60 |
| Canada | 35,051 | 60 |
| United States | 275,000 | 46 |

*Source:* International Pharmaceutical Federation 2012. *Global Pharmacy Workforce Report*. The Netherlands: International Pharmaceutical Federation.

place over time and to discuss the likely impact of the changes on the supply of, and demand for, pharmacy labour.

While the focus of this chapter is on pharmacists registered in Great Britain, many of the key workforce issues discussed are more generally applicable. Direct comparisons of international workforce data are not always possible, partly because of differences in terminology and non-comparable health care systems, but also because it is difficult to obtain data matched by year. Some of the available international data on the workforce are presented in Table 14.1.

## WORKFORCE PROFILE IN GREAT BRITAIN AND OTHER COUNTRIES

In Great Britain, the workforce is divided into registered pharmacists and pharmacy technicians and unregistered support workers (e.g. dispensing and counter assistants). Registration with the General Pharmaceutical Council (GPhC; the regulatory body for the pharmacy profession) has always been compulsory for pharmacists, but it became mandatory for technicians only in July 2011 (Seston and Hassell 2012a).

Since the first edition of this book, four census surveys of the entire British pharmacist workforce have been conducted (see Hassell and Shann 2003a; Seston and Hassell 2009a,b) and the first pilot census of pharmacy technicians took place in 2010 (Seston and Hassell 2012a,b). Annual secondary analyses of the register of pharmacists have also been conducted (e.g. Hassell and Eden 2006; Seston and Hassell 2013). More recently, the GPhC commissioned a survey of registrants, which included a full census of technicians and a sample survey of pharmacists (Phelps et al. 2014). Thus, uniquely among the British health care professions, a large data set regarding the current and changing socio-demographic characteristics and the work and employment patterns of pharmacists and the technician workforce is now available. As of July 2013, when the most recent registrants' survey was conducted, there were 45,751 pharmacists registered with the GPhC. At the same point in time, the registered pharmacy technician workforce stood at 21,672.

In 2011, the non-practicing category of registration was removed, so all of these registrants are employed, although not everyone will be in a patient-facing role. The majority of registrants in Great Britain (90% of pharmacists and 95% of technicians) work in a pharmacy-related job. The majority are employed in their main job in the community sector (64% and 52% of pharmacists and technicians, respectively), while 22% of pharmacists and 38% of technicians work in a hospital setting in their main job (Phelps et al. 2014).

Given the marked shift within community pharmacy over the last 20 years or so from independent contractors to large multiple pharmacies, it is not surprising that the majority of pharmacists are now employees; for example, at the time of the last pharmacist census in 2008, only around 8% of posts held by pharmacists were independent owners, while more than half (54%) of pharmacists working in the community sector worked for one of the large multiples (Seston and Hassell 2009a).

Data from the Department of Health confirm the growing trend towards 'corporatization'. The proportion of community pharmacies in England belonging to large multiples (defined as those with more than five stores) has grown from 17% in 1969 to 61% in 2012. In Canada, the growth in the number of multiples is similar to trends witnessed in Great Britain. In New Zealand, on the other hand, the majority of retail pharmacies, because of legal restrictions on ownership, remain small, independently owned outlets (Norris 1997).

The recent pharmacy workforce surveys in Great Britain have, for the first time, provided accurate data about the extent to which pharmacists are employed (whether full-time, part-time or not in employment at all) and about how many jobs and the type of jobs (i.e. grade) they have. In 2008, the mean number of hours worked was just over 35 hours a week, although this is skewed somewhat by the large proportion (32%) of pharmacists working part-time (defined as 32 hours a week or less). While the majority (59%) of women pharmacists on the register in paid employment work full-time, most (77%) part-timers are women. There is a demonstrable relationship between part-time work, gender and age: the majority of women who work part-time are aged between 30 and 39 years, while the majority of male part-timers are aged 55 and over. Similar trends to these have been observed in Australia (Anderson et al. 1990), New Zealand (Norris 1997) and the US (Knapp 1994).

Women are now the majority of registrants on the British register, accounting for 60.4% of all registered pharmacists and 89.7% of all pharmacy technicians. In a number of countries where data are available (see Table 14.1), women are also in the majority (International Pharmaceutical Federation 2012), especially in the younger age groups. The impact that an increasingly female membership might have on the pharmacy workforce is discussed below.

Whereas the exact composition of the pharmacy workforce varies across different countries, there are also several notable similarities. Women now comprise nearly half, or over half, of the pharmacy workforce in most of the countries listed in Table 14.1, with the exception of the US and Saudi Arabia. Most pharmacists work in community pharmacy and the percentage in active employment is relatively high in those countries for which data are available. Although the proportion of women pharmacists in the US (46%) is smaller than in Great Britain, the tendency for women with young families to work part-time is similar in the two countries. In view of the continuing increase in the number of women entering the pharmacy profession and the younger age profile of women pharmacists compared with men, the proportion of pharmacists working part-time has increased in Great Britain and elsewhere.

## FACTORS AFFECTING SUPPLY AND DEMAND IN THE PHARMACY WORKFORCE

### DEMAND FACTORS

A number of factors influence the supply of, and demand for, pharmacists (Table 14.2).

The increasing emphasis on primary care in Britain and new contractual arrangements for community pharmacy have resulted in changes to the nature of pharmacists' employment, and will continue to influence demand for pharmacists. Pharmacists are being employed in a number of different settings and taking on prescribing roles, while the drive towards enhancing safety and efficiency within health care has resulted in recognition for pharmacists as providers of health care alongside general practitioners and other health care workers (Hassell et al. 1997). In particular, UK health policy, which called for community pharmacists to be used as the 'first port of call' in the management of minor ailments, and more recently the drive for pharmacists to improve public health outcomes through other locally commissioned services, such as National Health Service health checks, sexual health and drug misuse services and the establishment of healthy living pharmacies, illustrate how demand for pharmacists to perform additional clinical roles in addition to their dispensing role has grown (Hassell et al. 2011).

### TABLE 14.2
### Factors Influencing Supply of, and Demand for, Pharmacists

| Supply | Demand |
|---|---|
| Increasing feminization | Shift towards a primary care-led |
| Increasing 'Asianization' | National Health Service |
| Age of practitioners | Increased patient throughput in hospitals |
| Retirement rates | Increasing corporatization |
| Migration rates | Practice and professional developments |
| Career satisfaction | Organizational changes – longer hours |
| Part-time working | |
| Career motivation | |
| Changes to the undergraduate pharmacy course | |
| Competition for posts | |
| Salary | |

While professional development factors such as these may have a positive impact on the growth in workforce demand, developments within the general population will also influence demand. Discussing pharmacy workforce issues in Australian pharmacy, Anderson et al. (1990) argued several decades ago, for example, that an increase in prescription volumes due to the ageing population would increase demand for pharmacists. Indeed, government data in England bear this out. The dispensing volume in England increased from 473.3 million items in 1995 to 1000.5 million items in 2012, representing more than a 110% increase over the time period. Skilled pharmacy technicians will be assisting with some of this dispensing workload, but the extent to which this is happening is unclear (Willis et al. 2011).

Commercial developments taking place within the retail sector have also impacted on pharmacy workforce demand. A growing number and proportion of pharmacies are owned by supermarkets and larger multiples. These pharmacies tend to have longer opening hours, provide a greater number of pharmaceutical services, especially Medicines Use Reviews, and have higher prescription volumes. Additional pharmacists are often required to fulfil the legal obligations for continual professional cover and to manage a heavy workload.

Changes have also taken place in the secondary care sector, with extended opening hours and 'out-of-hours' clinics introduced by many hospital pharmacies. The extent of these changes on the work patterns of hospital pharmacists is unclear, but is likely to increase the demand for pharmacists who are able and willing to work flexible hours.

## Supply Factors

While commercial developments and changes within primary and secondary care have been emphasized as increasing demand for pharmacists, concerns are often raised about supply, in the past, in terms of whether there are sufficient numbers of pharmacists, technicians and other pharmacy staff (Hassell et al. 2002), and more recently about whether there are too many (Centre for Workforce Intelligence 2013). Aside from the more conspicuous factors that can affect the overall size of the workforce, such as new registrations, deaths, retirements, migration (Hassell et al. 2008; Schafheutle and Hassell 2009) and removals from the register, other forces are likely to impact on workforce numbers. These factors, perhaps more complex in their impact on career motivation and practice patterns, arise from the demographic characteristics of pharmacy practitioners.

### Women's Entry into Pharmacy and Their Impact on Workforce Supply

In all but two of the countries listed in Table 14.1, women comprise greater than half of the registered pharmacy workforce. The number of women pharmacists has increased over a relatively short period of time in Great Britain (Hassell 2000a; Hassell et al. 2002). The first workforce survey in 1964 reported that women represented 19% of registered pharmacists. By 1981, they constituted a third, and by 2000, they were the majority of all registrants.

In Great Britain, increasing female participation in paid employment has been an important factor in the growth of overall labour resources over the past 30 years, so the increasing prevalence of women in the pharmacy workforce is unsurprising. As in other labour markets, female employment in pharmacy has certain distinctive characteristics. For instance, female pharmacists, particularly married women with dependent children, are much more likely to be involved in part-time work compared with men (Hassell and Shann 2003b), and although many women work in community pharmacy, they comprise the majority (78%) in hospital pharmacy (Seston and Hassell 2009a). They also tend to be concentrated at the practitioner level and do not occupy senior positions in proportion to their number in the profession.

In Great Britain, this so-called 'feminization' process has led to concerns about workforce shortages in pharmacy. If women have primary responsibility for childcare in their families, inevitably they are unable to participate full-time in paid employment. Thus, it may be assumed that an increasing proportion of women pharmacists may reduce the size of the labour force, leading to a shortfall in the supply of pharmacists. However, researchers in Canada challenge this assumption. Muzzin et al. (1994) speculate that female pharmacists are actually guaranteeing the survival of pharmacy. Because of their preference for employment in retail pharmacy in the larger corporate organizations, women are helping 'to reorient pharmacy away from its business base and towards its chosen new professional jurisdiction of "patient counselling"'. Muzzin et al. (1994) also point out that female pharmacists in Canada are more mobile than men, moving to geographical regions where staff shortages are greatest.

The growth in the number of women in pharmacy has led to some critical and theoretical sociological analyses exploring women's entry into pharmacy and into professional occupations generally. The concept of 'occupational segregation', which refers to the way women are distributed through occupational categories compared with men, is central to this debate, as is the concept of 'vertical integration'. Writing about pharmacy in Great Britain, Crompton and Sanderson (1990), while viewing the increased participation of women in the pharmacy workforce as one beneficial consequence of the rising qualification levels among girls, nevertheless argue that work patterns in pharmacy still reflect a 'gendered division of labour'. To support this view, they cite women pharmacists' subordination to men in terms of job hierarchies and their concentration in stereotypical 'female' niches and part-time work, which, although offering opportunities for flexible working, are perceived as bringing fewer rewards. Consequently, what appear to be better career opportunities for women are, in fact, simply an extension of women's disadvantage into new areas of work. This view is also associated with arguments that the professions in which women participate are those in which material rewards have decreased and work has become routinized and de-skilled (Reskin and Roos 1987).

Looking at British pharmacy, Bottero (1994) challenged this perspective; she argued that the increased prevalence of women in pharmacy coincided with a raising of educational entry requirements and with attempts to 'professionalize' the pharmacist's role. The privileged positions held by many women in pharmacy are an indication of success, not subordination. Similar arguments have been put forward by Norris (1997), writing about New Zealand pharmacy (see also Chapter 6). Norris argues that women's entry into pharmacy has coincided with an upgrading of the profession, which has seen pharmacy in New Zealand increase its science base and move from an apprenticeship entry model to one which requires higher-education qualifications in order to secure a university place. Moreover, Norris (1997), in refuting the dominance of the secondary labour market thesis put forward by Crompton and Sanderson (1990), has also pointed out that while many women do work part-time, the majority nevertheless maintain a full-time commitment to their work. Both Bottero (1994) and Norris (1997) urge a more in-depth analysis of the pharmacy workforce. They suggest that 'feminization' is an inadequate description of the process that has occurred, not least because analyses of workforce change have tended to overlook the changing identity and motivations of male recruits into pharmacy, as well as age differences between men and women.

## The Increasing Participation of Ethnic Minority Groups in Pharmacy

The contribution to pharmacy of pharmacists from black and minority ethnic (BME) backgrounds and the impact their presence is likely to have on wider workforce issues has largely been overlooked, although BME groups now make up a significant proportion of pharmacy students and the qualified pharmacy workforce (Hassell et al. 1998). In a survey that included in the sample all 1991 pharmacy graduates, almost a quarter (23%) were from ethnic minority groups. Data are now routinely collected by the GPhC and have been the subject of regular analyses in recent years. Analyses indicate that BME pharmacists represented 39% of all registrants in 2011, and almost 70% of new entrants onto the register that same year (Seston and Hassell 2013).

Empirical research (Hassell et al. 1998; Willis et al. 2006a,b) that has taken account of the ethnicity of pharmacists has highlighted a number of important differences between BME and white pharmacists regarding career motivation, practice intentions and employment patterns. Although ethnic minority group pharmacists are represented in all sectors of the profession, they are over-represented as independent business owners in the retail sector and under-represented in managerial positions. While several ethnic groups are represented, members of the Indian ethnic group, most of whom are 'twice migrants' from East Africa, predominate (Hassell 2000b).

Even in the relatively short time that ethnic minority groups have become significantly represented in pharmacy, changes with respect to the ethnic profile of practitioners have taken place. Older ethnic minority pharmacists are mostly East African–Indian, whose involvement largely reflects their cultural and socioeconomic class background and the economic opportunities that were available for independent pharmacy business development shortly after their migration to the UK. In seeking upward mobility after migration, they chose to enter a profession which provided them with opportunities to go into business for themselves. By so doing, they fulfilled a desire for status and a preference to remain independent and autonomous, and they made the best use of their ethnic resources and family expertise. As migrants, self-employment for the older Asian pharmacists is viewed as prestigious, and employment of any family labour in the business is viewed in relation to the long-term benefits this provides for all the family, rather than in terms of any benefits it gives to the owner personally.

Younger ethnic minority pharmacists, however, are beginning to diversify in terms of practice intentions, so that independent business is not as popular a choice as it was for their predecessors. Changing preferences among the younger groups in part reflect generational and ethnic group differences, as well as social class differences among the more recent ethnic minority recruits. Pakistanis as an ethnic minority group *per se* are increasingly represented, as are ethnic minority women. Attributes such as autonomy and independence, which business ownership affords, are not as important for these two groups, and they have a greater tendency to want to work in hospital and corporate pharmacy settings. However, there is some evidence to suggest that experiences of racial discrimination may push them back into areas of practice where they are less likely to encounter prejudice. So while culture and personal preference explains the presence of many of the older East African–Indians in the self-employed business sector, structural factors such as racial discrimination may be playing a small part in pushing the younger ethnic minority pharmacists into self-employment.

These changes may have important implications for the pharmacy workforce. Ethnic minorities – some groups more than others – are certainly influenced by the perceived business opportunities in pharmacy. However, this is against a background of falling opportunities for ownership and increasing employee status. Thus, any reluctance on the part of the pharmacy profession to encourage diversification, or any reluctance among ethnic minority pharmacists, at an aggregate level, to enter hospital or other areas of practice, could have serious consequences for the health service in the future. Ethnic minority pharmacy graduates – indeed, all graduates – may require more encouragement to move into sectors other than community pharmacy. The success of such encouragement will largely depend on the pharmacy profession's willingness to accept any such movement into new practice areas by the ethnic minority pharmacists. It will also depend on increasing the awareness among white and ethnic minority groups of where the job opportunities in pharmacy are, and encouraging new recruits to consider a diversified range of career alternatives. Whether this happens is also likely to depend on salaries in hospital practice matching those in community pharmacy. Moreover, if ethnic minority pharmacists are experiencing discrimination in hospital and corporate settings, there is a case for encouraging employers to eliminate any disadvantages experienced by their staff.

## The Significance of Part-Time Work in Workforce Issues

Part-time work in pharmacy is usually discussed within the context of other studies, such as those concerning women in pharmacy, where it is seen as an important facet of women pharmacists' working lives. Indeed, in the labour market as a whole, part-time work is perceived as 'women's work', as five out of every six part-timers in Great Britain are female. Most of the literature on part-time work characterizes it in this way, as 'women's work', where it is mostly viewed as 'marginal' (Myrdal and Klein 1956). It is often perceived as a 'trap' by means of which women are exploited as part of the secondary sector of the labour market or of the reserve army of labour (Tam 1997). Other studies have focused on part-time workers as being in some way different from full-time workers. There is reference to part-timers being, for example, less committed to their work (Hakim 1995). In general, part-time work is rarely considered as an issue in its own right, and furthermore, there is very little work on the nature of men's part-time working patterns.

Evidence suggests that pharmacy may be a special case. It represents a professional occupation where, in terms of salary, work conditions and status, part-timers might be relatively less disadvantaged. It also differs in that a significant proportion of those who work part-time are male. Part-time work patterns are also extremely varied. A workforce survey conducted in 1978 differentiated between regular part-time work and casual or locum work. A later survey undertaken in 1994 by the National Association of Women Pharmacists drew a distinction between employee and self-employed part-timers and between those working for independent or company pharmacies. A 'qualitative workforce' survey from 1995 has highlighted some part-time work as an 'additional' occupation; that is, work done in addition to other work.

An even greater variety of work patterns undertaken by part-time pharmacists has been described. They may work regular pre-arranged hours or work at short notice. They may have one pattern of working, or a combination of several, and the patterns usually change over time as domestic circumstances and career aspirations change (Shann and Hassell 2006; Symonds 1998). There are also some gender-related differences regarding part-time work patterns. Men are more likely to be self-employed, to work for independent pharmacies or for a variety of types of pharmacy and to work at short notice or have a mixture of working patterns. Women, on the other hand, are more likely to be employees, to work for a multiple pharmacy chain and to have pre-arranged work patterns. Symonds (1998) has also shown that the concepts of part-time work as either a 'bridge' or a 'trap', as described in previous employment studies (notably Tam 1997), were found to have some application to part-time work in community pharmacy. For some part-timers, their work is viewed as part of a long-term career plan which enables them to make the transition ('crossing the bridge') back into full-time work or into another occupation. Similarly, for older pharmacists approaching the end of their full-time career, part-time work is often seen as part of the 'winding down' process – a 'bridge' into retirement. However, where part-time work is seen as a 'career break', it is often perceived as a 'trap', which may have a disadvantageous effect on long-term career and promotion opportunities. On the other hand, this employment pattern does allow women, in particular, to pursue a 'practitioner' career and to care for a family. For these pharmacists, a return to full-time work may not be envisaged.

There is also a third concept of part-time work – as a 'balance' – which can be applied in the particular case of pharmacy. Some part-time pharmacists stress the importance of having the freedom to choose where and when they work. They are often, but not always, self-employed pharmacists rather than employees, and often are taking advantage of favourable labour market conditions in pharmacy. They prioritize their different commitments to family, work, study, leisure pursuits and community activities, describing this prioritization as a 'balancing act'. They generally express a high degree of satisfaction with their work pattern, seeing themselves as having the best of all worlds.

Factors previously mentioned, such as the legal requirements that necessitate the presence of a registered pharmacist on the pharmacy premises at all times and the extended opening hours of many pharmacies, mean that pharmacies, especially in the community sector, may still rely heavily on the services of part-time pharmacists.

So whereas the general assumption is that part-time work reduces the supply of pharmacists, it may well be that part-time workers are actually filling a very real need.

While research has shown that part-time workers have different and complex work patterns which are interpreted as having positive or negative outcomes for them as individuals, how part-time work is viewed by pharmacy employers has not yet been investigated. There are other occupations where workers taking a career break or working part-time are seen as creating a labour market 'problem' with which managers have to deal. However, it may be that in the case of pharmacy, employers see part-time workers as a valuable and flexible labour supply with the ability to adapt to different work situations.

## Other Factors Affecting Supply

Other factors which affect the supply of pharmacists include the competition for posts (both within different geographical locations and within professional 'specialities'), the demands of training in a given speciality and recruitment and retention policies in different practice areas. In Great Britain, pharmacists' job dissatisfaction due to a number of issues, including long hours and stress (Jacobs et al. 2014), role expansion (Gidman et al. 2007), high workload (Hassell et al. 2011) and career expectations (Willis and Hassell 2008), have all been shown to impact on supply. High levels of staff turnover within community pharmacy in the US have similarly been explained by the poor conditions under which pharmacists are expected to work and dissatisfaction with features of their job, leading to the decision of many pharmacists to leave their positions (Schulz and Baldwin 1990). Work on job satisfaction in Great Britain and on occupational stress and workload indicate that pharmacists here are also increasingly concerned about their well-being, to such an extent that leaving the profession is a real consideration (Eden et al. 2009; Seston et al. 2009).

## CONCLUSION

Despite workforce planning being fundamental to the continuing development of any profession, robust empirical and detailed evidence about pharmacy workforce issues is scarce in some countries. However, in Great Britain, there is a growing body of primary and secondary research relating to the employment of pharmacists and support staff, and there now exists a far greater appreciation of the issues relating to pharmacy workforce recruitment, training and development. Although pharmacist numbers did increase steadily for a number of years, there has been a fall in numbers of registrants in the last four to five years, mostly due to changes in eligibility for registration and pharmacists retiring and leaving the register, rather than a drop in the number gaining registration. Graduation, migration, retirement and death are among the more obvious factors that alter the size of the pharmacy workforce. Others include individual career expectations and preferences, job satisfaction and career commitment and a raft of other interconnected factors.

Forecasting future supply and demand is thus enormously complex and difficult. While the factors mentioned above interact to decrease supply, the growth in schools of pharmacy and increasing student numbers could serve as a counterbalance to any loss elsewhere in the system. Greater 'corporatization', the growth in services being delivered by pharmacists and technicians, the expansion of clinical roles and an increasingly ageing population and a greater reliance on medicines all serve to increase demand for pharmacists; however, demand could be managed or diminished by the greater use of technology, with the emergence of Internet pharmacies and by future policy interventions.

## FURTHER READING

Willis, S., Shann, P. and Hassell, K. 2009. Pharmacy career deciding: Making choice a "good fit". *Journal of Health Organisation and Management*, **23**(1), 85–102.

## REFERENCES

Anderson, R.A., Bickle, K.R. and Wang, E. 1990. Pharmacy labour market assessment 1989. *Australian Journal of Pharmacy*, **71**, 492–501.

Bottero, W. 1994. The changing face of the profession? Gender and explanations of women's entry to pharmacy. *Work, Employment and Society*, **6**, 329–346.

Centre for Workforce Intelligence 2013. *A Strategic Review of the Future Pharmacist Workforce: Informing Pharmacist Student Intakes*. London: Centre for Workforce Intelligence.

Crompton, R. and Sanderson, K. 1990. *Gendered Jobs and Social Change,* London: Unwin Hyman Ltd.

Eden, M., Schafheutle, E.S. and Hassell, K. 2009. Workload pressure among recently qualified pharmacists: An exploratory study of intentions to leave the profession. *International Journal of Pharmacy Practice*, **17**, 181–187.

Gidman, W., Hassell, K., Payne, K. and Day, J. 2007. The impact of increased workloads and role expansion on female community pharmacists in the UK. *Research in Social and Administrative Pharmacy*, **3**, 285–302.

Hakim, C. 1995. Five feminist myths about women's employment. *British Journal of Sociology*, **46**, 429–455.

Hassell, K. 2000a. The impact of social change on professions – Gender and pharmacy in the UK: An agenda for action. *International Journal of Pharmacy Practice*, **8**, 1–9.

Hassell, K. 2000b. Ethnic diversity among pharmacy practitioners: A description and explanation of ethnic group participation in pharmacy, and implications for workforce issues. In: P Gard (Ed.), *A Behavioural Approach to Pharmacy Practice*. Oxford: Blackwell Science, 41–55.

Hassell, K. and Eden, M. 2006. Workforce update: Joiners, leavers, and practising and non-practising pharmacists on the 2005 Register. *Pharmaceutical Journal*, **276**, 40–42.

Hassell, K., Fisher, R., Nichols, L. and Shann, P. 2002. Contemporary workforce patterns and historical trends: The pharmacy labour market over the last forty years. *Pharmaceutical Journal*, **269**, 291–296.

Hassell, K., Nichols, L. and Noyce, P. 2008. Part of a global health care workforce: Emigration of British-trained pharmacists. *Journal of Health Services Research and Policy*, **13**(Supplement 2), 32–39.

Hassell, K., Noyce, P. and Jesson, J. 1998. A comparative and historical account of ethnic minority participation in the pharmacy profession. *Work, Employment and Society*, **12**, 245–271.

Hassell, K., Noyce, P., Rogers, A., Harris, J. and Wilkinson, J. 1997. A pathway to the GP: The pharmaceutical 'consultation' as a first port of call in primary health care. *Family Practice*, **14**, 498–502.

Hassell, K., Seston, E.M., Schafheutle, E.I., Wagner, A. and Eden, M. 2011. Workload in community pharmacies in the UK and its impact on patient safety and pharmacists' well-being: A review of the evidence. *Health and Social Care in the Community*, **19**(6), 561–575.

Hassell, K. and Shann, P. 2003a. *British Pharmacist Work Patterns: Summary of the 2002 Pharmacy Workforce Census*. Report for the Royal Pharmaceutical Society of Great Britain. London: RPSGB.

Hassell, K. and Shann, P. 2003b. The National Workforce Census: (3) The part-time pharmacy workforce in Britain. *Pharmaceutical Journal*, **271**, 58–59.

International Pharmaceutical Federation 2012. *Global Pharmacy Workforce Report*. The Netherlands: International Pharmaceutical Federation.

Jacobs, S., Hassell, K., Ashcroft, D., Johnson, S. and O'Connor E. 2014. Workplace stress in community pharmacy in England: Associations with individual, organisational and job characteristics. *Journal of Health Services Research and Policy*, **19**(1), 27–33.

Knapp, K.K. 1994. Pharmacy manpower: Implications for pharmaceutical care and health care reform. *American Journal of Hospital Pharmacy*, **5**, 1212–1220.

Muzzin, L., Brown, G.P. and Hornosty, R.W. 1994. Consequences of feminisation of a profession: The case of Canadian pharmacy. *Women and Health*, **21**, 39–56.

Myrdal, A. and Klein, V. 1956. *Women's Two Roles*, London: Routledge and Kegan Paul.

Norris, P. 1997. Gender and occupational change: Women and retail pharmacy in New Zealand. *Australian and New Zealand Journal of Sociology*, **33**, 21–38.

Phelps, A., Agur, M., Nass, L. and Blake, M. 2014. *GPhC Registrant Survey 2013: Findings*. London: NatCen.

Reskin, B. and Roos, P. 1987. Status hierarchies and sex segregation. In: C. Bose and G. Spittz (Eds.), *Ingredients for Women's Employment Policy*. New York: SUNY, Albany, 3–21.

Schafheutle, E.S. and Hassell, K. 2009. Overseas-trained pharmacists in Britain: What do registration data tell us about recruitment of overseas pharmacists? *Human Resources for Health*, **7**(51), 1–10.

Schulz, R.M and Baldwin, H.J. 1990. Chain pharmacists' turnover. *Journal of Administrative and Social Pharmacy*, **7**, 26–33.

Seston, E.M. and Hassell, K. 2009a. *The 2008 Pharmacy Workforce Census: Main Findings*. A report for the Royal Pharmaceutical Society of Great Britain. London: RPSGB.

Seston, E.M. and Hassell, K. 2009b. An overview of the main findings from the 2008 pharmacy workforce census. *Pharmaceutical Journal*, **283**, 419–420.

Seston, E.M. and Hassell, K. 2012a. First census of pharmacy technicians: 1. Demographics and working patterns. *Pharmaceutical Journal*, **288**, 140–141.

Seston, E.M. and Hassell, K. 2012b. First census of pharmacy technicians: 2. Qualifications, CPD activities, reasons for joining and plans to change work life. *Pharmaceutical Journal*, **288**, 141–142.

Seston, E.M. and Hassell, K. 2013. Workforce update – Joiners, leavers, and practising and non-practising pharmacists on the 2011 register. *Pharmaceutical Journal*, **290**, 619–620.

Seston, E.M., Hassell, K., Ferguson, J. and Hann, M. 2009. Exploring the relationship between pharmacists' job satisfaction, intention to quit the profession, and actual quitting. *Research in Social and Administrative Pharmacy*, **5**, 121–132.

Shann, P. and Hassell, K. 2006. Flexible working: Understanding the locum pharmacist in Great Britain. *Research in Social and Administrative Pharmacy*, **2**(3), 388–407.

Symonds, B.S. 1998. *Part-Time Work in Community Pharmacy: A Bridge, a Trap, or a Balance?* PhD Thesis (unpublished). Nottingham: University of Nottingham.

Tam, M. 1997. *Part-Time Employment – A Bridge or a Trap?* London: Ashgate Avebury.

Willis, S.C. and Hassell, K. 2008. Career intentions of pharmacy students. *Journal of Health Services Research & Policy*, **13**, 45–51.

Willis, S.C., Seston, E.M. and Hassell, K. 2011. *Identifying the Risks and Opportunities Associated with Skill Mix Changes and Labour Substitution in Pharmacy*. Report for the Centre for Workforce Intelligence. London: Centre for Workforce Intelligence.

Willis, S.C, Shann, P. and Hassell, K. 2006a. Career choices, working patterns and the future pharmacy workforce. *Pharmaceutical Journal*, **277**, 137–138.

Willis, S.C., Shann, P. and Hassell, K. 2006b. Who will be tomorrow's pharmacists and why did they study pharmacy? *Pharmaceutical Journal*, **277**, 107–108.

# 15 Pharmacists and the Multidisciplinary Health Care Team

*Christine Bond*

## CONTENTS

---

### KEY POINTS

- Contractual frameworks for community pharmacy increasingly emphasize the cognitive rather than the purely technical supply function of pharmacists.
- The medical profession has questioned pharmacy's ability to deliver an extended role.

- A triumvirate of doctor, nurse and pharmacist (as the experts in medicine and therapeutics) could be a very powerful and efficient combination for providing a high level of service to patients.
- Developments in information technology raise the possibility for 'read-and-write' access for pharmacists to an electronic patient record, which would improve communication between pharmacists and other members of the multidisciplinary health care team.

## INTRODUCTION

This chapter will consider the common background of pharmacy and medicine and its impact on the development of pharmacy as it is practised today. New extended roles and professional opportunities are also discussed.

## HISTORICAL DEVELOPMENT OF PHARMACY AND MEDICINE

At a time when the blurring of roles across different health care professionals is increasing, it is interesting to look back and reflect that general medical practitioners and pharmacists, in the UK at least, have a common ancestor in the mediaeval spicers. The spicers formed themselves into the Society of Apothecaries in 1617. They competed with the physicians, who by royal decree were the only group licensed to give, and charge for, medical advice. The apothecaries dispensed medicines for physicians and recommended medicines for those members of the public unable to afford physicians' fees. However, they were not themselves permitted to charge for this advice, but only for the medicines which they sold.

In 1815, the Apothecaries Act allowed a charge to be made specifically for the provision of advice, as well as for the medicine which was dispensed. As a result of this legislation, the two distinct professions of general practice – medicine and pharmacy – emerged and diverged. A further bill before parliament, which sought to reform the law and prevent the chemists and druggists giving advice and recommending treatments for purchase, posed a threat to the future pharmacy profession. A leading group of chemists and druggists came together and argued that this would not be in the public's best interest. Parliament was convinced and the bill was defeated.

In 1840, the Society of Apothecaries and College of Surgeons agreed on a joint curriculum of study for general practitioners, and proposed that likewise the chemists and druggists should be compelled to undergo an examination in order to receive a licence to carry out their business. In 1841, Jacob Bell, son of a leading chemist, formed the Pharmaceutical Society of Great Britain. The medical profession itself became united when the Medical Act of 1858 established the Medical Register, which included the names of surgeons and apothecaries alongside those of physicians. A fuller exposition of the historical development of pharmacy is given in Chapter 1.

## PHARMACISTS' CURRENT AND FUTURE ROLES

Recognition that the profession of pharmacy within the UK was not realizing its full potential was first officially identified in 1979 (Merrison 1979) and described in official reports, such as the *Nuffield Report* (1986) and subsequent Government White Papers. Extensive consultation both within and outside the profession resulted in a definitive description of the future role of community pharmacy, *Pharmaceutical Care: The Future for Community Pharmacy*, produced jointly by the Department of Health and the Royal Pharmaceutical Society of Great Britain (1992). This document considered various aspects of the community pharmacist's working practice under nine broad headings, including services to general practitioners, the over-the-counter (OTC) advisory role, health promotion and services to special needs groups such as the housebound. Thirty specific tasks were recommended to be either introduced nationally or on a pilot basis. While some of these tasks merely formalized ongoing practice and were generally welcomed, others were innovative, covering areas as diverse as simple health care advice, therapeutic drug monitoring and prescribing following agreed protocols. The report was received with some reservations by medical bodies and welcomed as 'pragmatic, prosaic and progressive' by the pharmaceutical profession.

The reality of the pharmacist's 'extended role' (i.e. those activities additional to traditional dispensing activities) has been reinforced by successive policy papers. Recent examples of these are *Prescription for Excellence in Scotland* and *Improving Health and Patient Care through Community Pharmacy – A Call to Action* in England. Pharmacists are also increasingly recognized in other strategic documents not focused on pharmacy but with a wider agenda, such as the management of drug misuse or improving adherence. Further, as will be referred to in more detail later, legislative and regulatory changes have allowed pharmacists to prescribe all prescription-only medicines (POMs), including controlled drugs, when practising within their own levels of competence. Finally, new contractual frameworks for community pharmacy have increasingly emphasized the cognitive as opposed to the technical supply function of pharmacists.

Most new roles for pharmacists are concerned directly or indirectly with medicines management and the optimization of prescribed and non-prescribed medication. Thus, there are interfaces with general medical practitioners and other health care professionals, as well as with the public. This unique, two-faceted role for the pharmacist has been contrasted with that of other health care professionals. The needs of the patient will be central to all such interactions, which may cause problems when the patient's needs appear to conflict with the general medical practitioner's instructions. Many of the 'new' roles may not be new, but merely new to pharmacy, with resultant perceptions of boundary encroachment by the existing suppliers of a particular service. For example, a wider role in the treatment of symptoms of minor ailments will inevitably require an element of diagnosis. Diagnosis is often considered to be an activity solely reserved for the medical profession, and any attempt by community pharmacists to participate in this may be regarded as encroaching on medical territory. Thus, objective evaluation of pharmacists' new roles is very important. The relatively new academic discipline of pharmacy practice research, a branch of health services research, has a central part to play in the development of the profession (see also the chapters in Section V of this book) by generating robust evidence of the effectiveness and efficiency of new pharmacist roles.

This chapter will look at the effects of three key issues in influencing the above developments, namely the influence of power and status in inter-professional relationships, channels and barriers to effective communication and pharmacists' input into prescribing.

## POWER AND STATUS IN INTER-PROFESSIONAL RELATIONSHIPS

### MEDICINE, PHARMACY AND OTHER HEALTH CARE PROFESSIONS

The main argument for maintaining the two professions of medicine and pharmacy and thereby separating the prescribing and dispensing functions has been the acknowledged conflict which would otherwise exist when income is related to the quantity and cost of a medicine prescribed. For example, in Japan, where doctors are commonly responsible for both prescribing and dispensing, drug costs are said to be higher than anywhere else in the world.

However, unlike the rest of Europe, pharmacists in the UK never quite achieved a monopoly over dispensing. There is a historical precedent allowing general medical practitioners to dispense, a right which is maintained, which has resulted in repeated bitter controversy between the two professions. This reality is expressed graphically by Kronus (1976) as:

> Given a common origin, how did physicians come to dominate one set of work tasks (prescribing and diagnosis) and retain the right to engage in drug dispensing activity, whilst pharmacists lost any claim to medical practice as well as a monopoly over their own task territory?

Once the distinct professions of medicine and pharmacy had emerged in the mid-nineteenth century, the main role of the community pharmacist increasingly became that of dispenser. This change underwent a further acceleration after the National Health Service (NHS) Act in 1948. Once there was free public access to medical advice, there was a reduced advisory role for the community pharmacist, whose task became increasingly technical (see also Chapter 1).

A reversal of this trend depends on the public's perception of pharmacists. Over 30 years ago, it was suggested that the mission of all pharmacists should be to 'move the boundary of responsibility from the practice of a technique (the dispensing of medicines) to the patient' (Brodie 1981). Today, the boundary has shifted closer to that ideal, but much remains to be done. New pharmacy roles may encroach on other boundaries, such as the roles of other health care professions, particularly medicine. In the past, the medical profession has refused to allow boundary encroachment by groups seeking to establish new roles for themselves.

However, a general recognition and acceptance by other professionals, patients and the public of the need for, and value of, direct pharmacist-led patient counselling alongside the increased range of OTC medicines has contributed to this shift (Blenkinsopp and Bond 2005). More recently, other roles such as Medicine Use Reviews (England), the New Medicines Service (England), the Chronic Medicines Service (Scotland) and the near-universal use of patient medication records (PMRs) for both prescribed and increasingly non-prescribed medicines have further established direct links between the patient and the pharmacist. Furthermore, these changes have been shown to be supported by the large majority of the public in the UK.

Health care is delivered by a range of professions who share a commitment to the welfare of their patients and clients, and a prohibition on exploiting their dependency. However, relations between these professions are often strained because of the dominance of medicine over all others. This dominance is attributed to the fact that medicine was the first profession to develop within the nineteenth century's rapidly expanding health care sector. Thus, although many of the allied health professions and nursing have many of the core features of a profession, they have not achieved all of the benefits, such as autonomy, remunerative rewards or equity of status. This pattern is replicated in varying degrees in other professions, such as physiotherapy, chiropody and pharmacy (see also Chapter 12).

This is exemplified by the development of the sub-profession of medical/clinical pharmacology by the medical profession in response to the challenge from pharmacy. Another example is the establishment of the obstetricians and gynaecologists in response to the developing role of midwives. There have, however, been some exceptions, such as the successful emergence of the dental profession and the partial success of clinical psychologists. In other settings (e.g. in third-world countries and on ships, expeditions and oil rigs), medical care has been successfully devolved to paramedics (e.g. allowing the treatment of minor symptoms following agreed protocols), and this has gradually been introduced into the UK. There is now extensive proliferation of extended and often autonomous new roles for many health care professions, including advanced nurse practitioners, physician associates and non-medical prescribers, including pharmacist prescribers. There are nurse-led specialist clinics in primary care (e.g. asthma, cholesterol measurement and immunizations) and consultant nurses practising in secondary care (e.g. leading colposcopy clinics). This may then be an opportune time for pharmacy to restate its professional role as the specialist expert in medicines, to regain control over drug use and to offer an alternative to their medical colleagues. The roles of the medical and pharmaceutical professions may be about to converge again, and in primary care, the public will have an expectation and choice of either approaching the pharmacist or the general practitioner for advice and treatment.

However, as is shown in various sections of this chapter, it has been more challenging for community pharmacists to gain respect from patients and health care colleagues than for pharmacists working in other settings, such as secondary care. The profession of community pharmacy was said by Hamilton and Dunn (1985) to be held in low esteem because:

- The commercial side of the work leads to a storekeeper-like image.
- Pharmacists can, if they wish, do no more than dispense, which is essentially a technical activity.
- Community pharmacy is seen as the career option for pharmacists for whom hospital or industry is not to their liking.

There has been some improvement in all three of the above in the past 30 years, but nonetheless, all three issues remain challenges which must be resolved before another 30 years have elapsed. The commercial environment in which community pharmacy is based is often perceived to undermine pharmacists' ability to provide unbiased advice which is solely in the patient's best interest; under current community pharmacy contractual frameworks, the majority of remuneration is linked to the volume of dispensing, whereas to succeed in industry and secondary care, there is a requirement for postgraduate qualifications and a greater cognitive contribution.

Thus, in primary care, there are a range of barriers to overcome if the pharmacist is to gain his/her rightful role. While the functions of the community pharmacist and the general medical practitioner may often overlap, the community pharmacist should be seen as providing a complementary rather than a competing service to the general public. General medical practitioners should welcome the contribution that community pharmacy could make to a reduction in its workload and the improved overall service that is made available to patients. Notwithstanding this, the response of the medical profession to an extended role for the community pharmacist has not always been totally supportive, and pharmacists' ability to deliver it has been questioned. Early surveys of medical practitioners conducted at the time that extended roles were first proposed indicated that while formalization of traditional roles may be supported by doctors, the introduction of more innovative tasks was not (Begley et al. 1994; Bond et al. 1995). While attitudes have become more positive as extended roles become established, there remains ambivalence when any new role is proposed (Hughes and McCann 2003).

## SEPARATION OF HOSPITAL AND COMMUNITY PHARMACY

It has been said that pharmacy differs from many, although not all, professions in that it is divided into two major areas of practice on the basis of location rather than activity. Thus, the community and hospital branches of pharmacy have become almost mutually exclusive, and their practice paths have increasingly diverged. Within the hospital category, several further subgroups have emerged, each with a different professional status. Of these, the clinical pharmacist who has a greater involvement with both patients and medical prescribers, as opposed to the more technically orientated compounding and distribution tasks, may be perceived to have the higher rank.

Until recently, there has not been a sufficient range of tasks offered in community pharmacy for any similar differentiation to emerge. However, the 'extended' role provides an opportunity both for specialized subgroups of community pharmacy to develop and for a new category of pharmacy itself to develop, namely primary care pharmacists, based on those pharmacists working directly within the general practice setting. Different models of delivering pharmaceutical care should be encouraged to facilitate the maximum contribution of pharmacy to health care.

## THE PRIMARY HEALTH CARE TEAM AND PHARMACY

The primary health care team was first described in 1979 by the Royal Commission on the NHS. In 1988, Professor Michael Drury, Department of General Practice Birmingham, wrote: 'One thing that can be said about team work in general practice is that there is not a lot of it about' (Drury 1988). There is evidence that this has changed in recent years, probably motivated by radical changes in the delivery of health care. However, unlike other paramedical groups and professions, the community pharmacist is still not seen to be part of the primary health care team, certainly not part of the core team, and often not part of the wider team as defined by Martin (1992). This does not reflect the wishes of the pharmaceutical profession. A survey of a sample of community pharmacists in Scotland showed that, with respect to drivers for undertaking extended roles, they placed the highest value on organizational aspects of their work and being well integrated with primary and secondary care; while total income was important, there were indications that pharmacists would be prepared to forgo income to attain their preferred job (Scott et al. 2007). These findings were interestingly similar to those of a much earlier English survey of community pharmacists which had shown that 95% were overwhelmingly in favour of being part of a multidisciplinary primary health care team (Sutters and Nathan 1993). Thus, despite increased roles and some wider recognition from other health care professionals in the intervening years, pharmacists still do not feel well integrated into the primary health care team.

## CHANNELS AND BARRIERS TO EFFECTIVE COMMUNICATION

### PRINCIPLES OF TEAM WORKING

Good professional communication in health care is an essential component of team working. Many professionals, each with their own specific expertise, may be involved in the care of a single patient. This approach has the potential to deliver optimum care, yet to realize fully the health care benefits, the potential pitfalls must be recognized and addressed. The key components of effective team working are summarized in Box 15.1.

Effective communication is central to achieving all of these components, whether at a superficial operational level as in sharing patient data, or at a deeper level focused on an appreciation of another professional's *modus operandi* and professional standing. Openness and honesty are paramount, as well as effective team management, rather than leadership. Differing levels of remuneration among team members may cause tensions within the team. These tensions are historical and will not be changed easily. The ultimate goal is resolution of such tensions and more equitable remuneration based on skills and competences, rather than background professional

---

**BOX 15.1　KEY COMPONENTS OF EFFECTIVE TEAM WORKING**

- Sharing a common purpose to bind and guide
- Having a clear understanding of one's own role
- Recognizing common interests
- Understanding the roles and responsibilities of others
- Pooling knowledge, skills and resources
- Sharing a responsibility for outcomes

discipline; however, in the interim, it is important to ensure that all team members feel equally valued in other ways.

## INTER-PROFESSIONAL COMMUNICATION

Of the health professionals interacting with community pharmacy, general medical practitioners are probably most involved with the pharmacist. The extended role features fairly regularly in journals read by the large majority of general medical practitioners. In general, such articles support a wider community pharmacy role, but with caveats, and there is most support for the extension of traditional roles as opposed to the more innovative aspects. There is also some evidence that a lack of confidence in the potential 'professional welcome' offered by the general medical practitioners to community pharmacists could be a rate-limiting step to improved collaborative working practices.

## THE CURRENT POSITION

An important mismatch in the perceptions of community pharmacists compared to general practitioners is highlighted in a large study of medicine management by community pharmacists (Community Pharmacy Medicines Management Project Evaluation Team 2007). In total, 17% of participating general practitioners said community pharmacists were their professional equals, 46% said that they were members of the primary health care team and 83% said that they were professional colleagues. In contrast, only 11% of community pharmacists thought they were professional equals, 72% regarded themselves as members of the primary health care team and 76% regarded themselves as professional colleagues.

A survey of London community pharmacists carried out in the late 1980s (Smith 1990) showed that 43% had some contact with primary health care personnel other than general medical practitioners. The most frequently cited professionals were the district nurse and staff of residential homes, although 17 different professional groups were named, and the contacts were mostly initiated by the other profession, rather than the pharmacist. The frequency of contact was at least weekly, though contact with general medical practitioners was more frequent. The vast majority of these contacts were associated with prescriptions, with three-quarters of these contacts initiated by the pharmacist. The study gave an important insight into interactions with the primary health care team. A total of 60% of the responding pharmacists felt that, in spite of the level of contact, their contribution to the team was not acknowledged. This appears to be something that has not changed in the last 30 years, since extended roles were first muted. In the medicine management study referred to above, when communicating with the local general practice about medicines, communication was mostly with the general practitioner (87%), then the receptionist (79%) and then the nurse (45%). Interestingly, there was little contact with the practice pharmacist (12%).

Some community pharmacists have a dispensing base within a health centre and these pharmacists have good communication with the local general medical practitioners. When the community pharmacists are based in health centres, there is more collaboration and communication between the two professions than when the pharmacist is more traditionally based in the 'high street'. In an early example of this co-location, one of the medical participants in such a health centre commented that such pharmacists were 'in a privileged position in that none of their advice need be commercially orientated' (Harding and Taylor 1990). This reinforces the relevance of one of the barriers for community pharmacy identified by Dunn and mentioned earlier.

## EXAMPLES OF GOOD PRACTICE

Published work demonstrates an increasing number of examples of the community pharmacist being integrated into the health care team. For example, drug misuse is increasingly prevalent and the care of drug misusers has increasing resource implications. This problematic group of patients is not always welcomed by health professionals or their other clients, and their planned management is particularly important (see also Chapter 19). Taking on a role not widely valued by medical colleagues is one way to demonstrate the value and quality of pharmaceutical care that can be provided by pharmacists. When pharmacist prescribing was first introduced, it was often difficult to identify patient groups for whom the general practitioner was prepared to delegate prescribing responsibility to the pharmacist. However, when some general practitioners refused to prescribe for drug misusers and local NHS organizations sought to identify alternative service providers, community pharmacists with prescribing rights provided an ideal option. Already used to supervising the daily administration of the opioid substitute methadone, prescribing was a natural extension to that role. Similarly, the increased emphasis on smoking cessation, the need to provide advice to a large percentage of the population and the availability of nicotine-replacement products from community pharmacy have combined to make the community pharmacy an ideal location. Smoking cessation services are now a core part of the Scottish community pharmacy contractual framework, and almost three-quarters of all services and the majority of quits are provided in this way. These schemes invoke a common purpose, meet a health care need, acknowledge specific roles and involve the sharing of information and responsibility for outcomes.

## PRESCRIBING AND MEDICINES MANAGEMENT

An increased role for pharmacists is inextricably linked to 'medicines management', a fundamental role which reflects pharmacists' unique training and specialized knowledge. The term 'medicines management' covers a wide range of activities, including advice and recommendations for treatment to policy makers, professionals and the public, as well as the direct and appropriate supply of medicines. Pharmacists' input into prescribing is one facet of this.

Prescribing may be defined as a recommendation for the use of a drug or remedy. However, the word 'prescribing' was traditionally interpreted as the recommendation for a medicine by a doctor or dentist, and the vehicle through which this was mediated was the piece of paper known as the 'prescription'. Nonetheless, in its strictest definition, a pharmacist's role in providing OTC advice to a patient in a community pharmacy, which may include the recommendation of medication, is also prescribing. However, since the UK publication of the first Crown Report (Crown 1999), these two 'prescribing functions' have been blurring to the extent that now about 2% of the pharmacy profession have acquired accredited independent prescribing status. More information on this issue follows later.

## PHARMACISTS' INFLUENCE ON GENERAL PRACTITIONERS' PRESCRIBING

When the NHS was first established and free medical advice and treatment was made available to all UK citizens, the OTC advisory role of the pharmacist appeared to be obsolete. Pharmacists were utilized more as suppliers of medicines and their role became very technical. However, with the advent of potent drugs that are formulated, produced and packaged by mass production methods, traditional dispensing skills became increasingly redundant:

> The pestle and mortar days of preparing medicines have been overtaken by pharmaceutical industrial technology which accurately and aseptically produces complex medicines, pills and ointments. Only occasionally, following consultant directions, are complicated medicines made up in the pharmacy. The mixing role of the chemist has thus been eliminated. (Roberts 1988)

Today, the dispensing task is not just restricted to the technical formulation and compounding of a prescription. It is more concerned with verifying the prescription, taking into account patient factors and previous drug histories (as far as is available from the PMRs) and then, when the dispensed medication is handed to the patient, providing appropriate counselling on medication use. The actual selection of the correct medicine pack from the shelf is normally only a small part of this process and is often done by a pharmacy technician, dispenser or even robot. Although there will still be the rare occasion when traditional compounding skills are required, this is likely to decrease even further due to increased concerns over product integrity, issues of liability and quality control and the increasing availability of commercial manufacture of what are known as 'specials'.

This change in what has come to be understood as dispensing has allowed pharmacists to develop a more proactive role in the prescribing process at the interface with the patient. This role is increasingly recognized by other health care professionals. Thus, community pharmacists are expected to identify dosage errors, prescribing errors and drug interactions. They are also at the forefront of the need to support adherence with prescribed medication regimes through concordant consultations, often as part of the Medicines Use Reviews, New Medicines Service and Chronic Medicines Service referred to earlier.

A further future proactive involvement for pharmacists in the prescribing process is in the management of repeat prescribing. Repeat prescribing accounts for approximately 75% of all general practice prescribing in the UK, and many patients are on poly-pharmacy regimes. Current practices for generating repeat prescriptions – either computer or receptionist written – are generally acknowledged to provide inadequate control, resulting in over-prescribing, stockpiling of drugs and infrequent review of therapy, which may lead to failure to identify issues such as drug interactions, adverse drug reactions, poor compliance and inappropriate treatment.

An early randomized study demonstrated that pharmacists can appropriately manage repeat prescribing with a resultant increase in the detection of problems (e.g. adherence problems and the identification of adverse drug reactions and drug interactions). There is also a reduction in drug wastage and cost avoidance by patients, as well as improved clinical benefits (Bond et al. 2000). Since then, a multiplicity of local pilot schemes confirmed that, when implemented in a real-world context, these same benefits were realized. Now known as repeat dispensing, this service has again become core to many community pharmacy contracts.

## PRIMARY CARE PHARMACISTS

In separate but parallel moves, pharmacists have also had an impact on prescribing at the professional interface. Across the developed world, drug costs have risen relentlessly and there has been a range of policy decisions and strategies introduced to address this. One such change in the UK was the introduction of pharmacist advisory posts within local NHS management structures and general practice-based pharmacists, often working with several different practices. These posts have a remit to review general practice prescribing through interpretation of the computerized feedback provided by the NHS at area and practice levels, respectively. On the basis of this, subsequent advice would be given and areas of 'poor' prescribing targeted for support and review. There is a growing body of anecdotal and research evidence which demonstrates that pharmacists based in general practice – known as primary care pharmacists – are highly regarded, have influence and have improved prescribing patterns.

One highly cited example of such a role is the PINCER trial (Avery et al. 2012), which showed that a pharmacist-led information technology intervention was more effective than computer-generated simple feedback targeted at 'at-risk' patients (i.e. those with a history of peptic ulcer disease receiving non-selective non-steroidal anti-inflammatory drugs without a co-prescription of a proton-pump inhibitor; those with a history of asthma prescribed a beta blocker; and finally those who are 75 years or older on a long-term prescription of angiotensin-converting enzyme inhibitor or loop diuretics without assessment of urea and electrolytes).

There are some ethical problems if the community pharmacist advising a doctor on prescribing is also the pharmacist who dispenses the prescription. Historically, the prohibition of links between community pharmacists and general medical practitioners, in order to separate the two parts of the prescribing/dispensing process, has favoured the development of the pharmaceutical profession. It has now become a professional liability and is inhibiting links being made which are not centred on the distributive dispensing process.

## PHARMACIST PRESCRIBING

As mentioned earlier, the first UK Crown Review (Crown 1999) of the prescribing, supply and administration of medicine facilitated the further involvement of pharmacists as both dependent and independent prescribers. The initial review recommended that individual groups of professionals should be able to apply for the authority to prescribe certain medicines under what became known as a 'patient group direction'. These are still widely used, mostly by nurses and pharmacists, to allow the supply of POMs to groups of patients who cannot be identified individually before they present for treatment. For example, they might be introduced in the event of an influenza pandemic to increase convenient and safe access to appropriate medicines not normally available without a prescription. However, for leading-edge pharmacists, full prescribing rights were the ultimate goal. In 2006, legislation was finally passed with equivalent NHS regulatory changes that meant that accredited pharmacists, alongside some other health care professionals such as nurses, could prescribe under the NHS any medicine, including controlled drugs, as long as they were practising within their perceived levels of competence. As noted earlier, implementing this within NHS structures and financial frameworks has not been simple, and progress has been frustratingly slow at times. Research has suggested that patients are supportive, and pharmacists enjoy the role. Currently, most prescribing in pharmacy is done by those working in primary care and community pharmacy. Few studies have critically reviewed the clinical outcomes of pharmacist prescribing compared to usual care, but one small randomized controlled trial conducted in patients with chronic pain showed that 6-month pain outcomes were significantly improved in patients whose analgesic drugs were prescribed by the pharmacist compared to those who were managed as usual by the general practitioner (Bruhn et al. 2013).

In recent changes to the undergraduate pharmacy curriculum, prescribing competencies will now become a core component, and all pharmacy graduates will potentially have prescribing rights. At that point, it is likely that prescribing will allow a multi-factorial role to emerge, encapsulating the Medicines Use Review, New Medicines Service, Chronic Medicines Service, repeat dispensing and prescribing.

In all of this, it is important not to forget that other professions, especially nurses, are extending their roles and acquiring similar authority. While many skills and competences are not the prerogative of a single profession, each profession will bring to the team their own professional paradigm. For example, the doctor may contribute diagnostic skills and the art of medicine, the nurse might contribute the caring dimension and the pharmacist might contribute the expertise in medicines and therapeutics. Such a triumvirate of doctor, nurse and pharmacist could be a very powerful and efficient combination for providing a previously unparalleled level of service to patients.

## INFLUENCES ON CHANGES IN OTC PRESCRIBING

The prescribing pharmacist may become the focus of the 'extended' profession; this is consistent with the recommendation of the Nuffield Committee of Inquiry into Pharmacy (1986) that the core function of the pharmacist is the sale and supply of medicines, and with Sogol and Manasse (1989), who have said, 'Pharmacy is a professional service that promotes and assures rational drug therapy in order to maximize patient benefit and minimize patient risk'.

However, we must not forget that the sale of OTC drugs as recommended treatments for patients who seek advice for the management of symptoms in community pharmacies remains one of the key roles of the pharmacist providing 'health care on the high street' on a drop-in basis. This role has been made more effective in recent years through the change in status of a range of previously POMs. This change in status from 'POM' to 'P' (pharmacy medicine) or even GSL (general sales list) is variously called 'reclassification', 'deregulation', 'switching' or 'depomming'! Although of benefit to the pharmaceutical profession, the main driving force has been the meeting of several agendas, which include the pharmaceutical profession, but also the pharmaceutical industry and the government. The move to reclassification of a wide range of medicines has been supported both by the pharmaceutical profession and the industry. However, there was some early ambivalence from the medical profession (see Chapter 9), although with time, early fears regarding issues such as misdiagnosis or delayed diagnosis of serious disease have proven unfounded.

The drivers of making more drugs available OTC were not solely or even primarily to make more effective use of the pharmacists' expertise and knowledge. The change came through a convergence of various agendas. First, the pharmaceutical industry had been suffering as a result of the moves to curb NHS spending on drugs and was looking to the OTC market to extend the brand life of existing products. Second, governments worldwide were looking at ways to reduce prescription drug costs. In the UK, the cost of general practitioner prescriptions has risen by over 50% in real terms over the past decade, although they have remained relatively constant at three-quarters of all drug costs and approximately 10% of the total health budget. The average 'real' cost per prescription has increased by 16.7%, and the number of prescriptions written by 30%. Reasons proposed for this are the ageing population, an increased rate of diagnosis and the increased use of drugs in preference to other treatments. It was thought that increased self-medication, supported by community pharmacists, could help reduce the drugs bill.

However, the full potential for self-medication was previously limited because of legal restrictions on the range of drugs available for sale. In the 1990s, there were worldwide moves to change this by the reclassification of a range of drugs. Hence, European directive 92/26/CEE states that medicines should only be POMs if they are dangerous when used other than under medical supervision, frequently used incorrectly, new and need further investigation or are normally injected. The consensus criteria for deregulation are currently said to be that the drug should be of proven safety, of low toxicity in overdose and for the treatment of minor 'self-limiting' conditions.

In 1989, Denmark was among the first of the Northern European countries to deregulate a large number of medicines, including cimetidine. The process started slowly in the UK with the deregulation of ibuprofen and loperamide (1983), terfenadine (1984) and hydrocortisone 1% cream (1985), but it has continued steadily with the support of the government, the Royal Pharmaceutical Society and, to a limited extent, the Royal College of General Practitioners. Other target preparations have included the 'morning after' pill, with the support of both the Royal College of General Practitioners and the General Medical Services Committee of the British Medical Association. At this time, the UK probably has one of the widest ranges of drugs legally available OTC in the Western world.

If costs are defined to include both monetary and non-monetary elements, it has been shown that the OTC availability of one of the first deregulated medicines, topical

1% hydrocortisone, saved patients in the UK £2 million pounds in 1987 alone (Ryan and Yule 1990), and the NHS is also said to make savings. Savings from the deregulation of loperamide were estimated to be £0.13 million in 1985, £0.15 million in 1986 and £0.32 million in 1987 (Ryan and Yule 1990). Standard models of supply and demand can also be employed to demonstrate the theoretical economic advantages of deregulation (Ryan and Bond 1994). Given that the principle is now established, there has been little evidence since to demonstrate the economic advantages of the policy. However, it has been suggested that the deregulation of drugs to treat a short-term acute condition (e.g. aciclovir for herpes) has taken these drugs out of general practitioner budgets, but this is not likely to be true for drugs used longer term, such as the proton-pump inhibitors. Experience of their effectiveness when bought OTC may then trigger a request for a longer-term prescription from the GP. Indeed, the author is unaware of any study demonstrating cause and effect, but omeprazole is currently the single most prescribed drug in both England and Scotland.

The extension of the OTC prescribing role of the community pharmacist under the current system through increased availability of a wider range of medicines has caused some concerns about the appropriateness of provision and much publicized WHICH reports of miss-selling (WHICH 2013). However, a recent large study commissioned by the Royal Pharmaceutical Society – the MINA study (Watson et al. 2014) – showed that patients attending community pharmacy for the management of one of four targeted minor illnesses, and mostly receiving a 'depommed medicine', had similar outcomes compared to patients with the same conditions managed by emergency services or general practitioners. Furthermore, attending community pharmacies for treatment was significantly more cost effective than either alternative provider, and patients were highly satisfied. On the negative side, there was some indication from audio recordings that despite the right drug being sold and patients achieving good clinical outcomes, the process of the consultation could be improved. Pharmacists and their staff therefore need to be trained for this increased responsibility, especially by improving their communication and interpretation skills.

With such potent medicines now more widely used OTC, it would be advantageous if they could be added to a central patient drug record which could be accessed by both general practitioners and community pharmacists. For general practitioners, this would provide information on the treatments already tried/being taken by the patient, underpin future prescribing decisions and increase their awareness of the potential for drug interactions or therapeutic duplication. For pharmacists, access to a central medical record would inform their OTC prescribing decisions, as well as their role with respect to prescribed medicines. While electronic health records make this an ever-greater likelihood of becoming a reality, there are suggestions that general practitioners may not want to have the increased responsibility of knowing this information (Porteous et al. 2003).

Most recently, government funding for the provision of a restricted formulary of OTC products paid for by the NHS for the management of minor ailments has been introduced. This is known as a Minor Ailment Scheme. In Scotland, this is provided by all community pharmacists as a core component of their contract. In England, it is a locally commissioned service provided only in some areas by some pharmacists. In Scotland, the service is supported via an electronic health infrastructure. While currently standalone, all patients are identified by their unique NHS Scotland number, enabling subsequent linking with other NHS datasets. There is limited evidence (Paudyal et al. 2013) which demonstrates that these schemes are effective, cost effective and reduce the number of general medical practitioner consultations for minor ailments, wherein patients seek a prescription for a medicine for which they are exempt from payment, but which can also be bought from a pharmacy. While this service, to some extent, runs against the philosophy of encouraging patients to take more responsibility for their own health, and in effect transfers costs back to the NHS, it is a move towards directing patients to use the NHS service that is most appropriate to their needs.

## INFORMATION TECHNOLOGY

The use of information technology in the health service is currently relatively small compared to other industries, such as banking and tourism. However, in the UK, all general practitioners and community pharmacists, as well as other health care professionals, are linked to the NHS-net. There is now widespread, although not universal, electronic transfer of prescription information from general practitioners to community pharmacists, and the 'holy grail' of community pharmacists having at least selected access to the patient medical record is ever nearer. This should open up the possibility for 'read-and-write' access for pharmacists to an electronic patient record, which would facilitate many of the innovative developments described above and improve communication. Such a mechanism to improve communication and information flow in a controlled but relevant way will support the greater involvement of pharmacists in multidisciplinary patient care. It should also make possible the delivery of some aspects of the role described previously from the community pharmacy base, rather than by a primary care pharmacist based in surgeries. This could avoid the total partitioning of the profession into three main groupings and would actually promote a range of different models of involvement.

A completely different use of information technology is the increasing use of apps to support health care, such as the self-monitoring and reporting of clinical parameters back to health care teams and reminders to take medicines to improve adherence. E-pharmacy services also include online advice and Internet supply, raising new ethical and practical challenges for the profession to address.

## CONCLUSION

In the past decade, pharmacists have had an opportunity to extend their role in multidisciplinary health care because of external factors resulting from the agendas of the pharmaceutical industry and the government, pressures on the workforce, changing patient demography and increasing demands for health care. The pharmacy profession has responded positively to this opportunity, and looking back, the profession's role in secondary and primary care has dramatically changed since the end of the twentieth century. Pharmacists' expertise in medicines and therapeutics has been central to this shift in role.

Looking to the future, it might be expected that the technical dispensing role will be further separated from the cognitive, largely medication-related services provided by pharmacies. Scenarios for an extended pharmacy role might be for a 'community' pharmacist to be based full-time in a general medical practice, developing a range of services which could include activities such as advice on formulary development, patient medication review and asthma clinics, as well as pain and warfarin clinics. Development of a role for pharmacists within the general medical practice base would not obviate the need for 'high street' pharmacies. Rather, it would be an additional model for delivering pharmaceutical care which would allow the utilization of a wider range of pharmacists' skills.

Removal of community pharmacists from the commercial setting would allow them to provide advice that is untainted (imagined or otherwise) by possible commercial pressures, and barriers between general medical practitioners and community pharmacists have been blurring, with a general recognition of the role of teams rather than individuals in the provision of health care. This is already the case in the hospital setting where pharmacists' advice is highly valued by medical colleagues at all levels. The future for pharmacy is bright, and today's graduates have the skills and competences to deliver the vision so many have been working for.

## FURTHER READING

Adams, T. 1999. Dentistry and medical dominance. *Social Science and Medicine*, **48**, 407–420.

Ashley, J. 1992. Pharmacists and the 'D' word. *Pharmaceutical Journal*, **248**, 375.

Blane, D. 1991. Health professions. In: G. Scrambler (Ed.), *Sociology Applied to Medicine*. London: Balliere Tindall, 221–235.

Bond, C.M. and Grimshaw, J.M. 1994. Clinical guidelines for the treatment of dyspepsia in community pharmacies. *Pharmaceutical Journal*, **252**, 228–229.

Bond, C.M., Grimshaw, J.M., Taylor, R.J. and Winfield, A.J. 1998. An evaluation of clinical guidelines for community pharmacy. *Journal of Social and Administrative Pharmacy*, **15**, 33–39.

Bond, C.M., Sinclair, H.K., Taylor, R.J., Williams, A., Reid, J.P. and Duffus, P. 1995. Pharmacists: An untapped resource for general practice. *International Journal of Pharmacy Practice*, **3**, 85–90.

Comptroller and Auditor General 1993. *Repeat Prescribing by General Medical Practitioners in England*. London: HMSO.

Comptroller and Auditor General 1994. *A Prescription for Improvement*. London: HMSO.

Cotter, S.M., Barber, N.D. and McKee, M. 1994 Professionalisation of hospital pharmacy: The role of clinical pharmacy. *Journal of Social and Administrative Pharmacy*, **11**, 57–66.

Crown, J. 1999. *A Review of the Prescribing, Supply and Administration of Medicines*. London: Department of Health.

Cunningham-Burley, S. 1988. Rediscovering the role of the pharmacist. *Journal of the Royal College of General Practitioners*, **38**, 99–100.

Department of Health 1987. *Promoting Better Health, CM249*. London: HMSO.

Department of Health 1989. *Working for Patients, CM555*. London: HMSO.

Department of Health 1997. *The New NHS – Modern, Dependable, CM3807*. London: HMSO.

Dowell, J., Cruickshank, J., Bain, J. and Staines, H. 1999. Repeat dispensing by community pharmacists: Advantages for patients and practitioners. *British Journal of General Practice*, **48**, 1858–1859.

Drury, M. 1991. Doctors and pharmacists – Working together. *British Journal of General Practice*, **41**, 116–118.

Edwards, C. 1992. Liberalising medicines supply. *International Journal of Pharmacy Practice*, **1**, 186.

Ford, S. and Jones, K. 1995. Integrating pharmacy fully into the primary care team. *British Medical Journal*, **310**, 1620.

Freidson, E. 1972. *Profession of Medicine*. New York: Mead and Co.

Harris C.M. and Dajda, R. 1996. The scale of repeat prescribing. *British Journal of General Practice*, **46**, 643–647.

Jepson, M. and Strickland-Hodge, B. 1993. Patients' choice of pharmacy, the importance of patient medication records and patient registration. *Pharmaceutical Journal*, **251**, R35.

Macarthur, D. 1992. Professions at war: A look at the uneasy relationship between dispensing doctors and pharmacists in the UK. *Australian Journal of Pharmacy*, **73**, 870–871.

Marsh, G.N. and Dawes, M.L. 1995. Establishing a minor illness nurse in a busy general practice. *British Medical Journal*, **310**, 778–780.

Matheson, C. and Bond, C.M. 1995. Lower gastrointestinal symptoms. *Pharmaceutical Journal*, **253**, 656–658.

Matthews, L.G. 1980. *Milestones in Pharmacy*. Egham: Merrell Division.

NHS England 2013. Improving Health and Patient Care Through Community Pharmacy – A Call to Action. Gateway Reference: 00878. Available at: http://www.england.nhs.uk/wp-content/uploads/2013/12/community-pharmacy-cta.pdf

Porteous, T., Bond, C., Duthie, I. and Matheson, C. 1997. Guidelines for the treatment of hayfever and other allergic conditions of the upper respiratory tract. *Pharmaceutical Journal*, **259**, 62–65.

Porteous, T., Bond, C.M., Duthie, I. and Matheson, C. 1998. Guidelines for the treatment of self limiting upper respiratory tract ailments. *Pharmaceutical. Journal*, **260**, 134–139.

Rogers, P.J., Fletcher, G. and Rees, J.E. 1992. Recording of clinical conditions by community pharmacists in patient medication records. *Pharmaceutical Journal*, **249**, 723–727.

Scott, A., Bond, C.M., Inch, J. and Grant, A. 2007. Preferences of community pharmacists for extended roles in primary care – A survey and discrete choice experiment. *Pharmacoeconomics*, **25**(9), 783–792.

Scottish Government 2013. Prescription for Excellence. Available at http://www.scotland.gov.uk/Resource/0043/00434053.pdf.

Scottish Office Department of Health 1997. *Designed to Care – Renewing the National Health Service in Scotland, CM3811*. London: HMSO.

Spencer, J. and Edwards, C. 1992. Pharmacy beyond the dispensary: General practitioners' views. *British Medical Journal*, **304**, 1670–1672.

Taylor, R.J., 1986. Pharmacists and primary care. *Journal of the Royal College of General Practitioners*, **36**, 348.

Wain, C. 1992. The primary care team. *British Journal of General Practice*, **42**, 498–499.

Welsh Office 1997. *Putting Patients First, CM3841*. London: HMSO.

Whitehouse, C.R. and Hodgkin, P. 1985. The management of minor illness by general practitioners. *Journal of the Royal College of General Practitioners*, **35**, 581–583.

# REFERENCES

Avery, A. et al. 2012. A pharmacist-led information technology intervention for medication errors (PINCER): A multicentre, cluster randomised, controlled trial and cost-effectiveness analysis. *Lancet*, **379**, 1310–1319.

Begley, S., Livingstone, C., Williamson,V. and Hodges, N. 1994. Attitudes of pharmacists, medical practitioners and nurses towards the development of domiciliary and other community pharmacy services. *International Journal of Pharmacy Practice*, **2**, 223–228.

Blenkinsopp, A. and Bond, C. 2005. *Over the Counter Medicine*, London: BMA.

Bond, C.M., Matheson, C., Williams, S., Williams, P. and Donnan, P. 2000. Repeat prescribing: A role for community pharmacists in controlling and monitoring repeat prescriptions. *British Journal of General Practice*, **50**, 271–275.

Bond, C.M., Sinclair, H.K., Taylor, R.J., Williams, A., Reid, J.P. and Duffus, P. 1995. Pharmacists: An untapped resource for general practice. *International Journal of Pharmacy Practice*, **3**(2), 85–90.

Brodie, D.C. 1981. Pharmacy's societal purpose. *American Journal of Hospital Pharmacy*, **38**, 1893–1896.

Bruhn, H., Bond C.M., Elliott, A.M. et al. 2013. Pharmacist led management of chronic pain in primary care: Results from a randomised controlled exploratory trial. *BMJ Open*, **3**, e002361.

Community Pharmacy Medicines Management Project Evaluation Team (C. Bond Principal Investigator) 2007. The MEDMAN study: A randomized controlled trial of community pharmacy-led medicines management for patients with coronary heart disease. *Family Practice*, **24**(2), 189–200.

Crown, J. 1999. *A Review of the Prescribing, Supply and Administration of Medicines*. London: Department of Health.

Department of Health and Royal Pharmaceutical Society of Great Britain 1992. *Pharmaceutical Care: The Future for Community Pharmacy*. London: Royal Pharmaceutical Society of Great Britain.

Drury, M. 1988. Teamwork: The way forward. *Practice Team*, **1**, 3.

Hamilton, D.D. and Dunn, W.R. 1985. *Report Submitted to the Post Graduate Education Committee of the Royal Pharmaceutical Society of Great Britain, Paper 1*. London: Royal Pharmaceutical Society of Great Britain.

Harding, G. and Taylor, K. 1990. Professional relationships between general practitioners and pharmacists in health centres. *Journal of the Royal College of General Practitioners*, **40**, 464–466.

Hughes, C.M. and McCann, S. 2003. Perceived interprofessional barriers between community pharmacists and general practitioners: A qualitative assessment. *British Journal of General Practice*, **53**, 600–606.

Kronus, C.L. 1976. The evolution of occupational power. *Sociology of Work and Occupations*, **3**, 3–37.

Martin, C. 1992. Partners in practice: Attached, detached, or new recruits. *British Medical Journal*, **305**, 348–350.

Merrison, A.W. 1979. *Royal Commission on the National Health Service, CM7615*. London: HMSO.

Nuffield Committee of Inquiry into Pharmacy 1986. *Pharmacy: A Report to the Nuffield Foundation*. London: Nuffield Foundation.

Paudyal, V., Watson, M.C., Sach, T. et al. 2013. Are pharmacy-based minor ailment schemes a substitute for other service providers? A systematic review. *British Journal of General Practice*, **63**(612), e472–e481.

Porteous, T., Bond, C., Robertson, R, Hannaford, P. and Reiter, E. 2003. Electronic transfer of prescription related information: Comparing the views of patients, GPs and pharmacists. *British Journal of General Practice*, **53**, 204–209.

Roberts, D. 1988. Dispensing by the community pharmacist: An unstoppable decline? *Journal of the Royal College of General Practitioners*, **38**, 563–564.

Ryan, M. and Bond, C. 1994. Dispensing doctors and prescribing pharmacists. *Pharmacoeconomics*, **5**, 8–17.

Ryan, M. and Yule, B. 1990. Switching drugs from prescription-only to over-the-counter availability: Economic benefits in the United Kingdom. *Health Policy*, **16**, 233–239.

Smith, F.J. 1990. The extended role of the community pharmacist: Implications for the primary health care team. *Journal of Social and Administrative Pharmacy*, **7**, 101–110.

Sogol, E.M. and Manasse, Jr. H.R. 1989. The pharmacist. In: A.I. Wertheimer and M.C. Smith (Eds.), *Pharmacy Practice: Social and Behavioural Aspects*, Baltimore: Williams and Wilkins, p. 59.

Sutters, C. and Nathan, A. 1993. The community pharmacist's extended role: GPs and pharmacists' attitudes towards collaboration. *Journal of Social and Administrative Pharmacy,* **10**, 70–84.

Watson, M.C., Holland, R., Ferguson, J., Porteous, T., Sach, T., Cleland, J. and Bond, C.M. 2014. *Community Pharmacy Management of Minor Illness: The MINA Study*. London: Pharmacy Research.

WHICH 2013. Can you trust your local pharmacy's advice? Consumers Association. Available at: http://www.which.co.uk/news/2013/05/can-you-trust-your-local-pharmacys-advice-319886/.

# 16 Pharmaceutical and Health Care Needs of Older People and Their Carers

*Nina Barnett and Ruth Goldstein*

## CONTENTS

### KEY POINTS

- Ten million people in the UK are aged more than 65 years and this number is projected to increase by 5.5 million in 20 years, and to 19 million in 2050.
- People aged 75 years and over are more likely to take prescribed or purchased medicines and are more susceptible to drug-related problems than the general population.

- A combination of written and oral advice, together with repetition and reinforcement, is a particularly effective method for older people to improve the ability to recall important information.
- Residential homes in the UK are required to register with a pharmacy and the pharmacist is required to provide an appropriate level of pharmaceutical care to residents and carers.
- The New Medicines Service introduced in 2011 makes provision for at least two telephone consultations with the pharmacist for older people in their own homes who have been newly prescribed certain drugs.

## INTRODUCTION

This chapter deals with the delivery of pharmaceutical services to older people. Older people deserve particular attention in the context of pharmaceutical care for two reasons. First, as the body ages, it ceases to function as efficiently as previously, and physical and cognitive disabilities may develop. Second, access to services may be problematic due to these physical and cognitive disabilities, so the standard service provision may not be adequate for older people. This chapter will cover, in general terms, the physical and cognitive effects of ageing which result in this sector of the population being 'in need'. It will then explore why access to services is particularly problematic for the older population and methods of identifying older people who need additional support with medicines. The final section will consider particular interventions and services that have been, and are being, developed for older people.

## THE OLDER POPULATION

It is recognized that people aged 75 years and over are more likely than the general population to take prescribed or purchased medicines. Ageing results in altered pharmacokinetics and pharmacodynamics, and consequently older people have a greater susceptibility to drug-related problems. Furthermore, poly-pharmacy and iatrogenic disease are more prevalent in the older population. These factors, together with impairment of cognitive and physical function, may result in their failure to use medications appropriately.

When medicines are prescribed, the intention is to improve the patient's quality of life. There is, however, always an element of risk associated with medicine taking, which may result in a diminished quality of life or a less-than-optimal pharmaceutical outcome. Suboptimal pharmaceutical outcomes can lead to hospital admission and these have been found to be most prevalent among older people living alone, those taking two or more medications or those receiving no assistance with their medication.

Five main causes of suboptimal outcome following the incorrect use of medicines have been identified (Box 16.1). The provision of specific pharmaceutical services, such as medication reviews and domiciliary visits, can help to ensure that these potential problems do not lead to poor outcomes.

BOX 16.1    FIVE MAIN CAUSES OF SUBOPTIMAL OUTCOMES
FOLLOWING THE INCORRECT USE OF MEDICINES

- Inappropriate prescribing
- Inappropriate delivery (e.g. medicine not available when needed or a carer fails to administer the medicine)
- Inappropriate behaviour by the patient (e.g. compliance-related problems)
- A patient idiosyncrasy
- Inappropriate monitoring (e.g. failure to monitor the effects of the treatment regimen on a patient)

Adapted from Hepler, C.D. and Strand, L.M. 1990. *American Journal of Hospital Pharmacy,* **47**, 533–543.

## Older People and Their Medication: The Potential Problems

Many older people and their carers cannot cope with the complexity of medication regimes and this can lead to poor medicines adherence, which in turn will reduce the benefit from medicines. The advent of evidence-based medicine, where multiple conditions are treated with multiple guideline-based therapies, often leads to poly-pharmacy. A King's Fund report (Duerden et al. 2013) suggested that while some poly-pharmacy is appropriate, it can be problematic for some people. Moreover, purchased over-the-counter (OTC) medicines can increase poly-pharmacy and may interact with prescribed medication, especially as health professionals may not be aware of the OTC medicines being taken (Barber et al. 2000). Reduced visual and cognitive capacity, combined with memory loss, increase the likelihood of a medication error and of poor adherence, while child-resistant packaging may prove a problem among those lacking manual strength and dexterity. Additionally, the small size of printing on containers, closures and labels is a hindrance to those with reduced visual capacity. In addition to practical barriers, older people, in common with others, may have perceptual barriers to medicine taking. Beliefs and concerns about medicines, including side effects and questions about whether the medicines are necessary, are known to contribute to poor adherence. Many of these factors contribute to the need for a carer to assist an older person with medication taking.

It seems reasonable to assume that people are more likely to use medicines correctly if they are given information in a form and a language that they understand. Explanation and reinforcement of dosage instructions on container labels are essential to avoid the misinterpretation of instructions, leading to uneven and inappropriate spacing between doses. However, when consulting with an older person, it is as important to address their beliefs and concerns about medication if they have the capacity to decide what they want to take. A carer's requirement for information about prescribed medication begins once the general medical practitioner (GP) writes a prescription. It may be worthwhile encouraging patients and carers to prepare questions about medicines before a consultation and write down information during consultations to aid recall. Certainly, the combination of written and oral advice, together with repetition and reinforcement, is generally considered to be a most effective method for improving the ability to recall important information, as is the establishment of a medicine-taking routine.

## IDENTIFYING OLDER PEOPLE WHO NEED SUPPORT WITH MEDICINES

There are a number of factors that make older people more vulnerable to medicines-related problems than their younger counterparts. The National Service Framework (NSF) for Older People was the first time that a national document recognized the contribution of pharmacists in support of older people, through the medicines booklet that accompanied the publication of the NSF. The publication of the NSF, which included recommendations for a single assessment process between health and social care, led to the development of four validated medicines 'trigger questions' which explore key areas of concern for older people (Box 16.2). These have been adapted and incorporated into many medicines assessment templates since publication.

Many practitioners have tried to devise checklists for the identification of older people at risk of medicines-related problems and there is broad agreement regarding

---

**BOX 16.2   GOOD QUALITY PHARMACEUTICAL CARE – IMPLICATIONS FOR CARERS WITH ELDERLY DEPENDENTS**

This represents two key aspects of supporting medicines optimization for older people – their knowledge of their medicines and the roles of the health care team (where to get more information) and the how easily they can get access to the medicines they need through current systems. This can be represented in other ways, for example organizational and individual, practical and perceptual or in a number of other ways.

- Access: do you need help getting a regular supply of your medicines?
- Compliance: people can forget to take their medicines. When, during the last week, did you forget to take your medicines?
- Day to day: do you ever have difficulty swallowing or using your medicines, or getting medicines out of their containers?
- Clinical: do you think (realistically) that some of your medicines could work better?

If there is a positive answer to any of the above questions, refer to a pharmacist for support.

Medicines Trigger Questions: Rosenbloom, E.K. and Goldstein, F.R. 2007. *International Journal of Pharmacy Practice*, **15**, 21. Adapted for *North West London Hospitals Trust* by Nina Barnett, August 2011.

content (Barnett and Seal 2013). However, it is difficult to create a definitive checklist as high-risk situations are multi-factorial, constantly changing and require consideration of individual circumstances. For example, an older person with poor sight who is prescribed warfarin could be considered as high risk, but this is mitigated by living with their spouse who organizes their medicines. If their spouse is no longer present, their risk increases. The PREVENT tool (Table 16.1) was developed from

## TABLE 16.1
## PREVENT Tool for the Identification of Medicines Risks for Older People

| Aspect | Examples |
|---|---|
| Physical impairment (PHY) | Swallowing difficulty, nil by mouth, impaired dexterity, poor vision, hard of hearing, poor mobility where this will impact them taking medication |
| Risk from specific medicines/medicines-related admission (RIS) | High risk medicine: *Antipsychotics, anticoagulants/antiplatelets, insulin /oral hypoglycaemics, Non-Steroidal Anti-Inflammatory Drug (NSAID), benzodiazepine, antihypertensives, opiates, methotrexate, injectable medicines, cytotoxic drugs, drugs requiring therapeutic drug monitoring with no monitoring,* steroids |
| | Complex of medicine regimen including problematic polypharmacy, recently stopped, started or changed medicines where unmanaged |
| | Drug interaction causing harm identified |
| Adherence issues (ADH) | Poor adherence e.g. various dispensing dates on medicines, no recent dispensing of medication |
| | Poor medicine knowledge e.g. cannot give names of medicines they are taking |
| | Patient stopped taking all or some of their medicines which has lead or could lead to worsening of their clinical condition. |
| Cognitive impairment (COG) | Unable to take medication regularly without support as they have a condition which affects their memory e.g. delirium, dementia |
| New diagnosis/exacerbation of disease (EEC) | Admission is related to poor management of medication for a long term clinical condition or deterioration of organ system function e.g. renal, hepatic, cardiac |
| | Previous admission or A&E attendance within 30 days |
| | Depression, high level of life stress, uncontrolled mental health condition, alcoholism. Smoker |
| | Multiple new medication prescribed where adherence challenges identified |
| Compliance support (COS) | Refer all new requests |
| Societal/social (SOC) | Difficulty managing activities of daily living independently or has carers to help with daily activities but not medicines |
| | Evidence of social difficulty e.g. no fixed abode, unkempt on admission which impacts them taking medication. Smoker |

*Source:* Adapted from Barnett, N., Athwal, D. and Rosenbloom, R. 2011. *Pharmaceutical Journal,* **286**, 471.

a literature review and the collective experience of pharmacy practitioners as a risk-assessment tool which acts as a guideline to the identification of people at risk of preventable medicines-related problems.

In order to use the tool effectively, identified risks must then be considered in light of whether the risk is currently managed (and what happens if this changes) and whether it is modifiable through pharmacy intervention or whether signposting is needed. While this tool has mainly been used in a hospital setting, it is easily adaptable to the community environment.

## Living Conditions of the Elderly

Older people live in a range of different types of accommodation, including their own homes, supported accommodation (warden controlled, residential and nursing homes) and may live alone or with a spouse, family or carers. The type of accommodation largely reflects an individual's physical and cognitive status. Most people who live in their own homes are generally able to cope for themselves, with possibly some daily or weekly support from family members, friends or formal carers, such as home carers and community nurses. As a person becomes more frail or socially isolated, perhaps following the death of a partner, supported accommodation, such as the home of a family member or warden-controlled accommodation, provides the advantage of maintaining the older person's independence while giving access to low-level assistance by the 'warden'. As older people become increasingly frail (i.e. lose weight, become easily fatigued, weak, slow and reduced in ability to be physically active), the more physically and cognitively impaired tend to move to more caring residential settings, where carers, including home carers, nurses and doctors, will take a larger active role in looking after the older person. As frailty increases, so do the demands on health and social services.

The domiciliary arrangements for older people can impact on how they receive pharmaceutical services. If a person lives at home, they are likely to control their own health care provision, although they may rely upon services which are accessible from their own home, such as domiciliary visits by health personnel. Older people in residential care settings tend to rely on the staff in the institution to monitor their health care needs, and access to pharmacy services is often through a carer. The effects of this on the type and nature of pharmaceutical services provided for an older person are discussed throughout the remainder of this chapter.

## Carers of Older People

Most of us are reliant on the support of carers as we go through life. With regards to medicine taking, prompting one another to take medication is a familiar part of cohabiting. Older people require a variety of support from carers, depending on their own health status and the care available to them. Informal carers, such as partners, siblings, children and friends, fulfil a major role in supporting older people. However, the level and type of support are often more complex in terms of time commitment and necessary skills, such as nursing care, than informal carers can provide. Furthermore, as marriages fail and family structures break down, older people whose partners are no

**TABLE 16.2**
**Formal Carers Supporting Older People**

| Type of Carer/Service | Type of Support Provided |
|---|---|
| Home carers | Personal care, social support and domestic support |
| Nurse | General health care, including bathing, changing dressings and supporting incontinence problems |
| Chiropodist | Foot care |
| Counsellor | Bereavement support |
| Social worker | Housing issues, financial advice and social issues |
| Doctor | Medical care |
| Occupational therapist | Mobility care |
| Pharmacist | Medicines optimization, including supply, review and advice |

longer alive place a great demand for support on the formal care service. A summary of formal carers and services that most often support older people is provided in Table 16.2.

Older people also encounter difficulty in accessing a community pharmacy, despite the fact that, as a group, they are the highest users of medicines. In such circumstances, pharmacists should consider the needs of carers and assess whether a domiciliary service should be provided and how that can be accessed.

## ACCESS TO PHARMACEUTICAL SERVICES

There has never been an accurate figure placed on the numbers of people who access pharmacy services on a daily basis. However, in the late 1980s, it was estimated that in excess of six million people visited a community pharmacy daily in the UK. This figure does not take account of the telephone enquiries received by pharmacists, nor any of the additional services that pharmacists provide that result in pharmaceutical services being delivered outside the pharmacy premises. The main reasons patients use the services from pharmacies are listed in Box 16.3.

### ACCESSING PHARMACEUTICAL SERVICES

Pharmacies are situated in the majority of hospitals, in some health centres and on most high streets. So why is access a problem? It is not a problem in terms of the spread of services. In fact, in some places, there is a choice of pharmacies within a very short distance, but access requires patients to go to the pharmacy. The patient, carer or other professional health or social care worker is expected physically to attend the pharmacy to receive any of the services outlined in Box 16.3. People can, of course, telephone a pharmacist to receive pharmaceutical support, and this method has been utilized to support medicines optimization as part of the New Medicines Service in England, which started in 2011 and is especially useful for housebound patients. However, there are some patients for whom there are other barriers, such as speech difficulties (aphasia) and language, which make pharmacy support more difficult.

> ### BOX 16.3  PATIENTS' MAIN REASONS
> ### FOR USING PHARMACIES
>
> - To purchase over-the-counter medication
> - To obtain medication which has been ordered on a prescription
> - To seek advice about prescribed or purchased medication (including information about dosages, adverse effects, drug interactions, prices and methods of obtaining supplies)
> - To gain health-promotion advice (e.g. on diet control or smoking cessation)
> - To discuss treatments and medications advertised on television, radio, the Internet, etc.
> - To discuss their concerns about health, finance, family matters and general social issues
> - To confirm, or otherwise, information they have received from others, such as doctors, nurses and next-door neighbours

The problem of access may appear only to be relevant to a small proportion of the population, but it is important to get a perspective on the size of that proportion: 10 million people in the UK are aged over 65 years, and this is projected to increase by 5.5 million in 20 years and to 19 million in 2050. It is generally this group for whom there can be such a problem, as they receive 75% of all prescribed medications and are particularly in need of pharmaceutical support, yet they may experience the most difficulty in accessing pharmacy services.

## PHARMACEUTICAL SERVICES

### MEDICINES OPTIMIZATION

Hepler and Strand (1990) identified five key elements to pharmaceutical care. More recently, the Royal Pharmaceutical Society has produced guidelines to support medicines optimization, with four key principles (Figure 16.1). A health-related problem needs to be identified and the patient's understanding and experience of that problem understood from their perspective, as well as from the health perspective. If medication is part of a solution to the problem, choice should be evidence-based. Safety of medicines prescribing and use is key in managing and minimizing the problem to provide medicines optimization for the older person. There are a series of stages following this identification that may be carried out by a patient or carer alone rather than by a health professional, though often in collaboration. For example, this may be a husband-and-wife team with one prompting the other to complete the course of prescribed medication. Alternatively, a carer may take full responsibility for their dependant's medication management in administering medicines. It is important to explore issues of capacity to agree to medicine taking with health professionals where there is cognitive impairment. Some carers may wish to conceal medicines in

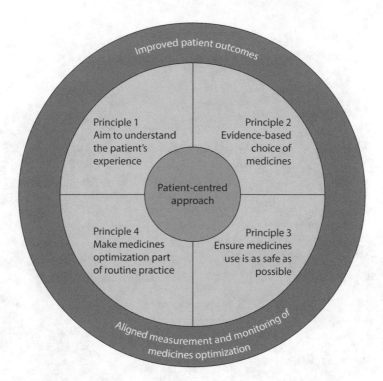

**FIGURE 16.1**  Four principles of medicines optimization. (From Royal Pharmaceutical Society 2013. Medicines Optimization: Helping Patients to Make the Most of Medicines. Good Practice Guidance for Healthcare Professionals in England. Available at: http://www.rpharms. com/promoting-pharmacy-pdfs/helping-patients-make-the-most-of-their-medicines.pdf.)

food to aid adherence. Advice from the GP or mental health professional and reference to appropriate guidance is key, especially when formal (e.g. social services) carers are administering medicines. Effective medication optimization requires not only a knowledge of the treatment prescribed, but also of the services available to older people in their locality. A summary of the aspects of 'knowledge and usability' are included in Figure 16.2.

If an older person resides in a residential or nursing home or in hospital, managing medicines is most often the responsibility of the staff. Pharmaceutical services to residential homes are different from those offered to people in their own homes and will therefore be dealt with as a separate section within this chapter.

## PHARMACEUTICAL SERVICES TO OLDER PEOPLE

Pharmaceutical services have traditionally been supplied either from registered premises in a community environment or from a hospital setting. The services have been limited in that services are usually provided from within the building. In the community, patients and/or carers must enter the pharmacy to receive their care. In a hospital environment, pharmacists may consult with patients on the wards or from a clinic or dispensary setting.

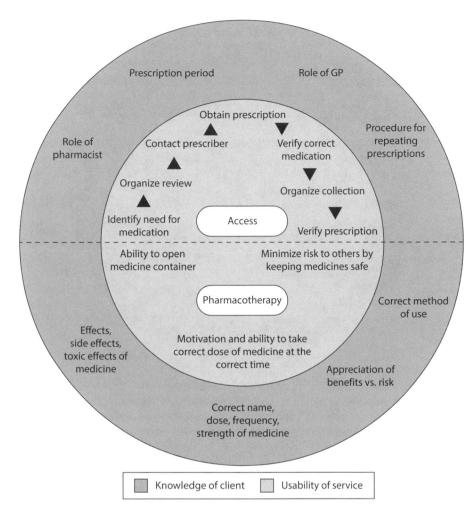

**FIGURE 16.2** The inter-relationship between service usability and the knowledge of the client. (From Goldstein, R., Rivers, P. and Close, P. 1993. *International Journal of Pharmacy Practice*, **2**, 65–70.)

Hospital pharmacy began the development of ward-based pharmacy services in the 1970s and now all hospitals in the UK largely offer a ward-based pharmacy service. In essence, this means that while the pharmacy itself is the point at which medicines are supplied, pharmaceutical advice is provided to the patient wherever they are in hospital.

Pharmaceutical services in the community differ from the hospital model, and although there are examples of services being offered away from the pharmacy itself, the current position is that community pharmacies remain the focus of pharmaceutical advice and support in the community. Examples of services that are helping community practices to get closer to patients are provided. However, it should be recognized that not all community pharmacists offer these services. There is no obligation for community pharmacists (other than maintaining their position as community-based experts) to accept the extended roles described below. However, for older patients and their carers, the provision of such services is advantageous.

## EXTENDED PHARMACEUTICAL SERVICES TO OLDER PEOPLE

### Domiciliary Visits

Older people who are unable to access pharmaceutical services may not have the opportunity to discuss their health and medication-related issues face-to-face with a pharmacist. Rather, they must rely upon information and advice being provided through their carer. Residential homes in the UK are required to register with a pharmacy, and the pharmacist in turn is mandated to visit the home to ensure that residents and carers are provided with appropriate levels of pharmaceutical care. Unfortunately, for patients living in their own homes, there is no formal system for pharmacist home visits. While carers may visit pharmacy premises for advice, new services, such as Medicines Use Reviews and the New Medicines Services, are not available through carers.

The advent of the New Medicines Service in 2011 has moved some way towards supporting people in their own homes as people who are newly prescribed certain new drugs are eligible (under certain conditions) for at least two telephone consultations with a pharmacist, for which the pharmacist is remunerated. Unfortunately, the Medicines Use Review service is still not routinely available by telephone. Neither service is routinely available in people's homes, though some localities have commissioned domiciliary Medicines Use Reviews. Evidence suggests that although domiciliary visits may be beneficial to patients and carers, there still tends to be a poor uptake (Schneider and Barber 1996). Possible reasons for this are listed in Table 16.3.

### Repeat Prescribing Services

The process of repeat prescribing allows patients who are on regular treatment to obtain a specified number of supplies of medication without the necessity of seeing

---

**TABLE 16.3**

**Reasons Patients and Carers are Hesitant to Take Up the Offer of Domiciliary Pharmaceutical Services**

| Reason | Further Explanation |
|---|---|
| Identify need | Patients and carers have to know domiciliary services are available and have to accept that they may require such a service. |
| Accepting support | As domiciliary services are 'new', patients and carers have to be willing to accept the service, which may appear to be tailored for particularly 'dependent' people. Few would want to be classed as dependent. |
| Non-traditional | This whole role is new to pharmacists; not all are willing to become involved with their patients outside the supportive structure of their shops. |
| Emotion | Some people who accept that they may benefit from the service are deterred as they feel uncomfortable allowing the pharmacist access to their home. |

their doctor. This is popular among patients, as they do not spend time making and attending appointments for routine, regular prescriptions. Recent research indicates that nearly 50% of patients receive repeat prescriptions, and that this proportion increases with age, with more than 90% of patients aged 85 years and older receiving their medication via repeat prescriptions (Harris and Dajda 1996). The repeat prescribing service is now linked with the more recently introduced Electronic Transfer of Prescription (ETP) service in England, which further facilitates access to medications where people choose a named pharmacy for prescription dispensing.

Although repeat prescribing is frequently used as a way of dealing with regular requests for prescribed medication, there is concern that the process for issuing prescriptions does not incorporate adequate controls to ensure that patients are regularly reviewed so that they always receive appropriate medication. For example, one study identified that 66% of repeat drugs were prescribed without the apparent authorization of GPs, and that for 72% of the drugs prescribed, there was no evidence of a review by a doctor within the previous 15 months (Zermansky 1996). While documentation of medication reviews every 15 months is required as part of the Medicines Indicators in the GP contract Quality and Outcomes Framework (General Practitioners Committee, NHS Employers and NHS England 2013), there is no measure as to the type or quality of the review.

In addition to clinical issues such as reviewing the appropriateness of medication, there is evidence that a considerable amount of prescribed medication is unused (Rees et al. 1993, 1995; Woolf 1996). Within Derbyshire, for example, 1.25 tonnes of unused medicine is collected quarterly from community pharmacies. A review of medicines waste in 2010 recorded that wastage of prescription medicines was estimated to be around £300 million per year, with up to half being avoidable (Trueman et al. 2010).

There is a discrepancy between medication that is prescribed and supplied and patients' drug usage. Since it is accepted that a high proportion of medication is prescribed via the repeat prescribing process, it is a logical conclusion that a proportion of prescribed medication is not used by patients.

There are a range of issues which may be revealed by involving the pharmacist in the repeat prescribing process (Box 16.4). The problems listed in Box 16.4 show why pharmacists' involvement in repeat prescribing can be important, particularly for older people, and the advent of ETP has made this easier. Such involvement has yet to become commonplace, although there are moves to support information technology integration between pharmacists and GPs, which will facilitate pharmacists being able to access GP notes to support medication review. Many pharmacists are already involved in home delivery services and provide Mew Medicines Services and Medicines Use Reviews, so they may have information about the older person's circumstances to contribute to the GP's knowledge of the person.

## Pharmacy Clinics in Non-Pharmacy Premises

The supply of medicines classed as either prescription-only medicines or pharmacy medicines is restricted to pharmacy premises. However, the provision of 'pharmaceutical advice' can occur from any site. For instance, pharmacists have occasionally offered 'clinic-like' services to older persons' day centres and the offices of charities for older people, such as Help the Aged. The advantage of such a service is that

> **BOX 16.4   POTENTIAL PROBLEMS IDENTIFIED BY PHARMACISTS MONITORING REPEAT PRESCRIBING**
>
> - Drug interactions: common when patients are receiving poly-pharmacy (a frequent problem with older people).
> - Drugs causing adverse effects: particularly prevalent among older people due to pharmacokinetic and pharmacodynamic changes resulting from the ageing process.
> - Medicines being ordered in inconsistent quantities: results in the patient or carer having to make unnecessary trips to the pharmacy to get supplies. This may cause particular problems for older patients with access problems.
> - Medicines labeled with inappropriate or inadequate directions: this may be an additional problem when a carer or carers are in charge of administration.
> - Medicines being prescribed which are no longer needed.

older people who have limited mobility can receive pharmaceutical information and advice from a location that they regularly visit. Although there is no remuneration available to pharmacists for the provision of such a service, the benefit is in the building up of goodwill and customer contact for the future.

## Pharmacy Telephone Helplines

The advantages of a telephone service to an older person who is unable to attend a pharmacy or a busy carer are obvious. Access to a health care professional without physically being present at the pharmacy can be beneficial. However, such a service is not financially viable for all community pharmacies, and therefore a dedicated telephone service is offered only in a few locations. Additionally, older patients seeking support through this mechanism may speak to a pharmacist who they do not know and who does not have access to their medication records. Many hospital medicines information services now provide a patient helpline for medicines for patients in their National Health Service Trust or locality.

## Services to Residential Homes

Since the mid-1980s, there has been a requirement in the UK for residential homes to be provided with the services of a named community pharmacist. For this, pharmacists receive an annual fee for the support they provide above and beyond the standard supply of prescribed medication. Pharmacists who serve residential homes must undergo specific accredited training prior to claiming a fee for these services. Each pharmacist determines the exact nature of the services delivered. Some of the most common services are outlined in Table 16.4.

The home staff and the pharmacist negotiate the precise nature of services to be provided. As it is a competitive market, pharmacies often lobby residential home

**TABLE 16.4**

**Range and Description of Services Pharmacists Provide to Residential Homes**

| Type of Service | Details of Service |
|---|---|
| Medication reviews | Pharmacists review the actual medication being prescribed by going through the home's records and offering advice to the staff accordingly. |
| Drug chart reviews | Pharmacists check the drug charts, looking for unusual dosages, drug interactions and drugs being administered on a long-term basis when not necessary. |
| Administration reviews | Pharmacists check through the home's administration records to advise staff of any administration issues which may be causing problems, such as eye drops being administered at inappropriate times or sedatives being given too early in the evening. |
| Medication storage review | Pharmacists review how medication is stored to ensure that drugs are stored under correct temperature and light conditions. They also check that the potential for drugs to be mixed up between patients is avoided. |
| General practitioner clinics | Pharmacists attend general practitioner consultations with residents in the homes and offer advice at the point of prescribing (similar to ward rounds in hospital environment). |
| Over-the-counter clinics | Pharmacists offer advice sessions to residents and staff to discuss over-the-counter medication. Purchases are not possible, but information and guidance is given. |
| Repeat prescription services | Pharmacists organize with home staff and the general practitioner surgery that they will take responsibility for the ordering and supply or repeat medications for residents. |
| Staff training | Pharmacists provide educational programmes for staff covering issues such as identifying side effects, correct administration procedures and common over-the-counter preparations. |

staff for their business, and it is up to the individual homes to choose the pharmacy that they feel will best suit their needs. This area of a pharmacist's service has become very competitive. Some pharmacies have specialized into providing these services and others have chosen not to offer such services.

## CONCLUSION

This chapter has drawn attention to the specific needs of older people in terms of medicine usage, identified people who may need more support and highlighted the potential for services in supporting these needs. This area of pharmacy service delivery is constantly being developed in response to research evidence. Furthermore, structural changes in health care delivery (e.g. the current emphasis on primary rather than secondary care specialized services) has created opportunities to develop new and innovative services.

## FURTHER READING

Audit Commission 1994. *A Prescription for Improvement: Towards More Rational Prescribing in General Practice*. London: HMSO.

Barber, N.D., Alldred, D.P., Raynor, D.K. et al. 2009. Care homes' use of medicines study: Prevalence causes and potential harm of medication errors in care homes for older people. *Quality and Safety in Health Care*, **18**, 341–346.

Barnett, N.L. and Oboh, L. 2008. Target old people with medication risks. *Pharmaceutical Journal*, **280**, 276.

Buetow, S.A., Sibbald, B., Cantrrill, J.A. and Halliwell, S. 1996. Prevalence of potentially inappropriate long term prescribing in general practice in the United Kingdom, 1980–96: Systematic literature review. *British Medical Journal*, **313**, 1371–1374.

Department of Health (England) 2001. National Service Framework for Older People. Available at: https://www.gov.uk/government/publications/quality-standards-for-care-services-for-older-people.

Department of Health (England) 2001. National Service Framework for Older People: Medicines and Older People. Available at: http://webarchive.nationalarchives.gov.uk/20130107105354/http://www.dh.gov.uk/prod_consum_dh/groups/dh_digitalassets/@dh/@en/documents/digitalasset/dh_4067247.pdf.

Goldstein, R. and Rivers, P. 1996. Informal carers medication role. *Health and Community Studies*, **4**, 142–149.

Goldstein, R., Rivers, P. and Close, P. 1993. Assisting elderly people with medication – The role of home carers. *Health Trends*, **25**, 135–139.

McDermott, D., Carter, P., Deshmukh, A., Carter, D. and Schofield, J. 1997. General practitioners' attitude to additional services by community pharmacists. *Pharmaceutical Journal*, **259**, R39.

Mental Welfare Commission for Scotland 2013. Good Practice Guide: Covert Medication. Available at: http://www.mwcscot.org.uk/media/140485/covert_medication_finalnov_13.pdf.

National Care Forum 2013. Medicines Safety Resources, Including: Making the Best Use of Medicines Across All Care Settings, Risk Assessment Tool for Medical Conditions and Medication. Available at: http://www.nationalcareforum.org.uk/medsafetyresources.asp.

National Institute for Health and Care Excellence 2009. Medicines Adherence CG 76. Available at: http://guidance.nice.org.uk/CG76.

National Institute for Health and Care Excellence 2014. Managing Medicines in Care Homes. Available at: http://www.nice.org.uk/guidance/sc/SC1.jsp.

Secretary of State for Health 1996. *Choice and Opportunity. Primary Care: The Future*. London: HMSO.

Social Care Institute for Excellence 2014. Assessing the Mental Health Needs of Older People: Mental Capacity. Available at: http://www.scie.org.uk/publications/guides/guide03/law/capacity.asp.

## REFERENCES

Barnett, N., Athwal, D. and Rosenbloom, R. 2011. Medicines-related admissions: You can identify patients to stop that happening. *Pharmaceutical Journal*, **286**, 471.

Barnett, N. and Seal, R. 2013. Medicines optimisations from principles to practice: Risk assessment tools. *Pharmaceutical Journal*, **291**, 49.

Barnett, N.L., Deham, M.J. and Francis, S.A. 2000. Over-the-counter medicines and the elderly. *Journal of the Royal College of Physicians of London* **34**, 445–446.

Duerden, M., Avery, T. and Payne, R. 2013. *Polypharmacy and Medicines Optimization: Making it Safe and Sound*. London: King's Fund.

General Practitioners Committee, NHS Employers and NHS England 2013. http://www. nhsemployers.org/~/media/Employers/Documents/Primary%20care%20contracts/ QOF/2015%20-%2016/2015%2016%20QOF%20guidance%20for%20stakeholders. pdf.

Goldstein, R., Rivers, P. and Close, P. 1993. Good quality pharmaceutical care – Implications for carers with elderly dependants. *International Journal of Pharmacy Practice*, **2**, 65–70.

Harris, C.M. and Dajda, R. 1996. The scale of repeat prescribing. *British Journal of General Practice*, **46**, 640–641.

Hepler, C.D. and Strand, L.M. 1990. Opportunities and responsibilities in pharmaceutical care. *American Journal of Hospital Pharmacy*, **47**, 533–543.

Rees, J.A., Collett, J.H. and Asher, D.M. 1993. Quantifying the costs of repeat prescribing on multiple item prescription forms. *Pharmaceutical Journal*, **251**, 636–638.

Rees, J.A., Collett, J.H. and Asher, D.M. 1995. Cumulative costs of inadvertent excess prescribing on multiple item prescription forms. *International Journal of Pharmacy Practice*, **3**, 209–212.

Rosenbloom, E.K. and Goldstein, F.R. 2007. The development of trigger questions to support the case finding of people with unmet medicines-management needs. *International Journal of Pharmacy Practice*, **15**, 21.

Royal Pharmaceutical Society 2013. Medicines Optimization: Helping Patients to Make the Most of Medicines. Good Practice Guidance for Healthcare Professionals in England. Available at: http://www.rpharms.com/promoting-pharmacy-pdfs/helping-patients-make-the-most-of-their-medicines.pdf

Schneider, J. and Barber, N. 1996. Provision of a domiciliary service by community pharmacists. *International Journal of Pharmacy Practice*, **4**, 19–24.

Trueman, P., Lowson, K., Blighe, A. et al. 2010. Evaluation of the Scale, Causes and Costs of Waste Medicines. York Health Economics Consortium and School of Pharmacy, University of London, London. Available at: http://eprints.pharmacy.ac.uk/2605/1/ Evaluation_of_NHS_Medicines_Waste__web_publication_version.pdf.

Woolf, M. 1996. *Residual Medicines: A Report on OPCS Omnibus Survey Data*. London: OPCS Social Survey Division, HMSO.

Zermansky, A.G. 1996. Who controls repeats? *British Journal of General Practice*, **46**, 643–647.

# 17 Pharmaceutical and Health Care Needs of People with Mental Health Problems

*Sally-Anne Francis*

## CONTENTS

---

### KEY POINTS

- Mental illness has been reported to be the most common single cause of disability adjusted life years lost in the Western World.
- People with long-term physical health conditions commonly also experience mental health problems, resulting in significantly poorer health outcomes and reduced quality of life.
- Factors which contribute to, and result from, mental health problems include family problems, childhood sexual abuse, domestic violence, stress, loss, social isolation and a variety of social and economic pressures.
- There is considerable stigma associated with mental health problems.

- For many severe mental health problems, drug therapy is the most common form of treatment, and patients have to cope with managing their medication and the potentially quite disabling adverse effects.
- Factors affecting non-adherence with medication include a patient's beliefs about their illness and perceived costs–benefits of treatment, cultural and ethnic influences, poor therapeutic relationship with professionals and compulsory admission to hospital.
- Pharmacists can help people's non-adherence to medication by providing information and advice, encouraging patients' involvement in prescribing decisions, liaising with members of the community mental health team to contribute to medication review, improving the continuity of supply and providing compliance aids.

## INTRODUCTION

Mental health problems are common in the general population. Approximately 450 million people worldwide have been estimated to have a mental health problem (World Health Organization 2001). Mental, emotional or psychological problems, many of which do not meet standardized criteria for diagnosable mental illness, together account for more disability than all physical health problems combined (Stewart-Brown and Layte 1997). Furthermore, many people with long-term physical health conditions also have mental health problems. These co-morbidities can lead to significantly poorer health outcomes and reduced quality of life (Naylor et al. 2012).

The Global Burden of Disease Study (2010) reported that while life expectancy has improved worldwide, disability is more prevalent. Mental disorders are responsible for little more than 1% of deaths, but account for almost 11% of the disease burden worldwide. Mental illness is the most common single cause of disability-adjusted life-years lost in the Western world (23%, compared to 16% each for cardiovascular disease and cancer) (Murray and Lopez 1996). Disability-adjusted life-years as an indicator of a population's health is discussed elsewhere (see Chapter 26).

Within the National Health Service in England, mental illness accounts for more than 12% of the total budget, and with respect to responding to future demands, it is anticipated that mental health services will have some significant challenges (McCrone et al. 2008) (Box 17.1).

## MENTAL HEALTH SERVICES AND POLICY

Mental health services available in the UK include primary care services (e.g. the general practitioner [GP], community nurse and community pharmacist), specialist services such as the community mental health team (structured locally according to local policies) and highly specialized hospital services. The primary care services provide the majority of mental health care. One in four of a GP's patients will need treatment for a mental health problem in primary care (Joint Commissioning Panel for Mental Health 2013).

**BOX 17.1    FUTURE SIGNIFICANT CHALLENGES
TO MENTAL HEALTH SERVICES**

- Increase in dementia and a rise in the population of older people.
- Greater need for help for people with mental health problems, as it is estimated that many people with needs are not in touch with services and therefore remain undiagnosed and untreated.
- Greater understanding of when and whether mental health promotion works in reducing the prevalence of mental illness.

Adapted from McCrone, P. et al. 2008. *Paying the Price. The Cost of Mental Health Care in England to 2026.* London: The King's Fund.

The most common mental health problems are depressive and anxiety disorders. The vast majority will be treated effectively in primary care; others will require referral to specialist services. Most people with severe mental health problems, such as schizophrenia, will be in contact with specialist services. Medication and psychological approaches are the most common forms of treatment used, either alone or in combination.

In Great Britain, GPs prescribe most psychotropic medications, and most moderate anxiety and depressive disorders are entirely and successfully managed in primary care using medication. A range of psychological treatments (e.g. cognitive behavioural therapy and anxiety management techniques) has also been shown to be effective in the treatment of mental health problems. Evidence indicates that this therapeutic approach is effective in relieving symptoms and improving functioning. While patients generally prefer psychological interventions, there is limited availability.

## POLICY GUIDANCE ON SERVICES FOR PEOPLE WITH MENTAL HEALTH PROBLEMS

In the UK, the shift of care for people with mental health problems from large institutions to the community started in the 1950s and was influenced by a number of factors (Box 17.2).

From the 1980s, there have been three distinct phases to the transformation of mental health services (Gilburt et al. 2014):

- A period of rapid de-institutionalization
- Development of comprehensive models of care (including care coordination and extended community services)
- Evolving service provision and delivery to meet local needs

Significantly, in 1999, the National Service Framework for Mental Health (Department of Health 1999) proposed a coordinated programme for improving mental health services. It set seven standards for the delivery and monitoring of mental health services. Standard 1 was concerned with mental health promotion, reducing the discrimination experienced by people with mental health problems and promoting social inclusion. Standards 2 and 3 addressed the identification,

**BOX 17.2   HISTORICAL INFLUENCES ON THE SHIFT TO COMMUNITY-BASED MENTAL HEALTH SERVICES**

- The less restrictive social climate of the 1960s and 1970s
- The exposure of poor conditions and standards of care in some of the large institutions
- Social psychiatry and the impact of psychosocial interventions
- The advent of drug therapy
- The (mistaken) political assumption that community care would be cheaper

Adapted from Lelliott, P. et al. 1997. *London's Mental Health. The Report of the King's Fund London Commission.* London: The King's Fund, pp. 33–44.

assessment and meeting the needs of individuals with mental health problems in primary care. Standards 4 and 5 focused on the care and needs of people with severe mental health problems. Standard 6 addressed the needs of individuals who provided care for people with severe mental health problems (carers). Standard 7 summarized the action required to meet a target reduction in suicide rates. Adoption and implementation of the core standards of the National Service Framework fostered a period of change during which major improvements to services for people with mental health problems across England occurred. Local requirements were considered and services were adapted to meet local needs.

More recent policy documents have led to the continued development of mental health services in terms of the structure of services and improving the physical health of people with mental health problems. More specifically, there has been enhanced access to psychological therapies, implementation of the National Institute for Health and Care Excellence-approved treatments for depressive and anxiety disorders and development of service provisions for older people, in particular for those with dementia.

## Living with Mental Health Problems

Many adverse factors seem to contribute to, and result from, mental health problems. These may be cumulative and may interact with genetic vulnerability. Such factors may include family problems, childhood sexual abuse, domestic violence, stress, loss, social isolation and a variety of social and economic pressures. Illicit drug taking and excessive intake of alcohol can exacerbate mental health problems.

Consistently, people with severe mental health problems and their relatives have reported preferring community to hospital care. However, one disadvantage of living in the community is the absence of social contacts. Other issues, such as coping with the potential stigma of mental health problems and acknowledging their illness, are also pertinent to individuals living in the community. For many severe mental health problems, drug therapy is the most common form of treatment and patients have to cope with managing their medications and their potentially quite disabling adverse effects. Consequently, current providers of care are challenged to develop suitable services in the community to address these concerns.

## Social Isolation

Many studies have illustrated the social isolation experienced by people with mental health problems living in the community and the subsequent association with a poor outcome. For example, isolation in the home, as well as poor housing, polluted neighbourhoods, crime and inadequate benefits, have been factors associated with depression and anxiety in women (Payne 1991). Many people with serious mental health problems experience disintegration of family relationships, but the greatest effects are evident with other social contacts. The size of social networks has been shown to diminish with continued readmissions to hospital.

## The Stigma of Mental Health Problems

Psychiatric illness can have a negative image, impacting considerably on the lives of people with mental health problems. Failure to understand the causes of mental health problems and the associated stigma can result in discrimination and social exclusion. Stigma is an aspect of a patient's self-conception represented by feelings that other people think less of them, avoid them or feel uneasy with them because of their illness (Hyman 1971). The social order defines stigma by imposing its values of what is deemed acceptable or deviant, and such criteria of stigma may vary over time and between cultures (Scambler 1984).

> Stigma is thus a social phenomenon that implies a person, an audience, and a set of powerful negative images that connect the two. There is no measurement procedure… that allows one to establish stigma and differentiate it from social undesirability. (Fabrega 1990)

Although discharge from hospital may remove an initial 'label', it still promotes the individual as having a psychiatric history. People with serious mental health problems living in the community who are socially isolated and do not have the opportunity for social interaction with others have limited means by which to rationalize the feelings of suspicion, hostility and anxiety that may develop.

Stigma is a major issue for those suffering mental health problems and their families (Box 17.3). A systematic review of the impact of mental health-related stigma

---

### BOX 17.3 THE STIGMA OF MENTAL HEALTH PROBLEMS

Wahl and Harman (1989) reported the results from a postal questionnaire survey of a self-help and advocacy organization of families of individuals with mental health problems. Over three-quarters of the respondents (77%) reported that the stigma of mental health problems affected their ill relative. The three most unfavourable consequences were to self-esteem, to the ability to make and keep friends and to success in acquiring a job. Perceived contributors to the stigma of mental health problems were most commonly reported as movies about mentally ill killers, news coverage of tragedies caused by mentally ill people and violence by mentally ill people. The authors concluded that there was consistent evidence that stigma was an enormous burden for the families of people with mental health problems, as well as to the sufferer him or herself.

on help-seeking behaviour found that stigma had a negative effect on seeking help and was a disproportionate deterrent for ethnic minorities, youth, men and those in military and health professions (Clement et al. 2014). When comparing the public stigma attitudes towards schizophrenia, depression and anxiety, it was found that stigma attitudes comprised the same three factors, irrespective of diagnostic label: negative stereotypes, patient blame and inability to recover. However, schizophrenia was significantly associated with the most negative stereotypes, was least blamed and was viewed as least likely to recover when compared to anxiety and depression (Wood et al. 2014).

## Medication Adherence

It has been estimated that up to 50% of patients are non-adherent with their oral anti-psychotic medication within a few months of discharge from hospital (Weiden and Olfson 1995). A double-blind controlled study also showed that patients with schizo-phrenia who defaulted on oral medication were also very likely to default on depot (intramuscular injections) medication and that both forms of maintenance medica-tion had similar rates of relapse (Falloon et al. 1978).

Adherence with antipsychotic medication is related to a patient's beliefs about their illness (insight) and the benefits of treatment (perceived decrease in symp-toms), personal variables such as culture and ethnic group, patient's experiences, severity of illness, attitudes to treatment, perceived costs of treatment (e.g. side effects), poor relationship between patient and professionals, compulsory admission to hospital and barriers to treatment (e.g. access or a lack of family/social support) (Perkins 2002).

Lewis (1934) rejected the assumption that those people with mental health prob-lems who had greater insight were more likely to accept treatment. In a long-term follow-up study of people with schizophrenia, McEvoy et al. (1989) found that patients who were supported by people with an interest in the patient's treatment were more likely to be medication adherent, whether or not they had insight (i.e. whether they perceived themselves as ill or not).

Non-adherence not only represents a patient that resists or lacks the motivation to accept the medication or treatment plan that a clinician offers, it may also represent the failure of the practitioner to offer an appropriate clinical intervention that allows a better therapeutic outcome for that individual (see Chapter 11). Non-adherence can be an expression of independence and a judgement about the utility of an intervention.

> The quality of one's life is a personally defined concept and so too are the reasons why a patient refuses to do what is recommended. Appropriate health behavior should be thought of as a behavior that meets the person's goals and achieves some mutually definable outcome (Liang 1989).

## MEETING THE NEEDS OF PEOPLE WITH MENTAL HEALTH PROBLEMS

Due to the heterogeneity within specific mental disorders, patients may present with widely different symptoms and may experience different outcomes despite the treat-ment prescribed. Therefore, treatment programmes need to be individualized for patients so that they receive the most appropriate care. When measuring the outcomes of drug therapy, Marder and May (1986) warned that using 'not relapsed' as an indicator of functioning in the community is unacceptable. Many patients experience severe impairment in the community due to personality and environmental influences which reflect the need for other therapeutic approaches alongside drug therapy (e.g. psychotherapy, vocational rehabilitation, family therapy and social skills training). They recommend that drugs should only be used where they are demonstrably effective for an individual and at the minimum effective dose. Psychosocial and pharmacological approaches used together have been shown to have cumulative effects.

Patients and their carers should be encouraged to be involved in their drug therapy and the role of medication, and the goals of treatment should be understood. Similarly, the limitations of drug therapy should be clearly explained (i.e. it does not always cure the illness and it does not necessarily alleviate psychosocial and interpersonal difficulties). Donoghue (1993) investigated the problems, concerns and needs that 81 patients with mental health problems experienced with their medicines while living in community settings. Most patients reported that they received inadequate information concerning their medicines, and that greater access to information would improve their confidence in their medicines. The most frequently cited sources of information were friends or other unqualified people. Patients had reservations concerning their medicines, and more than half reported having stopped their treatment in the past, most frequently because of adverse or unexpected effects that had affected their quality of life. It was recommended that pharmacists could address these needs through providing information and advice, promoting adherence to treatment, encouraging patients to become involved in prescribing decisions, liaising with members of the community mental health team to contribute to prescribing decisions and medication review, improving the continuity of supply, providing compliance aids where appropriate and providing information and support to patients and carers on obtaining, storing and the administration of medicines.

## Examples of Pharmacists Meeting the Needs of People with Mental Health Problems

Kettle et al. (1996) reported on the positive contributions of a pharmacist to the pharmaceutical care of patients as a member of a hospital-based community mental health team. Clinicians actioned 120 of the 185 recommendations made by the pharmacist during the 4-month project. The pharmacist also liaised between the carers of a supported residence and their community pharmacist, resulting in the introduction of compliance aids for residents' medications. The results of this project led to a change in the provision of clinical pharmacy services at the hospital, with pharmacists consequently participating as members of nine community mental health teams. This has involved these pharmacists taking on a number of roles (Box 17.4).

Watson (1997) reported on two local initiatives that had been designed and evaluated to address the pharmaceutical care needs for people discharged from psychiatric hospitals. During this study, community pharmacists completed a training programme prior to providing extended services. One of the most valued outcomes of this project was the advisory sessions held by pharmacists in mental health day centres. Taking the advisory role away from the pharmacy was perceived to have

> ## BOX 17.4    PHARMACISTS' ROLES AS MEMBERS OF
> ## THE COMMUNITY MENTAL HEALTH TEAM
>
> - Provision of drug information to all prescribers
> - Contributing to drug treatment plans and regular medication review
> - Liaison where appropriate with community pharmacists
> - Provision of information and training on drug-related issues to other health care professionals
> - Provision of information and counselling on medicines to individuals and their carers where appropriate

additional benefits. The pharmacist did not have to contend with distractions, more reticent members of the group could be encouraged to participate and people were less inhibited in their discussions. In addition, the pharmacist was viewed as 'independent' from the psychiatric team, which was deemed an additional advantage.

The above examples are local projects where enthusiastic pharmacists with a particular interest in meeting the needs of people with mental health problems have demonstrated the positive contributions that they can make to this patient group. However, evidence is limited on service models that may be implemented on a wider scale. Maslen et al. (1996) investigated the routine involvement of a sample of community pharmacists with people with schizophrenia and their perceived competence in advising this client group. Few pharmacists reported being routinely asked for medication-related advice. The pharmacists also reported being significantly less confident about advising patients with schizophrenia regarding their medication compared with other chronic illness groups, such as those with asthma, diabetes, hypertension, depression or drug addiction.

## DEVELOPING CURRENT SERVICES

Pharmacists have a major role in helping individuals with mental health problems and their families to understand their illness and its treatment and to enable individuals to seek local self-help groups (e.g. SANE, MIND, Depression Alliance, Rethink Mental Illness and Young Minds). The physical health of patients with mental health problems can also be poorer due to weight gain, cardiovascular disease, self-neglect, poor diet and high levels of smoking. Pharmacists have opportunities to offer further support and advice to address these physical health needs.

Maslen et al. (1996) acknowledged that while community pharmacists are likely to be in frequent contact with people having mental health problems, they are also likely to have received little formal education or training since registration that focuses on the treatment of people with mental health problems. In the UK, a College of Mental Health Pharmacy has been established, whose objective is to advance education and research in the practice of mental health pharmacy (www.cmhp.org. uk/). In 2010, the Royal Pharmaceutical Society of Great Britain published a mental health toolkit to support the integration of pharmacy into care pathways for mental health. It provides a framework to demonstrate the contribution of pharmacy to the care of people with mental illnesses as part of the wider health care team in community pharmacy, GP practices, hospitals or prison services. The key points of the toolkit focus on promoting mental health and well-being, communicating with people about mental health issues, improving medication adherence and supporting people at risk of suicide.

## CONCLUSION

Mental health problems contribute to a large proportion of the disease burden worldwide. The majority of people with mental health problems live in the community and are in contact with primary care services. The community pharmacist is one of the primary health care professionals in a position to contribute to the care of this client group. About one in ten people who consult their general practitioner with a mental health problem will be referred to specialist services, where specialist mental health pharmacists can further contribute to the care of this client group.

People living with mental health problems may have to contend with problems such as social isolation and stigma. Pharmacists can contribute to reducing the impact of these factors through forging positive relationships with this patient group. Medication is a common form of treatment for many people with mental health problems. Studies have demonstrated strategies that pharmacists may adopt to help this patient group with their medication, such as the provision of information and the opportunity for discussion to help people and their carers understand their medication and cope with adverse effects, monitoring of drug therapy and lifestyle advice to support their physical health needs.

## FURTHER READING

Department of Health 2009. *Living Well with Dementia: A National Dementia Strategy*. Available at: www.gov.uk/government/publications/living-well-with-dementia-a-national-dementia-strategy.

Department of Health 2011. *No Health Without Mental Health: A Cross-Government Mental Health Outcomes Strategy for People of All Ages*. Available at: www.gov.uk/government/publications/no-health-without-mental-health-a-cross-government-outcomes-strategy.

National Institute for Health and Care Excellence 2011. *Common Mental Health Disorders: Identification and Pathways to Care*. NICE guidelines 123. Available at: www.nice.org.uk/guidance/CG123.

National Institute for Health and Care Excellence 2011. *Quality Standard for Service User Experience in Adult Mental Health. NICE quality standards [QS14]*. Available at: www.nice.org.uk/guidance/qs14.

Royal Pharmaceutical Society of Great Britain 2010. *Mental Health Toolkit*. Available at: www.rpharms.com/support-resources-a-z/mental-health-toolkit.asp.

## REFERENCES

Clement, S., Schauman, O., Graham, T. et al. 2014. What is the impact of mental health-related stigma on help-seeking? A systematic review of quantitative and qualitative studies. *Psychological Medicine* **26**, 1–17.

Department of Health 1999. *A National Service Framework for Mental Health.* London: Department of Health.

Donoghue, J. 1993. Problems with psychotropic medicines in the community. *Pharmaceutical Journal,* **251**, 350–352.

Fabrega, H. 1990. Psychiatric stigma in the classical and medieval period: A review of the literature. *Comprehensive Psychiatry,* **31**, 289–306.

Falloon, I., Watt, D.C. and Shepherd, M. 1978. A comparative controlled trial of pimozide and fluphenazine decanoate in the continuation therapy of schizophrenia. *Psychological Medicine,* **8**, 59–70.

Gilburt, H., Peck, E., Ashton, B., Edwards, N. and Naylor, C. 2014. *Service Transformation: Lessons from Mental Health.* London: The King's Fund.

Global Burden of Disease Study 2010. 2012. *Lancet,* **380**(9859), 2095–2128.

Hyman, M.D. 1971. The stigma of stroke. *Geriatrics,* **26**, 132–141.

Joint Commissioning Panel for Mental Health 2013. Guidance for Commissioners of Primary Mental Health Care services. Available at: http://www.jcpmh.info/good-services/primary-mental-health-services/.

Kettle, J., Downie, G., Paln, A. and Chesson, R. 1996. Pharmaceutical care activities within a mental health team. *Pharmaceutical Journal,* **257**, 814–816.

Lelliott, P., Audini, B., Johnson, S. and Guite, H. 1997. London in the context of mental health policy. In: S. Johnson, R. Ramsay, G. Thornicroft et al. (Eds.), *London's Mental Health. The Report of the King's Fund London Commission.* London: The King's Fund, pp. 33–44.

Lewis, A.J. 1934. The psychopathology of insight. *British Journal of Medical Psychology,* **14**, 332–348.

Liang, M.H. 1989. Compliance and quality of life: Confessions of a difficult patient. *Arthritis Care and Research,* **2**, S71–S74 (Abstract).

Marder, S.R. and May, P.R.A. 1986. Benefits and limitations to neuroleptics – and other forms of treatment – in schizophrenia. *American Journal of Psychotherapy* **40**(3), 357–369.

Maslen, C.L., Rees, L. and Redfern, P.H. 1996. Role of the community pharmacist in the care of patients with chronic schizophrenia in the community. *International Journal of Pharmacy Practice,* **4**, 187–195.

McCrone, P., Dhanasiri, S., Patel, A., Knapp, M. and Lawton-Smith, S. 2008. *Paying the Price. The Cost of Mental Health Care in England to 2026.* London: The King's Fund.

McEvoy, J.P., Freter, S., Everett, G. et al. 1989. Insight and the clinical outcome of schizophrenic patients. *Journal of Nervous and Mental Disease,* **177**, 48–51.

Murray, C.J.L. and Lopez, A.D. (Eds.). 1996. *The Global Burden of Disease: A Comprehensive Assessment of Mortality and Disability from Diseases, Injuries and Risk Factors in 1990 and Projected to 2020: Summary.* Harvard: Harvard School of Public Health.

Naylor, C., Parsonage, M., McDaid, D., Knapp, M., Fossey, M. and Galea, A. 2012. *Long-Term Conditions and Mental Health. The Cost of Co-Morbidities.* London: The King's Fund and Centre for Mental Health.

Payne, S. 1991. *Women, Health and Poverty.* London: Harvester Wheatsheaf.

Perkins, O. 2002. Predictors of noncompliance in patients with schizophrenia. *Journal of Clinical Psychiatry,* **63**, 1121–1128.

Scambler, G. 1984. Perceiving and coping with stigmatizing illness. In: R. Fitzpatrick, J. Hinton, S. Newman, G. Scambler, and J. Thompson (Eds.). *The Experience of Illness.* London: Tavistock Publications, pp. 203–226.

Stewart-Brown, S. and Layte, R. 1997. Emotional health problems are the most important cause of disability in adults of working age. *Journal of Epidemiology and Community Health,* **51**, 672–675.

Wahl, O.F. and Harman, C.R. 1989. Family views of stigma. *Schizophrenia Bulletin,* **15**, 131–139.

Watson, P.J. 1997. Community pharmacists and mental health: An evaluation of two pharmaceutical care programmes. *Pharmaceutical Journal*, **257**, 419–422.

Weiden, P.J. and Olfson, M. 1995. Cost of relapse in schizophrenia. *Schizophrenia Bulletin*, **21**, 419–429.

Wood, L., Birtel, M., Alsawy, S., Pyle, M. and Morrison, A. 2014. Public perceptions of stigma towards people with schizophrenia, depression and anxiety. *Psychiatry Research*, **220**, 604–608.

World Health Organization 2001. *The World Health Report 2001 – Mental Health: New Understanding, New Hope*. Geneva: World Health Organization.

# 18 Pharmaceutical and Health Care Needs of Ethnic Groups

*Mohamed Aslam, Farheen Jessa and John Wilson*

## CONTENTS

---

**KEY POINTS**

- There are distinct variations in mortality and morbidity between ethnic minority groups and the indigenous population.
- Pharmacists should identify subgroups with particular health needs and communication difficulties and modify the way health advice is disseminated accordingly.
- All cultures have a system of health beliefs that explain how illness occurs and can be treated.
- Ethnic groups may demonstrate pluralistic patterns of health care consumption.
- Pharmacists should be aware of the theory and practices of Ayurvedic and Unani medicines.
- Pharmacists should be aware of when Ramadan commences and finishes.
- Fasting during Ramadan may have an effect on specific disease states and drug adherence.

---

## INTRODUCTION

Ethnicity refers to variations in the human species created by the interplay of geography and heredity. Each ethnic group can be defined as a social group with a distinctive language, values, religion, customs and attitudes (Hillier 1991). In the United Kingdom, there are a wide range of these groups, including Turks, Greeks, Irish, Jews and West Indians. But those groups with a significant number of people include Chinese (mainly from Hong Kong), African–Caribbean and large numbers originating from the various countries of the Indian subcontinent, including Hindus, Sikhs and Muslims. For the purposes of this chapter, the term 'Asian' will be used to cover people originating from India, Pakistan, Bangladesh and East Africa.

The problems of complying with/adhering to a medication regime are common, and not specific to ethnic minorities. However, within this group, culture and religious faith, as well as literacy problems, are additional factors which may affect adherence. Culture refers to a group's religious values, attitudes, rituals, family structure, language and social structure (Rothschild 1981). In order to deliver optimal pharmaceutical care, pharmacists need to be aware of patients' cultures and religions, as well as their medical conditions. Cultural differences can affect perceptions of illness, treatment-seeking behaviour and responses to health care. This chapter will discuss the pharmaceutical implications of some religious and cultural beliefs, an understanding of which will help pharmacists respect the unique needs of clients from ethnic minorities and provide a more appropriate service. Failure to respect or be aware of these differences may well result in a failure of medications.

## ETHNIC DIFFERENCES IN DISEASE MORBIDITY AND MORTALITY

Epidemiological studies have shown that there are distinct variations in mortality and morbidity between ethnic minority groups and the indigenous population due to their different genetic and cultural backgrounds, suggesting different health service needs. For instance, Asians and African–Caribbeans have relatively high mortality rates for strokes and hypertension. Diabetes is very high in immigrants from the Indian subcontinent, while Asian women are at higher risk of osteoporosis. These are a few examples of which there are many more. Marmot (1989) suggests that:

> These variations may occur due to a variety of reasons; the conclusion may be that we should pay great attention to the social and economic position of immigrants but these are unlikely to be the only factors that determine their pattern of disease.

By focusing on cultural/lifestyle features, there is the prospect for enhancing the understanding of disease aetiology and for disease prevention. Social, cultural and dietary customs, for example, may directly contribute to some of the diseases suffered by Asians, such as rickets and osteomalacia. There are also instances where morbidity and mortality among an ethnic minority are lower than the national average. Inflammatory bowel disease, for example, is rare among Indian migrants, while multiple sclerosis is rare among migrants from Asia and Africa to Great Britain.

In the UK, the government's concerns about disadvantages which may affect all racial minority groups were acknowledged in a report in which the government set out to aim for an improvement in the rights and standards available to all patients: '... all health services should make provision so that ... your privacy, dignity, religious and cultural beliefs are respected' (Department of Health 1991). Additionally, the Commission for Racial Equality's (1992) Code of Practice in Primary Healthcare Services urged community pharmacists to ensure that services are delivered in a way that is both appropriate and accessible to ethnic minorities. Pharmacists therefore require an awareness of the ethnic population(s) they serve, together with an epidemiological grounding in the culturally diverse patterns of disease.

## PROVIDING CULTURALLY SENSITIVE HEALTH ADVICE

### THE PUBLIC'S PERCEPTION OF THE PHARMACIST

Ethnic minorities' expectations of health care may influence their use of pharmaceutical services. Those originating from countries with little access to Western-style medicine may, for instance, not regard the pharmacist as an appropriate source of health care advice. In order to try and overcome this, promotional campaigns are required to inform ethnic minorities of the pharmacist's advisory function.

LANGUAGE AND COMMUNICATION

Pharmacists should identify subgroups with particular health needs or communication difficulties. Literacy rates and dialects vary between ethnic groups, and hence will affect the types of problems experienced in providing a pharmaceutical service to those groups. The problem of communication could be addressed by employing staff from the local community.

Some people from ethnic minority groups may not be able to read English. Those who have difficulty in English usually also have difficulties in reading their 'mother' language. However, it is equally important to realize that a leaflet written in English is likely to be understood by at least one member of the family, even if the patient is unable to read it. Therefore, it is better to provide a leaflet written in English rather than none at all.

Providing translated material from the pharmacy requires careful consideration because of the large number of languages which may be spoken by ethnic groups. Leaflets written in English generally relate to the indigenous lifestyle and do not translate readily to meet the specific needs of ethnic minorities. To overcome the language and cultural barriers that are present in existing health promotion requires the production and dissemination of culturally sensitive and linguistically appropriate materials. Such materials should be made readily available to health and community workers and also distributed to community and religious centres. They might also include web-based resources, podcasts, etc., in addition to printed material.

An alternative approach to disseminating health advice is the use of suitable media coverage such as Asian satellite television and radio or magazines and newspapers read by ethnic minorities, which routinely feature items on health issues.

USE OF FAMILY AND FRIENDS

Pharmacists may be able to marshal family and friends in promoting pharmaceutical care among ethnic groups' health. A pregnant woman, for instance, will receive a lot of support from other members of her family, especially her mother, mother-in-law or an equivalent elder, who will feel that it is their responsibility to advise the younger woman about pregnancy.

Folic acid consumption by women pre-conception and in the first trimester of pregnancy is recommended to reduce neural tube defects in infants, a condition particularly prevalent among infants of mothers born in Pakistan and India. Instead of targeting only child-bearing women, pharmacists would be wise to include family members when giving health education and promotional advice. By informing the mother-in-law or husband, for example, about the importance of folic acid, the patient can be actively encouraged to follow the advice provided.

## TRADITIONAL SYSTEMS OF HEALTH CARE

All cultures have a system of health beliefs that explains how illness occurs, how it can be treated or cured and who should be involved in the healing process. Sensitivity to patients' health beliefs and cultural differences is important in delivering health care. Traditional medicine and its preparations and practices play major roles in the health care of the ethnic community. Strong ties to the traditional diets and religions brought from the mother country remain. Not surprisingly, comparable ties exist for health care and medicine. Ethnic minorities demonstrate pluralistic patterns of health care consumption. That is, the traditional health beliefs are integrated with those of the indigenous health care system. For example, consumers from ethnic minorities may adopt over-the-counter medication. However, the same consumers simultaneously maintain many of the cultural health beliefs of the culture of origin, such as the use of traditional remedies for ailments.

In many parts of the world, the only health care available to people is provided by traditional healers. Many groups of people now living in the UK retain their beliefs in traditional medicine to varying degrees, regarding it as an integral part of their culture, affecting diet and social behaviour (see also Chapter 7).

## TRADITIONAL MEDICINE FROM THE INDIAN SUBCONTINENT

The indigenous system of medicine in India is called the Ayurvedic system, while in Pakistan it is known as Unani-Tibb, or Unani for short. Both systems of medicine employ crude herbal drugs and these are normally administered in the form of pills, syrups, confectionery or alcoholic extracts. Ayurvedic medicine is solely of Hindu origin, while Unani derives from Ancient Greece, and that which is practised today has been influenced by Persian, Egyptian and African medicine.

The central figure in both systems of medicines is the traditional healer known as the Hakim. There are also associated pharmacopoeias akin to the British and European pharmacopoeias. The Hamdard pharmacopoeia, for example, lists over 3,000 different preparations supplied by a flourishing pharmaceutical industry based on traditional medicine.

## THE PHILOSOPHICAL BACKGROUND OF ASIAN MEDICINE

It is important that pharmacists are aware of the theory of Ayurvedic and Unani medicine. This section illustrates the importance of knowing about patients' belief systems in facilitating communication and support between the patient and health professional, which in turn enhances patients' confidence in their treatment.

### Ayurvedic System

The basis of all treatments in the Ayurvedic system is the balancing of the life energies within a person. It uses meditation as a primary and fundamental tool and also employs diets, mineral substances, aromas and herbs. The components that are used in Ayurveda do not originate from scientific concepts or experiments but from 'direct observation' of nature. There are five elements of Ayurveda; ether, air, water, fire and earth. These are meant to communicate the essential universal principle that is inherent in a particular element.

### Unani System

The basis of the Unani system is humoral pathology, in which the four main humours of the body – blood, mucus and yellow and black bile – are combined with the four primary qualities – warmth (or heat), cold, moisture (or dampness) and dryness. Thus, the humours are categorized as blood (damp and hot), mucus (damp and cold), yellow bile (dry and hot) and black bile (damp and cold). If the humours are in equilibrium, the person is healthy. If, however, one becomes dominant, then the equilibrium is disturbed, resulting in illness. Thus, by conserving the symmetry in a patient's life and maintaining the humoral balance, health is protected. The role of the Hakim is to teach the patient how to conserve or restore symmetry.

The Chinese believe in a similar 'yin–yang' theory in that *yin* stores vital strength inside the body while *yang* protects the outside and corresponds to the surface of the body. Diseases occur when there is an imbalance between *yin* and *yang*, and the fundamental principle, once again, is to restore balance and harmony.

## CONFLICTS WITH ALLOPATHIC MEDICINE (HOT/COLD THEORY CONFLICT)

The hot/cold imbalance appears prominently across various different cultures (e.g. Chinese and Asian). It emphasizes the importance of temperament and the humours and places great emphasis on the concept of hot and cold applied to medicines, herbs and food. This does not refer to the temperature of the material. Broadly, hot foods are those that are rich in protein, while cold foods are rich in vitamin C. In these traditional systems, all foods and medicines are classified according to their particular qualities as hot or cold and damp or dry, to varying degrees.

Treatment of disease with the Unani and Chinese medical systems is dependent on the principle that a hot disease is cured by a cold remedy, damp diseases require dry preparations, and so on. This concept brings conflict with allopathic medicine, as in Unani and Ayurvedic practice, it is believed that most Western medicines are 'hot' and therefore inappropriate for hot illnesses. Pregnancy, for example, is a 'hot' condition and, therefore, in pregnancy, one should not eat too many 'hot' foods. It would therefore be considered inappropriate to take 'hot' medicines during pregnancy. This could contribute to poor adherence with, for example, folic acid tablets taken before and during pregnancy, or iron preparations.

A similar philosophy is applied to disease states. In the absence of disease, the body humours are considered to be in balance; any disturbance in this balance results in morbidity. Some diseases are of 'hot' temperament (e.g. kidney ailments and warts). The body's balance is restored and the illness cured by the ingestion of medicine or food of the opposite temperament.

Both the Unani and Ayurvedic systems of treatment are now available in Great Britain. In Great Britain, the majority of Hakims, although offering a service to the Asian community, have no formal qualifications to practise. The holistic approach and the sympathetic ear are of undoubted psychological benefit, and some remedies do appear to work. Patients of alternative healers tend to rate highly the interpersonal skills of these healers and report a better healer–patient relationship (Ahmad 1992). Unfortunately, the benefits can often be outweighed by the potential hazards; therefore, it seems that before the positive benefits of traditional healers can be appreciated, the detrimental consequences of their practices must first be eliminated by imposing strict controls.

## HAZARDS OF TRADITIONAL PRACTICE

Pharmacists providing a service for ethnic minorities should be aware of traditional health concepts and their possible problems and associated dangers.

### Dual Treatment

Patients may be receiving dual treatment from both their Western medical doctor and their traditional healer. If they are given the same drug by both, this can lead to problems such as overdose.

### Toxicity

There have been cases of poisoning associated with the use of Chinese herbal remedies due to the ingestion of aconitine, anticholinergic agents and podophyllin. There is also a potential risk of exposure to heavy metals. Minerals such as gold, silver, tin, mercury, lead and arsenic are commonly used in Asian medicine in uncontrolled quantities (e.g. metal-containing or -coated pills known as kushtay are taken by adult Asian males for sexual dysfunction and are supposed remedies for psycho-sexual problems). Although there is no direct evidence for adverse reactions to the use of these materials, it is clear that the ingestion of materials containing several percent by weight of arsenic, mercury, lead and other heavy metals cannot be beneficial.

### Drug Interactions

Interactions may occur between Western drugs and the biologically active substances present in traditional medicines. An example of this is the fruit karela (*Momordica charantia*), which is used in curries, but is also used by the Hakim to lower blood sugar. It can interact with chlorpropamide and may produce hypoglycaemia in an otherwise stabilized diabetic patient.

### Adherence

Patients may be poorly adherent if prescribed a Western drug that is not compatible with the traditional concept of disease (e.g. pregnant women and 'hot' medicines).

### Adulteration

Western medicines may be present in uncontrolled quantities in 'traditional' remedies. Adulteration of Chinese herbal remedies with synthetic substances has also been reported.

## RAMADAN

During the month of Ramadan, the ninth month of the Islamic year, all adult Muslims are expected to fast between the hours of sunrise and sunset. The actual date for the commencement of this fast varies from year to year depending on the phase of the moon. During this period, all food and drink and, except in special cases, all medicines are excluded. When fasting, no food or water is consumed and smoking is prohibited. No medicines of the following forms are used: oral medications, injections, ear and nose drops, pessaries or suppositories and inhalations. Following sunset, the family meet together and the fast is broken with a light snack and a lot of fluid, often fizzy drinks.

After about 20 minutes, prayers are said and a large main meal, *'Iftar'*, is served. A further light meal, *'Suhur'*, is eaten early in the morning before dawn prayers, after which the fast continues until the evening. Fasting involves major changes in the pattern of physical activity and sleep patterns, as well as an alteration in the normal pattern of intake of food and fluid.

The Quran (the Muslims' holy book) says that health is promoted by fasting. Complete fasting is seen as a way of combining spiritual, physical and individual needs, while at the same time establishing a greater awareness of God, self-discipline and an empathy with the poor and needy.

Those who have acute or chronic diseases are exempt from the fast as well as menstruating, pregnant or lactating women. Individuals travelling long distances would be expected to make up the fast at a later date. Children and the elderly may or may not be expected to fast, depending on their age and health. Normally, children do not fast until they reach the age of puberty. Some devout Muslims still fast despite their pregnancies and ill health. Abstaining from fasting is difficult when the rest of the family observes the fast, due to feelings of isolation or social pressure to keep the fast.

In people who are fit and well, the fast seems to create no particular difficulties and the body's normal homeostatic mechanisms will usually cope. Urinary volume, electrolytes, pH and nitrogen excretion tend to remain within normal limits. Some studies, however, have indicated that some biological functions do change. Arousal, vigilance and memory may decrease during Ramadan, especially during the first few days. Studies of hormonal changes have given inconsistent results. Hakkou et al. (1994) concluded that even though Ramadan has been practised for 14 centuries and is followed by perhaps one billion people worldwide, there have been few well-conducted studies on its impact on health and disease.

## EFFECT OF RAMADAN ON SPECIFIC DISEASE STATES

Fasting during Ramadan has particular implications for health care workers, since in some cases fasting can result not only in general lethargy, but also in problems with drug adherence (Box 18.1). This highlights the need for pharmacists' awareness of the particular needs of these patients during this month.

---

### BOX 18.1   PROBLEMS OF DRUG COMPLIANCE AND LETHARGY DURING RAMADAN

A study of accident and emergency attendances showed a significant increase in the number of Muslims attending during Ramadan compared to non-Muslims (Langford et al. 1994). It was suggested that this increase was due to non-compliance and general fatigue resulting from fasting, leading to a lowered threshold for help-seeking advice.

**BOX 18.2    THE EFFECT OF FASTING ON PEPTIC ACID DISEASE**

Endoscopic examination conducted in the Kashmir Valley, an area with a prevalence of 4.7% for peptic ulcers, showed that it was not uncommon for patients to have both duodenal and gastric ulcers (Malik et al. 1995). During Ramadan of 1995, patients with peptic ulceration were instructed to take ranitidine twice daily, at '*Suhur*' and at '*Iftar*'. While patients with acute duodenal ulcers showed signs of healing during Ramadan, those with chronic peptic ulcers did not. Indeed, several patients with chronic peptic ulcers suffered bleeds during the study period. Ramadan fasting was concluded to be hazardous to patients with acid peptic diseases in general and those with chronic peptic ulcers in particular.

## GASTROINTESTINAL DISORDERS

Fasting would logically be expected to cause problems for patients with peptic acid diseases, particularly ulceration (Box 18.2).

## ASTHMA

Studies have shown that there are no chronobiological effects on the pharmacokinetics of sustained-release preparations of theophylline (Box 18.3).

## DIABETES

There have been a number of studies on the effects of fasting among diabetic patients (Box 18.4).

**BOX 18.3    PLASMA CONCENTRATIONS OF THEOPHYLLINE DURING FASTING**

Cherrah et al. (1990) showed that the area under the plasma concentration time curve and maximum plasma concentration for sustained-release theophylline (Armophylline-R) did not vary significantly with the time of administration, indicating that the drug could be taken outside daylight hours and still provide asthmatic control. In a study of a small group of men with stable asthma who wished to fast, sustained-release theophylline (Euphyllin CR) was given before dawn (0300 hours) (Daghfous et al. 1994). Blood samples taken over five days following dosing indicated considerable inter-patient variability. However, for individual patients, there was no significant difference between plasma concentration during and following Ramadan fasting. The study concluded that asthmatic patients could be allowed to fast if they were stabilized on a sustained-release theophylline preparation.

## BOX 18.4   THE EFFECTS OF FASTING IN DIABETIC PATIENTS

Salman et al. (1992) observed 21 insulin-dependent diabetic children aged between 9 and 14 years during Ramadan fasting. Doses of insulin were carefully adjusted and the insulin was given before both the evening meal and the pre-dawn meal. There were no significant complications and none of the patients developed symptomatic hypoglycaemia, indicating that Ramadan fasting is feasible in older and longstanding diabetic children and does not alter short-term metabolic control. Nevertheless, fasting should only be encouraged in children with good glycaemic control whose blood glucose levels are regularly monitored at home.

One study has concluded that most adult patients with type 2 diabetes can fast (Beshyah et al. 1990), but it is necessary to increase the dosage of hypoglycaemic medication in the evening to combat hyperglycaemia and reduce it in the morning to prevent hypoglycaemia. However, other studies have reported considerable problems with diabetic control during the fast (Tang and Rolfe 1989), while Barber and Wright (1979) found no convincing evidence to suggest that it is safe for all Muslims with diabetes to fast.

## Pregnancy and Breast-Feeding

Pregnant women who fast have lower glucose and insulin concentrations and higher triglyceride levels at the end of Ramadan. Women who fast during breastfeeding lose on average 7.6% total body fluids during the day and the milk concentrations of lactose, sodium and potassium are changed (Rashed 1992).

Pregnant, breastfeeding and menstruating women are exempt from fasting during Ramadan. However, they are often unaware of these exemptions. If informed of these exemptions, evidence suggests they choose not to fast (Reeves 1992).

## Drug Adherence and Ramadan

### Cessation of Therapy

Complying with prescribed medications may present problems during Ramadan, and evidence suggests that the majority of patients will modify their treatment (Aslam and Assad 1986), while some will stop medication completely or take all of their doses in a single intake (Aslam and Healy 1986). Stopping medication completely is potentially dangerous; for example, epileptic attacks have been reported in patients who ceased their medication while fasting (Aslam and Wilson 1992). Likewise, patients with chronic respiratory disease, normally managed with steroids and bronchodilators, have been admitted into intensive care as a result of not taking their medication during daylight hours (Wheatly and Shelly 1993).

### Change in Dosage Intervals

If doses are omitted during daylight hours, there is an increased likelihood that patients on multiple therapies will take medications together in a single dose, increasing the risk of drug interactions. As the plasma half-life is unaffected by dose size, the time period for which the blood concentration is above the minimum effective level will increase if multiple doses are taken together, while toxic adverse effects may be produced. To overcome this, sustained-release preparations are preferable, as they produce the required therapeutic effect without excessively high blood concentrations, which may lead to adverse effects. Similarly, drugs with a long half-life in the body will have a longer action and can therefore be taken less frequently. For instance, the non-steroidal anti-inflammatory drugs vary in half-life from 2 to 3 hours for ibuprofen, up to 36 to 38 hours for piroxicam.

## Antacids

Gastrointestinal disorders, ranging from constipation to peptic ulcers, are frequently treated by antacids. However, if during Ramadan they are taken immediately after breaking the fast with large quantities of milk or directly after the main meal, their efficacy will be substantially impaired.

## Fruit Juices and Carbonated Drinks

The large quantities of orange juice and carbonated drinks consumed at the conclusion of the fast may affect the bioavailability and pharmacokinetics of a number of drugs. Such drinks have a markedly acidic pH, in the order of 2–4. Consumption of large quantities of these of up to a litre at a time will affect the pH of the gastrointestinal tract, which may in turn interfere with the dissolution of enteric-coated (gastro-resistant) preparations, such as prednisolone, and affect the action of antibiotics such as erythromycin base and ampicillin. The activity of such antibiotics may also be reduced as they are frequently taken with meals during Ramadan.

## Pharmacists' Role in Patient Adherence during Ramadan

The implications of Ramadan for pharmacy and patient health are valid throughout the Muslim world. Pharmacists require an awareness of the potential difficulties Ramadan poses with respect to prescribed medication regimens. Pharmacists have a key role, not only in counselling patients on their medication and to ensure patient adherence to dosage regimens, but also in recommending to prescribers products such as slow-release preparations and drugs with longer half-lives, which enable continued treatment while fasting.

Faced with a fasting patient for whom one has just dispensed a medicine with a frequent dosing schedule, what does one do? Many patients will wish to fast even though they are technically exempt, and attempts to persuade them to break their fast by taking the medication may well prove futile. In such a situation, the pharmacist could, in addition to informing the patient's general practitioner, have recourse to religious advice from the local mosque.

## INFORMATION RESOURCES

Pharmacists should be aware of Muslim patients' informational needs during Ramadan. This requires an awareness of when Ramadan starts and finishes each year. This information can be obtained from the local mosque, along with the exact timings that the fast starts and finishes for each day for the whole month. Larger mosques, like Christian cathedrals, are fully staffed during office hours, and a mullah would be pleased to offer advice to pharmacists and patients. Information for pharmacists is also available on the Internet, for instance: http://psnc.org.uk/swindon-and-wiltshire-lpc/wp-content/uploads/sites/62/2013/07/pharmacy_guide_to_ramadan.pdf.

Given the implications of Ramadan to patient health, we believe that the start and finish dates of Ramadan could also usefully be published in appropriate medical and pharmaceutical journals.

## CONCLUSION

The concept of pharmaceutical care requires pharmacists to assume responsibility for ensuring optimal therapeutic outcomes for patients. To achieve this requires the flexibility to respond to patients' individual needs, which in turn requires pharmacists to be aware of the multicultural population they serve, promoting appropriate use of medicines.

A cultural and religious sensitivity is central to the adoption by pharmacists of a holistic model of primary care encompassing health promotion, health maintenance and disease prevention. Misunderstandings stemming from differences in language or cultural perspectives can result in suboptimal care and poor therapeutic outcomes.

## ACKNOWLEDGEMENT

Since publication of the first edition of this book, Mo Aslam sadly died. In his professional career, he was recognized for his enormous contribution to furthering the understanding of Asian medicine by pharmacists and pharmacy students. He is greatly missed by his many friends and colleagues.

## REFERENCES

Ahmad, W.I.U. 1992. The maligned healer. The 'Hakim' and Western medicine. *New Community*, **18**, 521–536.

Aslam, M. and Assad, A. 1986. Drug regimens and fasting during Ramadan: A survey in Kuwait. *Public Health*, **100**, 49–53.

Aslam, M. and Healy, M.A. 1986. Compliance and drug therapy in fasting Muslim patients. *Journal of Clinical and Hospital Pharmacy*, **11**, 321–325.

Aslam, M. and Wilson, J.V. 1992. Medicines, health and the fast of Ramadan. *Journal of the Royal Society of Health*, **112**, 135–136.

Barber, S.G. and Wright, A.D. 1979. Muslims, Ramadan and diabetes mellitus. *British Medical Journal*, **2**, 675.

Beshyah, S.A., Jowett, N.I. and Burden, A.C. 1990. Metabolic control during Ramadan fasting. *Practical Diabetes*, **9**, 54–55.

Cherrah, Y., Aadil, N., Bennis, A. et al. 1990. Influence of the time of administration on the pharmacokinetics of an SR preparation of theophylline during Ramadan. *European Journal Pharmacology*, **183**, 2122.

Commission for Racial Equality 1992. *Race Relations Code of Practice in Primary Health Care Services*. London: Commission for Racial Equality.

Daghfous, J., Beji, M., Louzir, B. et al. 1994. Fasting in Ramadan, the asthmatics and sustained release theophylline. *Annals of Saudi Medicine*, **14**, 523.

Department of Health 1991. *The Patients' Charter: Raising the Standard*. London: HMSO.

Hakkou, F., Tazi, A. and Iraki, L. 1994. Conference report Ramadan health and chronobiology. *Chronobiology International*, **11**, 340–342.

Hillier, S. 1991. The health and health care of ethnic minority groups. In: G. Scrambler (Ed.), *Sociology as Applied to Medicine*. London: Bailiere Tindall, 135–147.

Langford, E.J., Ishaque, M.A., Fothergill, J. and Touquet, R. 1994. The effect of the fast of Ramadan on accident and emergency attendances. *Journal of the Royal Society of Medicine*, **87**, 752–761.

Malik, G.M., Mubarik, M. and Hussain, T. 1995. Acid peptic disease in relation to Ramadan fasting: A preliminary endoscopic evaluation. *American Journal of Gastroenterology*, **90**, 2076–2077.

Marmot, M.G. 1989. General approaches to migrant studies: The relation between disease, social class and ethnic origin. In: J.K. Cruickshank and D.G Beevers (Eds.), *Ethnic Factors in Health and Disease*, London: Wright, 12–17.

Rashed, A.H. 1992. The fast of Ramadan. *British Medical Journal*, **304**, 521–522.

Reeves, J. 1992. Pregnancy and fasting during Ramadan. *British Medical Journal*, **304**, 843–844.

Rothschild, H. (Ed.) 1981. *Biocultural Aspects of Disease*. New York: Academic Press.

Salman, H., Abdallah, M.A., Abanamy, M. and Al Howasi, M. 1992. Ramadan fasting in diabetic children in Riyadh. *Diabetic Medicine*, **9**, 583–584.

Tang, C. and Rolfe, M. 1989. Clinical problems during fast of Ramadan. *Lancet*, **1**, 1396.

Wheatly, R.S. and Shelly, M.P. 1993. Drug treatment during Ramadan. Stopping bronchodilator treatment is dangerous. *British Medical Journal*, **307**, 801.

# 19 Pharmaceutical and Health Care Needs of Injecting Drug Users

*Janie Sheridan and Jenny Scott*

## CONTENTS

**KEY POINTS**

- Pharmacists should have a knowledge of the relevant services and an understanding of the structure and role of local services for injecting drug users.
- The provision of sterile injecting equipment to injecting drug users from community pharmacies is now recognized internationally as an important aspect of harm reduction.
- Psychoactive drugs, such as opiates and stimulants, have a number of drug interactions, some of which could increase the risk of overdose.
- There is a high incidence of psychological problems among injecting drug users which may be associated with the drug itself or where drug use may exacerbate a pre-existing psychological disorder.
- Prescribing doctors may require prescribed daily doses of methadone or buprenorphine to be consumed under the supervision of a pharmacist on the pharmacy premises.
- Traditional prescribing services for opiate users are unlikely to be appropriate for those injecting performance and image-enhancing drugs, though the sharing of injecting equipment or multi-dose vials carry an equal risk of blood-borne viruses to that for illicit drug users.

## INTRODUCTION

Community pharmacists usually encounter a relatively narrow spectrum of the drug-using population. By the nature of the services that they provide, they tend to see either people being dispensed medication to assist them to stop using illicit drugs, usually opiates, or people seeking sterile injecting equipment. However, not all illicit drug use leads to problematic drug use and dependence. The use of heroin and cocaine is, however, particularly associated with dependence. Injecting drug users (IDUs) face particular health risks and social problems. Additionally, they may be reluctant to access treatment or services. This can put pharmacists who operate needle and syringe programmes (NSPs) in a unique position, where they have regular contact with this hard-to-reach, vulnerable group. The provision of sterile injecting equipment is in itself an effective intervention to prevent blood-borne virus (BBV) spread. Additional advice and care can reduce or manage injecting-related complications, such as skin and soft-tissue infections. Signposting to specialist treatment services or general practitioners can lead to large reductions in risk to the individual and benefits for the wider public, especially through crime reduction. This chapter is focused on information for pharmacists to inform the delivery of effective pharmacy services for IDUs. Best practice guidance, updated in 2014, is published by the National Institute for Health and Care Excellence (NICE) in England (PH52).

In recent years, there has been a decline in illicit drug use in England. Data from 2010/11 suggested that the number of heroin and crack cocaine users fell below 300,000 for the first time since measurement began in 1996. The number of people injecting drugs also fell from 129,977 in 2005/06 to 93,401 in 2010/11.

## TABLE 19.1
## Health Care Issues of Injecting Drug Users

| Health Care Issues of Injecting Drug Users | Examples |
| --- | --- |
| Those which arise out of the route of drug administration (injecting) | Those relating to blood-borne viruses (e.g. human immunodeficiency virus and hepatitis) |
| | Venous and arterial damage causing vascular insufficiency |
| Those which are related to the drug being used or its microbiological or chemical contaminants | Skin and soft-tissue infections (e.g. abscesses and cellulitis) |
| | Granulomas (e.g. in lung or periphery) |
| | Respiratory problems in opiate users |
| | Constipation in opiate users |
| | Poor dentition |
| | Side effects from long-term performance- and image-enhancing drugs |
| | Drug interactions |
| | Drug overdose |
| | Psychological or psychiatric problems |
| Those which relate to the lifestyle of many drug users, including poly-drug use | Poor general health status |
| | Poor nutritional status |
| | Poor dentition |
| | Poor liver function |
| | Overdose |
| Special groups | Pregnancy |
| | Homeless |
| | Older drug users |

While IDUs will have the same health care needs as the general population, they may also incur health-related problems either due to the drug itself, through injecting, or through lifestyles associated with illicit drug use (Table 19.1).

This chapter is by no means exhaustive in content, but rather focuses on those issues particularly pertinent to UK pharmacists, though the issues covered here will also be applicable to other countries and other health care systems.

## ATTITUDE, STIGMA AND PARTNERSHIP WORKING

Drug misusers are often stigmatized in society and sometimes by health care professionals. An important ethical aspect of health care provision is a non-judgmental, professional service. Research shows that drug users feel stigmatized (Matheson 1998; Neale et al. 2008) and want to be treated like anyone else when they use pharmacies. Judgemental attitudes prevent engagement with services and ultimately marginalize IDUs even further, which can lead to greater risk-taking behaviours. Good therapeutic relationships promote engagement and recovery.

**TABLE 19.2**

**Agencies and Health Professionals Involved in the Care of Injecting Drug Users**

| Agency/Professional | Description/Example |
|---|---|
| Drug treatment centres | Provided by the National Health Service and third-sector organizations. Provide assessment of people with drug and alcohol problems, devise care plans and deliver care, including prescribing and psychosocial interventions. |
| General practitioners | Provide primary health care and, in some cases, management of drug dependence, commonly in partnership (known as 'shared care') with specialist drugs services. |
| Street agencies | May provide a 'drop-in' service for people with drug problems or other low-threshold services. Often focus on information, advice and advocacy. They may be targeted at specific groups such as young drug users, women, steroid users, stimulant users, etc. Some may be based within or as part of specialist drugs services. |
| Outreach workers | Go out into communities to make contact and provide help for those who would not normally contact traditional services, such as sex workers. |
| Social services | May lead on safeguarding concerns, particularly child protection issues. Also coordinate other social support. |
| Probation services | Drug intervention programmes, offering drug treatment as an alternative to prison for certain drug-related offending. |
| Needle exchange | May be offered by pharmacies but also by other agencies. |
| Mutual aid groups | For example, Smart Recovery, Narcotics Anonymous and family support groups. |

Pharmacists should develop good working relationships with general practitioners and with specialist drugs services. Either may be involved in prescribing for people with drug problems; the latter may also provide sterile injecting equipment. Knowing how to signpost or refer to relevant services is essential, and understanding the structure and role of local services will help. A good knowledge of local safeguarding procedures is essential. Examples of relevant local services are listed and described in Table 19.2.

## HARM REDUCTION AND HARM MINIMIZATION

Many individuals who use drugs may be unwilling or unable to stop using them. Harm reduction is a philosophy which underpins much of the treatment and advice given to IDUs (i.e. to minimize the harm that drug misusers incur while using drugs) in the UK. The following definition from Harm Reduction International encapsulates the intention: 'harm reduction' refers to policies, programmes and practices that aim primarily to reduce the adverse health, social and economic consequences of the use of legal and illegal psychoactive drugs without necessarily reducing drug consumption. Harm reduction benefits people who use drugs, their families and the community (Harm Reduction International 2010).

Providing clean needles and syringes and a facility for the safe disposal of used equipment through needle exchange programmes is a harm reduction approach which attempts to reduce the need to share used injecting equipment and therefore reduce the risk of contracting BBVs. Benefits extend to sexual partners of IDUs through reduced sexual transmission risks. Community pharmacy involvement in the provision of sterile injecting equipment is now recognized internationally as an important aspect of harm reduction (Matheson et al. 2007; Samitca et al. 2007; Vlahov et al. 2010). Prescribed methadone and buprenorphine, as part of opioid substitution therapy, contribute to harm reduction in that opioid injectors are given an oral dose of methadone or buprenorphine to prevent withdrawal symptoms. This reduces the need to inject illicit opiates and begins to help the client move away from the cycle of criminality and to reduce and possibly stop injecting drugs. Indeed, in the UK, Australia and New Zealand, for example, community pharmacists are widely engaged with the provision of such services (Lea et al. 2008; Matheson et al. 2007; McCormick et al. 2006; Sheridan et al. 2007).

## HEALTH NEEDS RELATED TO THE ROUTE OF DRUG ADMINISTRATION

### INJECTING

There are many hazards associated with injecting drug use. Those covered here are, for the most part, related to intravenous injecting. However, it should be noted that not all injecting drug use is intravenous: some users inject intramuscularly; for example, those who inject performance- and image-enhancing drugs (PIEDs). Others inject drugs just beneath the skin surface ('skin popping'), often once vascular damage is so severe that it prevents intravenous access. Pharmacists should be familiar with, and recognize the possible hazards/conditions associated with, injecting drug use, as they may be the only primary health care worker who has regular contact with the IDU.

### SKIN/VEIN PROBLEMS

A number of skin and vein problems result from injecting, and these are summarized in Table 19.3.

### VIRAL INFECTIONS

BBVs such as human immunodeficiency virus (HIV) and hepatitis B and C may be contracted by sharing contaminated needles and syringes, as infected blood may remain in the syringe when it is passed between users. IDUs should be discouraged from sharing not only needles and syringes, but also other 'injecting paraphernalia', such as spoons, filters or water used in the preparation of the drug for injecting, as these are possible sources of infection of BBVs, especially of hepatitis C.

### HIV/ACQUIRED IMMUNE DEFICIENCY SYNDROME (AIDS)

AIDS was first recognized in 1981, and is caused by HIV. In the UK, HIV is not common in people who currently or have previously injected drugs. They account

**TABLE 19.3**

## Skin and Vein Problems Associated with Intravenous Injecting

| Condition | Cause | Signs/Symptoms | Treatment |
|---|---|---|---|
| Phlebitis (can lead to 'track marks') | Painless inflammatory response to injecting | Inflammation | Use different injecting sites to give veins the chance to recover |
| Thrombophlebitis | Inflammatory response to injecting | Swollen vein. Possible fever and malaise | Rest the vein. Seek treatment if there is fever or malaise |
| Cellulitis | Bacterial infections of skin and subcutaneous tissues | Reddening of limb, swelling, heat and pain | Seek medical attention |
| Collapsed veins | Repeated use of same vein; inappropriate injecting technique | Injectors seek other veins. Dangerous if use is of the femoral vein as this is near the artery and nerve | If artery is hit by accident, remove needle, apply pressure and seek medical attention |
| Gangrene | Impaired blood supply. Can lead to amputation | Pain, loss of feeling in the area, swelling and discoloured skin and coldness, especially in the fingers and toes | Urgent medical attention needed |
| Abscesses | Injection of irritant substances and non-sterile injection | Raised lumps in skin – may be sterile or infected | Seek medical attention if there are signs of infection |
| Ulcers | Defective blood supply (repeated venous trauma). Impaired vascular supply | Craters of unhealed skin | Seek medical attention |
| Deep vein thrombosis | Caused by injecting into femoral vein. Periods of immobility | Blood clots formed – may end up in lungs and can lead to heart attack. In leg – hot, red and swollen. Soreness | Urgent medical attention needed |
| Emboli | Due to unfiltered particles being injected | Can end up in the lung, leading to breathing difficulties, and in the eye | Urgent medical attention needed |
| Septicaemia | Injection of bacteria into the blood stream | Malaise with unexplained fever | Urgent medical treatment needed |

for about 2% of all people living with HIV. Prevalence data from 2011 show 0.9% of IDUs outside of London are HIV positive and 3.9% within London are HIV positive (National AIDS Trust 2013). This low prevalence is due to the rapid response in the UK to introducing NSPs and the expansion of opiate substitution therapy in response to HIV from the 1980s onwards. Drug misusers, as a group, are often stigmatized, and in addition to this, an HIV-positive diagnosis can further increase feelings of isolation. Sterile injecting equipment and using condoms should always be recommended to prevent the transmission of HIV.

Drugs – prescribed or illicit – may have a detrimental effect on the immune system, which is an important consideration for HIV-positive drug users. However, not all IDUs who are diagnosed HIV positive will either want or be able to cease using either their illicit (or, in some cases, prescribed) drugs. What is important is that advice and practical help is available to enable these individuals to practise safer drug use and safer sex, alongside encouragement to attend appointments regularly at specialist HIV clinics, to ensure expert monitoring and support.

## Hepatitis

The term hepatitis means 'inflammation of the liver', and the forms of hepatitis most closely associated with injecting drug use are hepatitis B and C. It is important that IDUs are aware of their hepatitis B and C status in order to reduce the risk of transmission to others, to manage their health issues if they are positive for either and to understand and engage in practices which reduce the risk of contracting either disease. Indeed, it is possible to vaccinate against hepatitis B (see later). Screening for hepatitis B and C is thus important, and research indicates that community pharmacies are acceptable and cost-effective environments in which this can occur as part of a locally approved and integrated service (Hepatitis C Trust 2010).

## Hepatitis B

Hepatitis B is an inflammation and infection of the liver caused by the hepatitis B virus. Infection may occur following vaginal or anal intercourse, or as the result of blood-to-blood contact. The latter can occur by sharing blood-contaminated injecting equipment or by vertical transmission from mother to child. Generally, with an acute attack of hepatitis B, the person feels unwell, tired and loses their appetite, although some people have no symptoms, and infection can only be detected using serological testing. Jaundice occurs in some, but by no means all cases, and many cases may not be diagnosed at all.

In the majority of people, the virus is inactivated by the body's immune system. However, in about 5%–10% of infected adults, the virus persists, and these individuals became chronic carriers of the virus. Between 3% and 5% of people who have chronic hepatitis B infection go on to develop liver cancer each year. There are a number of ways of avoiding contracting or transmitting hepatitis B (Box 19.1), as well as harm-reduction strategies for chronic hepatitis B sufferers (Box 19.2).

## BOX 19.1   WAYS TO AVOID CONTRACTING OR TRANSMITTING HEPATITIS B

- Avoid unprotected sex.
- Use new sterile equipment (as attempts to clean used equipment may not kill the virus).
- Avoid sharing any paraphernalia associated with injecting (e.g. water, cups, spoons, filters, swabs, etc.).
- Infected individuals should cover up cuts and clean up any blood spillage safely using bleach.
- Do not share implements such as toothbrushes or razors, as these might provide direct contact with blood (e.g. through bleeding gums).
- Ensure that injecting drug users are vaccinated against hepatitis B. In the UK, this can be done free of charge by specialist drugs services.

## HEPATITIS C

It is estimated that around 250,000 people in the UK have chronic hepatitis C. Of these, 95% are thought to have been infected through past or current injecting drug use. IDUs are a particularly high-risk group for contracting hepatitis C through the sharing of blood-contaminated injecting equipment. Around half of all IDUs in the UK are positive for hepatitis C virus (HCV) antibodies, indicating current or past infection. Sexual transmission of the virus is believed to occur, but the risk is considered low.

The acute phase (1–26 weeks after infection) is a time when few, if any, symptoms are experienced. A minority of sufferers (about 5%) will have jaundice, and some may experience loss of appetite and feel sick and lethargic. However, some may exhibit no symptoms. Approximately 25% of those with acute hepatitis C become virus free and make a full recovery. A total of 75% go on to the chronic phase, when the virus grows in the liver. A very small minority of those with chronic hepatitis C appear to overcome the infection.

## BOX 19.2   HARM-REDUCTION MEASURES FOR CHRONIC HEPATITIS B SUFFERERS

- Keep generally healthy and maintain a balanced diet.
- Refrain from drinking alcohol at all, or keep intake to an absolute minimum.
- Take precautions to avoid contracting other blood-borne viruses, as prognosis is poorer with co-infection.
- When taking any drugs, whether prescribed, over the counter or illicit, advice should be sought about the possible effects these might have on the liver.

**BOX 19.3 HARM-REDUCTION MEASURES
FOR THOSE WITH HEPATITIS C**

1. Avoid alcohol consumption. This may be very difficult as it may require major changes in a person's lifestyle.
2. Avoid paracetamol consumption if liver function is poor.
3. Avoid co-infection with other blood-borne viruses (including other genotypes of hepatitis C).
4. Encourage clients to get vaccinated against hepatitis B.
5. Check use of other drugs – prescribed, over the counter and illicit. As with hepatitis B, certain drugs should be avoided in cases of impaired liver function.
6. Encourage those infected to seek treatment as the virus can be cleared in many people with appropriate management.

Estimates indicate that 10%–15% of those with chronic hepatitis C go on to develop cirrhosis and, in certain cases, cancer of the liver, both of which can prove fatal. No vaccination is currently available against hepatitis C.

Testing of IDUs for HCV could be much improved and therefore one role for pharmacists operating NSPs is to promote testing. Knowing where to refer locally is essential.

## How to Avoid Contracting/Transmitting Hepatitis C

All of the measures covered for hepatitis B apply to hepatitis C. Even though the risk of transmission of hepatitis C sexually is believed to be low, the practise of safer sex is still advisable. The main issue involves preventing risky injecting practices, in particular preventing the sharing of injecting paraphernalia. Drug users should also be encouraged to inject in a clean environment, free from blood spillages. Equally important is trying to prevent initiation into injecting and promote routes out of injecting (e.g. through the provision of foil through NSPs). Many injectors become infected in the first three months of their injecting career, so pharmacists should be particularly proactive in engaging new NSP clients in consultations. Harm-reduction measures for those with hepatitis C are shown in Box 19.3.

More information about all forms of hepatitis and leaflets and advice for IDUs can be obtained from the British Liver Trust and the Hepatitis C Trust (see below).

## NON-INJECTION ROUTES OF ADMINISTRATION

Drug misusers may choose to use alternative routes of administration which carry a number of associated risks, as outlined in Box 19.4.

## HEALTH NEEDS RELATED TO THE DRUG BEING USED

While it is accepted that IDUs are generally less healthy than the general population, not all IDUs suffer serious health-related consequences. Health-related issues may

**BOX 19.4    RISKS ASSOCIATED WITH NON-INJECTING ROUTES OF DRUG ADMINISTRATION**

Intranasal: nose bleeds, ulceration, rhinitis, septal perforation and risk of transmission of hepatitis C

Inhalation: asphyxiation, aspiration and peri-oral dermatitis

Smoking: respiratory infection, cough, cancer, accidental burns and chronic lung disease

Oral: gastric irritation

arise from the drugs being used. Complications/problems associated with the specific drug taken may be idiosyncratic or dose dependent. Idiosyncratic reactions are unpredictable, whereas dose-dependent reactions may be controlled. The purity of illicit drugs can be extremely variable, which makes accurate dosage estimates difficult. Furthermore, illicit drugs are usually diluted or cut with inert or, more rarely, active ingredients, the identity of which is usually unknown to the user, and their consumption may result in unintended consequences. For example, crack cocaine commonly contains phenacetin, which is harmful to the liver.

Some specific health problems associated with two groups of drugs – opiates and stimulants – are summarized in Box 19.5 and Box 19.6, respectively.

**BOX 19.5    HEALTH PROBLEMS ASSOCIATED WITH OPIATES**

Respiratory: opiates suppress the cough reflex, leading to increased risk of aspiration and bacterial infection. They also depress the respiratory centre in the brain, and respiratory depression is the cause of deaths due to heroin or other opiate overdose. In addition, foreign body embolization (caused by fibres from, for example, cotton wool filters – used to filter out particles before injecting – or particles mixed with the drug such as talc) is also a potential hazard.

Gastrointestinal: nausea, vomiting and constipation are all side effects of opiate use. Tolerance develops to all of these and other dose-related effects, with the exception of constipation.

Right-sided infection/tricuspid endocarditis: this has been linked to the injection of opiate (and other) drugs. The symptoms include fever, weakness and general fatigue and can also include headaches, night sweats and weight loss. Medical attention should be sought immediately.

Dental: Methadone suppresses saliva production. This, coupled with lifestyle factors such as poor diet, can lead to dental problems. Clients should be encouraged to drink water after taking methadone, clean their teeth regularly and register with a dentist if possible.

> ## BOX 19.6   HEALTH PROBLEMS ASSOCIATED WITH STIMULANTS (COCAINE AND AMPHETAMINE)
>
> Cardiorespiratory: stimulants activate sympathetic autonomic activity, resulting in increased blood pressure and force of myocardial contraction (and vasoconstriction with cocaine), so demand on the heart is increased, while the amount of blood it can receive is decreased. These drugs may also cause arrhythmias, and may precipitate tachycardia and myocardial infarction.
>
> Neurological: due to raised blood pressure, headaches, strokes and cerebral bleeds may occur. Association with convulsions has been suggested. Amphetamine can also induce a psychotic state in some users.
>
> Respiratory: cough, airway burns, problems with the nasal septum, sinus infections, shortness of breath, possible worsening of asthma and interference with gaseous exchange.

## DRUG INTERACTIONS

Psychoactive drugs, such as opiates and stimulants, have several drug interactions. These drugs may interact in a number of ways; for example, central nervous system depressants (e.g. alcohol, benzodiazepines and tricyclic antidepressants) may increase sedation and decrease respiration, increasing the risk of overdose. Interactions may also occur which alter methadone plasma levels through metabolism (e.g. rifampicin, which causes raised plasma levels). Drugs may affect the excretion of methadone by altering the urine pH. In addition, methadone at doses above 100 mg daily can occasionally affect the QTc interval of the heart's electrical cycle, increasing the risk of life-threatening arrhythmias. The use of methadone concomitantly with other drugs that can prolong QTc is not advocated. Details of drug interactions with methadone can be found in standard textbooks such as the British National Formulary and Stockley's Drug Interactions. Drug interactions involving illicit drugs are seldom well detailed (if reported at all), so it is often difficult to obtain accurate information. A recent review paper has summarized the clinical literature (Lindsey et al. 2012).

It is essential that pharmacists are aware of potential IDUs. Patients who access a needle exchange scheme or who purchase injecting equipment from a pharmacy are easily identified as potential injectors. However, they may not have informed their doctor about their illicit drug taking. Discreet questioning by the pharmacist may be required in order to ascertain what other drugs they are using and to make an appropriate intervention, being mindful of maintaining confidentiality.

## POLY-DRUG USE

Many IDUs will be using more than one drug. There may be additional complications associated with the combined adverse effects of using the drugs. For example, heroin users may also use benzodiazepines and drink alcohol. Such combinations put the client at greater risk of accidental overdose (see below). While one drug will probably be the primary drug of misuse, the use of other drugs must be taken into account when managing drug users' problems. If alcohol is taken in the presence of cocaine, coca-ethylene is formed, which is itself psychoactive, and cardiotoxic.

## PREMATURE DEATH

Using drugs not only causes direct physical and psychological harms to the individual, but also affects the user indirectly. Poor social welfare, legal problems, housing problems and problems with relationships are often present in the lives of drug users. These, in themselves, take their toll on the individual.

### OVERDOSE

While overdoses often prove to be fatal, some are not. Poly-drug use is a common factor, and drugs such as opiates, cocaine and prescription drugs are commonly detected (Hickman et al. 2007). In an Australian study, a quarter of a sample of heroin users had experienced a non-fatal overdose in the previous 12 months (Darke et al. 1996). These overdoses may be intentional (attempted suicide) or accidental. A number of factors are related to overdose, such as

1. Mixing heroin with other sedating drugs (e.g. benzodiazepines, methadone or other opiates or tricyclic antidepressants) and alcohol.
2. Loss of tolerance to the drug's effects, due to a break in drug taking (e.g. while in prison or after detoxification).
3. Variable drug content, particularly exposure to drugs with an increased content after a sustained period of low content.
4. Poor general health.
5. Gender, age and length of use – older males in their 30s and 40s who have been using opiates for some time and may be in poor health are at particular risk of fatal overdose.
6. Homelessness, possibly due to poor health or hurried injecting to avoid being caught in public places.
7. Lack of adequate response; for example. injecting alone or the use of ineffective interventions (such as slapping or drenching in cold water).

Because of drug users' poor physical health and often poor psychological health, they are particularly at risk of intentional overdose. One study in Melbourne, Australia, found 17% of survivors of non-fatal overdoses said their overdose had been intentional (Heale et al. 2003). The signs of overdose include those shown in Box 19.7.

Effective overdose prevention includes:

• The provision of information to increase awareness of overdose risks
• Provision of opiate substitution therapy with retention in treatment
• Improved through-care between prison and the community

> ## BOX 19.7 SIGNS OF OPIATE OVERDOSE
>
> - Pinpoint pupils unreactive to light.
> - Shallow respiration and/or snoring.
> - Low pulse rate and hypotension.
> - Varying degree of reduced consciousness/coma.
> - In an adult: a patient with a pulse, but who has stopped breathing, is almost always suffering an opiate overdose.

Pharmacists who provide NSPs should ensure that they have targeted, written advice that they can provide to NSP clients. They should also ensure that any person receiving methadone who misses three consecutive days of collection or more is not provided any further dosing until their situation can be discussed with their prescriber. This is because tolerance to opiates may be reduced, so the previous therapeutic dose could become toxic. Similarly, identification of suboptimal opiate substitution therapy dosing should be discussed with prescribers.

Many countries have introduced strategies to prevent overdoses being fatal. These include trying to ensure an effective response from others present when the overdose occurs and the provision of drug consumption rooms. An effective response to an opiate overdose includes the administration of naloxone. In many countries, this is supplied to IDUs for carrying on their person at all times. Friends and relatives are encouraged to administer the naloxone in the event of an overdose and administer cardiopulmonary resuscitation if the person is not breathing. If the person is breathing, they should be put in the recovery position. Training on administration is provided. There are apps that can be followed to guide the administering person. An ambulance should always be called if there is a suspected overdose, even if naloxone has been effective. Patients will normally be required to remain in hospital, since the half-life of naloxone is only 60–90 minutes, compared to 4–6 hours for heroin and 24–36 hours for methadone. Unless hospitalized, they may slip back into overdose once the effects of the naloxone have worn off.

Some pharmacies in the UK provide naloxone to IDUs. At present, this is usually done under a patient group direction. Pharmacists who are part of NSPs should discuss naloxone provision with commissioners and ensure that either they themselves provide naloxone or they know where to signpost the client to receive it.

## PSYCHOLOGICAL AND PSYCHIATRIC MORBIDITY

There is a high incidence of psychological problems among IDUs, particularly those with chaotic drug-taking habits. However, the direction of causality may be difficult to determine. Many drug users will have turned to illicit drugs as a form of 'self-medication' for conditions such as depression or post-traumatic stress disorder (e.g. following childhood abuse). On the other hand, certain drugs, such as cannabis, cocaine and amphetamine, are associated with psychotic episodes in some individuals. Psychological problems such as depression are also associated with the 'come down' after chronic use of cocaine, and chronic amphetamine use is associated with negative effects on social functioning. Community pharmacists may be ideally placed to refer individuals with such problems to specialist agencies.

## LIFESTYLE-RELATED HEALTH NEEDS

Drug users may suffer from a variety of conditions, such as asthma, diabetes, epilepsy, high blood pressure or hepatic or renal failure. Many drug users are not in contact with primary care professionals, often due to reluctance to access. They are a needy but under-resourced group. IDUs may be homeless and susceptible to health problems related to 'rough sleeping' (e.g. tuberculosis, hypothermia, skin conditions and infestations).

### POOR NUTRITIONAL STATUS

One of the contributing factors to the poor health status of drug users is poor nutrition. They often have limited financial resources, poor access to cooking facilities and a lack of knowledge about nutrition, with many obtaining most of their calorific intake from alcohol or sugary foods. Additionally, stimulant use reduces appetite. It is very important to take the time to discuss nutrition, persuade drug users to register with a general practitioner (if necessary) and to get a health check-up. Opiate users are also likely to be suffering from constipation, so advice on increasing the intake of fibre and fluids (not alcohol) and taking exercise is appropriate.

### POOR DENTAL HEALTH

Opiates reduce the amount of saliva produced. This has a negative effect on teeth. Coupled with this, depending on the formulation, methadone preparations may have a high sugar content and be of a low pH, which can have a detrimental effect on dental health. In all cases, encouraging IDUs to look after their teeth and register with a dentist is important. Pharmacists can help identify those with dental problems, provide advice and refer for dental treatment (Sheridan et al. 2001).

### ASTHMA

IDUs may also take drugs by other routes. Smoked or inhaled drugs are most likely to cause respiratory problems, and hypersensitivity to any drug of misuse (including adulterants) can result in bronchospasm. Smoking cannabis and tobacco impairs gaseous exchange and deposits tar in the lungs. Suppression of the cough reflex due to opiate use can predispose individuals to respiratory tract infections. Crack cocaine may produce chronic lung changes, impairing gaseous exchange. This condition is known as 'crack lung'.

### DIABETES

Stimulant drugs such as amphetamine, cocaine and ecstasy can all cause a decrease in appetite, which can result in hypoglycaemia if insulin levels are not reduced.

Conversely, cannabis may increase appetite and consumption of food. Drug users with diabetes should be referred for specialist advice.

### EPILEPSY

Convulsions may occur after benzodiazepine withdrawal, although this is rare and usually only takes place with shorter-acting benzodiazepines. Cocaine misuse has also been linked with seizures, and convulsions are a known symptom of cocaine overdose.

### HEPATIC AND RENAL FAILURE

Well-documented cases of hepatotoxicity have occurred with alcohol, ecstasy and anabolic steroids. As most illicit drugs are metabolized by the liver, hepatic failure may allow them to accumulate. Exceptions which are not metabolized wholly by the liver include ecstasy, cocaine and volatile solvents (except toluene). A metabolite of heroin and morphine is known to accumulate in patients with renal failure. Transferring heroin users to prescribed methadone is strongly advised.

## SPECIAL GROUPS

### PREGNANT DRUG USERS

While IDUs suffer stigma, this is accentuated for pregnant IDUs. Many may experience guilt and concern about the effects of their drug use on their baby. They may also have concerns about their child being taken into care. In the UK, being an IDU is not in itself sufficient reason for a child to be taken into care, and some IDUs are good parents and successfully raise children. However, drug use is a risk factor for child neglect and therefore it is important that all health care professionals who work with drug users are vigilant for signs of such. Pharmacists should ensure that their pharmacy has a child protection policy and should know the local safeguarding procedures that they should follow. Evidence shows that intensive intervention can help keep families together.

Pregnant heroin users are generally not advised to stop using opiates abruptly, because withdrawal in pregnancy can be dangerous. They should be encouraged to access opiate substitution therapy. Methadone or buprenorphine may be prescribed. Stopping injecting drugs and moving to orally administered drugs is advisable in order to minimize the risks of BBVs and other injecting-related harms. It also provides stabilization and therefore the ability to engage with antenatal care more successfully. Pharmacists may want to refer pregnant drug users to drug treatment centres.

One important consideration is that pregnant IDUs may not be in contact with other health care professionals. Pharmacists are in an ideal position to start a dialogue about antenatal care, the need for folic acid intake and good nutrition and smoking cessation, and they may also help a pregnant IDU to become registered with a general practitioner, where necessary.

## THE HOMELESS

Research indicates that homeless people experience more health problems than the general population and that they also find the greatest difficulty in obtaining appropriate health care (Bines 1994). Homeless people who are also drug users are even more prone to health problems (Morrish 1993), and those who inject drugs run additional risks of acquiring BBVs, with the problems being compounded by the lack of safe and private places to inject. They may also be at increased risk of overdose.

Drug misuse may have contributed towards an individual becoming homeless, or the drug problem may have occurred or been exacerbated as a result of homelessness, as many people use drugs or alcohol to escape the stress and misery of their situation. Finding safe and secure accommodation is an important facilitator in recovery.

Lack of a fixed address is not a barrier to registering with a general practitioner. However, some general practitioners are reluctant to register such patients and this, coupled with a reluctance by homeless people to approach services, means that many such individuals are not registered with a general practitioner. Community pharmacists are often their only contact with primary health care services. As such, pharmacists play a vital role in making contact with a hard-to-reach population. A helpful and non-judgemental attitude by pharmacists may facilitate the homeless drug user to access other services. Pharmacists should have an awareness of local services targeted at homeless people.

## SPECIFIC POINTS REGARDING THE COMMUNITY PHARMACIST'S ROLE

IDUs need a number of things in order to manage their drug use in a healthy manner, the most obvious being clean injecting equipment. Therefore, at the most basic level, meeting the health needs of drug injectors will involve providing them with sterile injecting equipment and a safe way in which to dispose of used injecting equipment (e.g. through NSPs, many of which operate through community pharmacies). In addition, IDUs will need harm-reduction advice, including information on how and why they should always use clean injecting equipment and paraphernalia. NICE advocates different levels of NSPs – see guidance for details.

Some injectors will be receiving treatment for their drug misuse, such as prescribed methadone or buprenorphine for the management of opiate dependence. Methadone and buprenorphine are prescribed as a substitute for opiates – usually heroin. Both drugs have good oral bioavailability and can be given by mouth and have long half-lives, and therefore can be given once a day. The prescriber may require the drug to be dispensed daily, and in some cases, pharmacists will also be asked to supervise the consumption of methadone or buprenorphine on the premises to ensure compliance. The consulting room should always be offered for supervised administration. In the UK, community pharmacists have been involved in needle exchange schemes for three decades. Equipment may be supplied in packs or bespoke, known as 'pick and mix'. Pharmacies have proved to be ideally placed to provide this service because they are accessible, and most are open for a greater number of hours than drug agencies. Clients might also be worried about being seen entering drug agencies, but using a community pharmacy carries no stigma. Pharmacists are available, often without appointment, to provide free and confidential advice on a whole range of topics, not just those related to drug misuse.

People who inject PIEDs may not see themselves as drug users. They are, however, at risk of BBVs if they share injecting equipment or multidose vials. They should be given specific information that focuses on their needs and should be referred to services that are able to address their particular drug use. Traditional prescribing services for opiate users are unlikely to be appropriate. Pharmacists may identify PIED users through requests for longer needles and larger syringes with larger barrels. Additionally, their appearance may be suggestive of PIED use (e.g. body-building image).

BBVs can be transmitted through unsafe sexual practices. For this reason, many needle exchange packs contain advice on safer sex and free condoms. It will be difficult to broach this subject with drug-using clients who do not wish to use the consulting room, so pharmacists should ensure that they also have adequate printed information leaflets on open display. For those being treated for conditions such as HIV, hepatitis and tuberculosis, pharmacists have an important role in monitoring and encouraging adherence. They may also have to explain complex medication regimes, and will have to be vigilant for drug interactions.

Pharmacy-based services should complement those of specialist services. In some cases, it may be appropriate to refer clients on to such agencies, and in some areas, formal referral systems are in place. Pharmacists should ensure that they are aware of local treatment and advice agencies and other NSPs. Ideally, they should make contact with such agencies and familiarize themselves with what they offer, and in turn, inform them of the services provided from the pharmacy.

## CONCLUSION

This chapter has highlighted a number of health issues relating to injecting drug misuse which are pertinent to pharmacists who provide services to IDUs. Some of these relate to drug use *per se* and others to the diverse consequences of a drug-misusing culture. These present a number of opportunities for community pharmacists, who may be responsive or proactive in their interventions. When dealing with IDUs, pharmacists have an opportunity to provide accurate and appropriate health promotion and harm-reduction advice and to provide or display written information about drug misuse, where to get help, HIV, hepatitis, etc. On a one-to-one level, pharmacists should also be aware of the immense impact that positive therapeutic relationships, including those with pharmacists, can have on a drug user.

## FURTHER READING

Derricott, J., Preston, A. and Hunt, N. The Safer Injecting Briefing. Liverpool: Hit Publications. Available at: http://www.exchangesupplies.org/article_the_safer_injecting_briefing_introduction.php.

Preston, A. The Methadone Briefing. London: Andrew Preston/ISDD. Available at: http://
www.exchangesupplies.org/drug_information/briefings/the_methadone_briefing/meth-
adone_briefing/contents.html.

Sheridan, J. and Strang, J. 2003. *Drug Misuse and Community Pharmacy*. London: Taylor &
Francis.

Wills, S. 2005. *Drugs of Abuse* (2nd Ed.). London: Pharmaceutical Press.


## CONTACTS

**British Liver Trust**
2 Southampton Road
Ringwood BH24 1HY (UK)
Information line: 0800 652 7330
General enquiries: 01425 481320
http://www.britishlivertrust.org.uk/

**The Hepatitis C Trust**
27 Crosby Row
London SE1 3YD (UK)
Office: 020 7089 6220
Email: admin@hepctrust.org.uk
http://www.hepctrust.org.uk/

**Terrence Higgins Trust**
314–320 Gray's Inn Road
London WC1X 8DP (UK)
Office: 020 7831 0330
http://www.tht.org.uk/

**Exchange Supplies**
http://www.exchangesupplies.org/


## REFERENCES

Bines, W. 1994. *The Health of Single Homeless People, Centre for Housing Policy*. New York:
University of York.

Darke, S., Ross, J. and Hall, W. 1996. Overdose among heroin users in Sydney, Australia: (I)
Prevalence and correlates of non-fatal overdose. *Addiction*, **91**(3), 405–411.

Harm Reduction International (formerly IHRA) 2010. '*What Is Harm Reduction?' A Position
Statement from the International Harm Reduction Association*. London: International
Harm Reduction Association.

Heale, P., Dietze, P. and Fry, C. 2003. Intentional overdose among heroin overdose survivors.
*Journal of Urban Health*, **80**(2), 230–237.

Hepatitis C Trust 2010. *Diagnosing Viral Hepatitis in the Community. A 3-Month Pharmacy
Testing Pilot*. London: Hepatitis C Trust.

Hickman, M., Carrivick, S., Paterson, S. et al. 2007. London audit of drug-related overdose
deaths: Characteristics and typology, and implications for prevention and monitoring.
*Addiction*, **102**(2), 317–323.

Lea, T., Sheridan, J. and Winstock, A. 2008. Consumer satisfaction with opioid treatment services at community pharmacies in Australia. *Pharmacy World and Science*, **30**(6), 940–946.

Lindsey, W.T., Stewart, D. and Childress, D. 2012. Drug interactions between common illicit drugs and prescription therapies. *American Journal of Drug and Alcohol Abuse*, **38**(4), 334–343.

Matheson, C. 1998. Views of illicit drug users on their treatment and behaviour in Scottish community pharmacies: Implications for the harm-reduction strategy. *Health Education Journal*, **57**(1), 31–41.

Matheson, C., Bond, C.M. and Tinelli, M. 2007. Community pharmacy harm reduction services for drug misusers: National service delivery and professional attitude development over a decade in Scotland. *Journal of Public Health*, **29**(4), 350–357.

McCormick, R., Bryant, L., Sheridan, J. and Gonzalez, J. 2006. New Zealand community pharmacist attitudes toward opioid-dependent clients. *Drugs: Education, Prevention, and Policy*, **13**(6), 563–575.

Morrish, P. 1993. *Living in the Shadows: The Accommodation Needs and Preferences of Homeless Heavy Drinkers*. Leeds: Leeds Accommodation Forum.

National AIDS Trust 2013. *HIV and Injecting Drug Use*. London: National AIDS Trust.

Neale, J., Tomkins, C. and Sheard, L. 2008. Barriers to accessing generic health and social care services: A qualitative study of injecting drug users. *Health and Social Care in the Community*, **16**(2), 147–154.

Samitca, S., Huissoud, T., Jeannin, A. and Dubois-Arber, F. 2007. The role of pharmacies in the care of drug users: What has changed in ten years – The case of a Swiss region. *European Addiction Research*, **13**(1), 50–56.

Sheridan, J., Aggleton, M. and Carson, T. 2001. Dental health and access to dental treatment: A comparison of drug users and non-drug users attending community pharmacies. *British Dental Journal*, **191**(8), 453–457.

Sheridan, J., Manning, V., Ridge, G., Mayet, S. and Strang, J. 2007. Community pharmacies and the provision of opioid substitution services for drug misusers: Changes in activity and attitudes of community pharmacists across England 1995–2005. *Addiction*, **102**(11), 1824–1830.

Vlahov, D., Robertson, A.M. and Strathdee, S.A. 2010. Prevention of HIV infection among injection drug users in resource-limited settings. *Clinical Infectious Diseases*, **50**(Suppl 3), S114–S121.

# Section IV

---

*Measuring and Costing Medicines Use*

# 20 Pharmacovigilance and Pharmacoepidemiology

*Corinne de Vries and Lolkje de Jong-van den Berg*

## CONTENTS

**KEY POINTS**

- Pharmacovigilance involves the detection of unexpected, usually undesirable adverse drug effects.
- Many countries have spontaneous reporting systems for the post-marketing surveillance of drugs: such systems are subject to considerable under-reporting of suspected adverse drug reactions.
- Several different types of adverse drug reactions can be distinguished.
- Pharmacoepidemiology attempts to quantify the frequency of adverse drug effects and identify subpopulations for which there are variations in the magnitudes of effects.
- Several study designs may be employed in pharmacoepidemiology, namely descriptive, case–control, cohort and experimental studies.
- In the analysis of pharmacoepidemiology data, due consideration should be given to sources of bias and confounding.

## INTRODUCTION

Pharmacovigilance involves the detection of unexpected, and often undesirable, adverse effects of drugs. Pharmacoepidemiology, often considered a subdomain in pharmacovigilance, attempts to quantify the frequency of these adverse effects, and to identify subpopulations for which there are variations in the magnitudes of effects.

Until relatively recently, adverse drug effects were of limited concern, as it was difficult enough to treat the disease. Reports of adverse drug effects began at the end of the nineteenth century when it was found that the use of chloroform led to an increased risk of cardiac arrest. Table 20.1 lists some examples of serious and unexpected adverse effects of drugs, identified after they had been marketed.

Some of the examples in Table 20.1 may be familiar; for example, most people will have heard of thalidomide. This product was advocated as safe and specifically suitable for use during pregnancy, but was found to cause limb defects in the newborn child when taken during the first trimester of pregnancy. In 1938, the revelation that diethylene glycol (used as a solvent for sulphanilamide) caused blindness prompted authorities in many countries to develop a system for monitoring drug safety. In the US, the Food and Drug Administration began to collect case reports of all adverse drug reactions (ADRs) in 1960. In the 1960s, the thalidomide tragedy and, subsequently, the discovery that oral contraceptives increased the risk of thromboembolic disease precipitated the foundation of the Committee on Safety of Medicine in the UK and similar spontaneous reporting systems in Europe.

In the 1990s, thalidomide was found to be beneficial in the treatment of leprosy and, in some cases, for the treatment of acquired immune deficiency syndrome. This demonstrates that even drugs that are known to be very toxic in certain subpopulations (e.g. the foetus) can be beneficial in others (e.g. people with human immunodeficiency virus infection or leprosy).

**TABLE 20.1**

**Examples of Adverse Drug Reactions**

| Year | Drug | Adverse Effect |
|---|---|---|
| 1880 | Chloroform | Cardiac arrest |
| 1923 | Cinchophen | Hepatitis |
| 1925 | Bismuth compounds | Nicolau syndrome |
| 1933 | Aminophenazone | Agranulocytosis |
| 1938 | Sulphanilamide (in diethyl glycol) | Renal failure |
| 1942 | Bismuth compounds | Hepatitis and renal failure |
| 1946 | Streptomycin | Deafness and renal failure |
| 1952 | Chloramphenicol | Aplastic anaemia |
| 1953 | Phenacetin | Nephropathy |
| 1958 | Isoniazid | Hepatitis |
| 1961 | Thalidomide | Phocomelia |
| 1962 | Procainamide | Systemic lupus erythematosus |
| 1964 | Phenylbutazone | Aplastic anaemia and agranulocytosis |
| | Aspirin and other non-steroidal anti-inflammatory drugs | Gastrointestinal ulcers and bleeding |
| 1965 | Barbiturates | Addiction |
| 1966 | Oral contraceptives | Thromboembolic disease |
| 1970 | Phenacetin | Urinary tract carcinoma |
| 1972 | Diethylstilboestrol | Vaginal adenocarcinoma |
| | Erythromycin | Cholestatic hepatitis |
| 1973 | Co-trimoxazole | Thromboembolic disease |
| 1974 | Practolol | Sclerosing peritonitis, corneal perforation |
| 1976 | Glafenine | Anaphylactic shock |
| 1979 | Triazolam | Psychosis |
| 1981 | Fenfluramine | Pulmonary hypertension |
| 1984 | Valproic acid | Spina bifida |
| 1996 | Mefloquine | Central nervous system side effects |
| 1997 | Indinavir | Haemolytic anaemia |
| 1997 | Terfenidine | Cardiac arrythmias |
| 1999 | Astemizole | Cardiac arrythmias |
| 2000 | Cisapride | Cardiac arrythmias |
| 2004 | Rofecoxib | Myocardial infarction, stroke |
| 2005 | Thioridazine | Cardiotoxity |
| 2009 | Efalizumab | Progressive multifocal leukoencephalopathy |
| 2010 | Sibutramine | Heart attack, stroke |

Drug safety is central to the role of pharmacists, whether they work in a pharmacy, a pharmaceutical company, a health authority or a medicines regulatory agency. They may have to advise on drug use or on the introduction or withdrawal of a drug from the market, or establish the likelihood that an adverse event is in fact an ADR. This chapter aims to provide insights into how ADRs are detected, how causality is established and how studies on drug safety should be interpreted and evaluated.

Pharmacovigilance has been defined by the World Health Organization (WHO) as 'the detection, assessment, and prevention of adverse drug effects in humans' (World Health Organization 1998). The major sources for pharmacovigilance are countrywide reporting systems for suspected ADRs and pharmacoepidemiology studies of specific drugs or adverse events. The major aims of pharmacovigilance are

- The early detection of hitherto unknown adverse effects and interactions
- The detection of increases in frequency of (known) adverse effects
- The identification of risk factors and mechanisms underlying adverse effects
- To establish quantitative aspects of risks
- The analysis and dissemination of information needed for drug prescribing and regulation

The main information sources for pharmacovigilance are patients, prescribers and pharmacists. It can be difficult to recognize an ADR. Therefore, once suspicion has arisen that an adverse event in a patient might, in fact, be an adverse reaction to a drug, how does one decide whether or not this should be reported to a spontaneous reporting system, and how can one establish whether the adverse event is in fact an ADR?

## SPONTANEOUS REPORTING SYSTEMS

Since the 1960s, many developed countries have implemented spontaneous reporting systems to perform post-marketing surveillance of drugs. These systems are mostly voluntary. Usually, report forms for ADRs are available in national drug formularies or drug bulletins. Typically, these systems will be able to detect serious and unexpected drug reactions. They can be seen as relatively inexpensive 'early warning systems' that can signal possible problems with drugs during their entire post-marketing phase. After they are marketed, the drugs are prescribed to a population that may differ to a great extent from the population in which it was tested during the clinical trials (e.g. elderly people, people with co-morbidity patterns that differ from the trial populations, pregnant women or children).

In the UK, the medicines regulator, the Medicines and Healthcare products Regulatory Agency (MHRA), collects spontaneous reports of ADRs through the 'Yellow Card Scheme'. Reports are collected for all medicines, including vaccines, blood factors, herbal medicines, homeopathic medicines and medical devices. Yellow Card reports can be made online via medicines information technology systems or by post, using a form available on the MHRA website or in the British National Formulary. Reports may be made by pharmaceutical companies, health care professionals (notably prescribing clinicians and pharmacists) and members of the general public. Information is collected on the name of the drug suspected of causing an ADR (route of administration, dose, etc.), suspected reaction (including time course), patient details (sex, age, etc.) and details of the reporter. Medicines which are being particularly monitored for ADRs by medicines regulatory authorities in the European Union have an inverted black triangle placed on their Summary of Product Characteristics and patient information leaflet.

With spontaneous reporting systems, no information is obtained about the number of people who have used a certain drug and the duration of therapy. Therefore, it is impossible to calculate the frequency of ADRs directly, and to compare risks of ADRs between drugs. For this, pharmacoepidemiological studies are needed. These are discussed later in this chapter. Unfortunately, there is a lot of under-reporting with spontaneous reporting systems: 90% of prescribers never report a suspected ADR, and reporting rates are rarely stable over time. Pharmacists report relatively more frequently, but they are less likely to become aware of an ADR because patients usually contact their prescriber and not their pharmacist about adverse events. The reasons for under-reporting have been called 'the seven deadly sins' (Inman 1986) (see Box 20.1).

Under-reporting leads to a number of problems that are characteristic of spontaneous reporting systems. First, the frequency of ADRs may be underestimated. Second, it may lead to the delayed detection of ADRs. Third, and probably most significantly, under-reporting may not be random, but is usually selective. For example, reporting rates for a new drug are usually highest during the first years after it has been introduced onto the market.

To improve reporting rates, many countries have developed ways of feeding back to reporters. This feedback may comprise a preliminary evaluation of a reported adverse case, therapy advice on how to deal with the adverse event, follow-up of the report by a telephone call, a personal visit, occasional publication of a case series in scientific medical journals or the regular publication of recently reported ADRs.

More recently, medicines regulators and pharmaceutical companies have been exploring the potential for mining data from social media sites, such as Twitter, to identify ADRs which might otherwise go unreported to a doctor, nurse or pharmacist (Sukkar 2015).

---

### BOX 20.1   REASONS FOR UNDER-REPORTING IN SPONTANEOUS REPORTING SYSTEMS ('THE SEVEN DEADLY SINS')

1. Complacency: the mistaken belief that only safe drugs are allowed on the market.
2. Fear of involvement in litigation.
3. Guilt because harm to the patient has been caused by the treatment that the doctor has prescribed.
4. Ambition to collect and publish a personal series of cases.
5. Ignorance of the requirements for reporting.
6. Diffidence about reporting mere suspicions which might perhaps lead to ridicule.
7. Lethargy: a person cannot be bothered to report the adverse drug reaction.

## When to Report a Suspected ADR

Specific guidelines for ADR reporting differ between countries and between spontaneous reporting systems. However, in general, all suspected ADRs should be reported if they are

- Unexpected, whatever their severity (i.e. not consistent with product information or labelling)
- Serious, whether expected or not
- Reactions to recently marketed drugs (i.e. less than five years on the market), irrespective of their nature or severity

Serious reactions are defined as a noxious and unintended response to a drug that

- Occurs at any dose and requires significant medical intervention, such as inpatient hospitalization or prolongation of existing hospitalization
- Causes congenital malformation
- Results in persistent or significant disability or incapacity
- Is life-threatening or results in death

## Establishing Whether an Adverse Event Is an ADR

Rarely can causality be proven when an adverse event coincides with drug use. Instead, several people have established criteria that can be applied to see how suggestive the potential association between an adverse event and drug use is of causality. Well known among these are the Bradford Hill criteria (Hill 1965) (Box 20.2).

This is best explained using an example. Suppose an individual takes indomethacin and develops a gastric ulcer. How do we know whether that gastric ulcer occurred as a consequence of indomethacin use? The answer is that we will probably never know for sure, but the Bradford Hill criteria can be suggestive of a causal association. Taking strength (criterion 1) as an example: if the individual has a history of gastric complaints, indomethacin may have been the final 'trigger' to developing an ulcer, but it may also be that the ulcer has developed irrespective of indomethacin use. However, the association has been found repeatedly in the literature (criterion 2), it is biologically plausible and coherent (criteria 6 and 7) and it is analogous to similar associations between other non-steroidal anti-inflammatory drugs (NSAIDs) and gastric complaints (criterion 9), for instance. The other criteria (e.g. temporality of the association) need to be established within the individual. If indomethacin use began after the development of the gastric ulcer, then obviously in this case it is unlikely that the gastric ulcer was an ADR.

After Hill, others developed rules for causality assessment, some of which are used at spontaneous reporting bureaus. The aim of applying such rules is to determine whether a causal association between the drug and the adverse event can be established, and to what degree (World Health Organization 1998).

## BOX 20.2 THE BRADFORD HILL CRITERIA (1965) TO ASSESS CAUSALITY BETWEEN DRUGS AND ADVERSE EVENTS

| Criterion | Explanation by Bradford Hill |
| --- | --- |
| Strength | Strong associations are more likely to be causal than weak associations because, if they could be explained by some other factor, the effects of that factor would have to be even stronger than the observed association and therefore would have become evident. However, weak associations are not necessarily non-causal. In addition, confounding can still be present. |
| Consistency | Consistency exists if the association is found repeatedly in different populations and under different circumstances. However, lack of consistency does not rule out causality. |
| Specificity | A true cause leads to a single effect, not multiple effects. This is not a very strong criterion: most drugs have multiple effects. This does not necessarily rule out causality. |
| Temporality | The cause (drug use) should precede the effect (the adverse drug reaction) in time. This does not mean that the adverse effect never happens by any other cause than drug use, however (i.e. it can happen due to other causes than drug use, as well). |
| Biologic gradient | Is there a dose–response relationship? If there is not, there may be a 'threshold' dose, and if there is, the association may still be confounded, but we often expect a dose–response relationship to exist in the case of causality. |
| Plausibility | This criterion refers to the biological plausibility of the hypothesis, although this is often not objective or absolute and is based only on current knowledge and beliefs. |
| Coherence | The cause-and-effect interpretation for an association should not conflict with what is known of the natural history and biology of the disease. Here, the same concerns apply as for 'plausibility'. |
| Experimental evidence | Does removal of the drug ('de-challenge') lead to disappearance of the adverse drug reaction, and does 're-challenge' lead to recurrence of the adverse drug reaction? If it does, then causality is more likely. |
| Analogy | Is the association similar to other well-known associations? If it is, then causality is more likely. |

## ADRs

There are a number of different classification systems of ADRs. Traditionally, ADRs have been classified into types A and B. Over the years, additional and rarer/harder-to-detect types of reaction have been added. Nowadays, ADRs are commonly classified into types A, B, C, D and E, though types F (failure of therapy), G (genetic reactions) and I (idiosyncratic) have also been described, along with alternative classification systems, such as DoTS, which incorporates dose-related, time-related and susceptibility factors.

### TYPE A (AUGMENTED)

These ADRs are usually detected during clinical trials, are typically dose related and are associated with the drug's pharmacological action. Hence, they are the most common ADR, they are predictable and are often less serious than other types. A typical example of a type A ADR is the development of extra-pyramidal symptoms ('Parkinsonism') after phenothiazine use. These drugs have anti-cholinergic properties that account for their beneficial effect in the treatment of schizophrenia. However, their anti-cholinergic properties also affect other parts of the central nervous system, leading to extra-pyramidal symptoms. Decreasing the dosage may eliminate the adverse effects. However, in some patients, this will result in a subtherapeutic dosage and, consequently, a recurrence of schizophrenia.

## Type B (Bizarre)

These ADRs result from an allergy-type reaction to the drug. They are usually very severe, often life threatening, and they stand out because they happen very rarely. Usually, the drug must be discontinued when such an ADR happens. A typical example is the development of anaphylactic shock after penicillin use. The body develops an immune response to the drug, and therapy must be discontinued immediately. This type of event is rare and it is usually not detected at the phase of clinical trials, but only at the post-marketing phase. However, because this type of event is so rare and unexpected, the link with the drug that caused it is usually made relatively easily. Therefore, like type A ADRs, type B ADRs are relatively easy to detect. Typically, type B reactions are the type of reactions that are reported to spontaneous reporting systems and published as case reports in the medical literature.

## Type C (Continuing)

These persist for a relatively long period of time (e.g. osteonecrosis of the jaw with prolonged use of bisphosphonates), the risk of which is linked to dose and duration of therapy.

## Type D (Delayed)

These ADRs are difficult to detect. They are characterized as an increased frequency of 'spontaneous' disease, occur at random intervals or after a long induction time and, although relatively common, can be serious. The connection between the drug and the adverse event, therefore, can be difficult to prove or refute. An example would be the possible association between breast cancer and the use of oral contraceptives. With this adverse event, the prevalence of breast cancer among the general population of women is relatively high, as is the use of oral contraceptives, there is a long time delay before the appearance of breast cancer, the effects are not experimentally reproducible, it is difficult to find a good comparator group and there are multiple causal factors.

## Type E (End of Use)

These are reactions that are associated with the withdrawal of a medicine. An example is the sleep disturbance, anxiety, panic attacks, etc., associated with discontinuation of treatment with benzodiazepines.

As previously stated, spontaneous reporting systems provide early warning signals of adverse drug effects. However, despite mechanisms to assess causality, such as de-challenge (observing the effect of withdrawing a drug) and re-challenge (observing the effect of reintroducing a drug following withdrawal), for instance, suspicions of adverse effects are difficult to prove and the frequency of ADRs cannot be established directly from spontaneous reporting. Additionally, not all ADRs are discovered through spontaneous reporting. To overcome these issues, pharmacoepidemiological studies are required.

# PHARMACOEPIDEMIOLOGY

Pharmacoepidemiology can be defined as the study of the use and the effects of drugs in large numbers of people. It is based on two disciplines: clinical pharmacology and epidemiology. Pharmacoepidemiology uses the techniques of chronic disease epidemiology to study the use and effects of drugs (i.e. the content area of clinical pharmacology). Its major application is after drug marketing to supplement any information about drug effects that is available from pre-marketing trials (Strom et al. 2012).

Pharmacoepidemiology addresses three main issues:

- What is the drug use in a specific population?
- What are the determinants of drug use?
- What are the outcomes of drug use (beneficial and adverse effects)?

## WHAT IS THE DRUG USE IN A SPECIFIC POPULATION?

Information on drug use in a population is accessed through prescribers, dispensers and drug users. These data sources have their own benefits and limitations, such as (in)completeness of data and the (non)availability of information on adherence, over-the-counter (OTC) drug use and the indications for which the drugs have been prescribed. Ideally, multiple information sources should be used in such a way that the data complement each other.

## WHAT ARE THE DETERMINANTS OF DRUG USE?

To achieve rational drug use, knowledge about the factors that determine drug choice or adherence to drugs is essential. For example, we could investigate why intervention methods vary in their effectiveness to influence prescribing, why women use more benzodiazepines than men and why adolescents are less likely to adhere to their insulin therapy than other diabetic patients. With such information and with insight into underlying health beliefs, interventions in drug use can be adequately targeted.

## WHAT ARE THE OUTCOMES OF DRUG USE (BENEFICIAL AND ADVERSE EFFECTS)?

Finally, we are interested in the effects of drug use. Are the drugs effective in treating the disorder for which they have been prescribed, and can we establish risk estimates

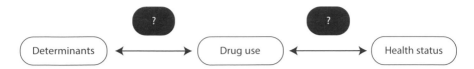

**FIGURE 20.1**   The concept of pharmacoepidemiology.

for the adverse effects associated with their use? Can we define subpopulations for which drugs are less appropriate? This provides the basis for decision making at several levels of health care: prescribing, drug formularies, reimbursement policies and market approval.

Figure 20.1 illustrates the basic approach in pharmacoepidemiology: we study the relationship between the exposure of individuals and subsequent outcomes. The exposure, in pharmacoepidemiology, is usually drug use, whereas the outcome is the adverse (or unexpected) effect. However, in studies of drug use determinants, drug use is the outcome, whereas determinants such as age, gender or socio-economic status can be the exposure of interest.

## RECORDS OF DRUG USE, DETERMINANTS AND OUTCOMES

To determine drug use, several information sources can be consulted: prescribers, dispensers and pharmacists. Each of these information sources has its strengths and limitations. This is illustrated in Figure 20.2 (Hartzema et al. 1998).

As seen in Figure 20.2, (in)correct information about drug use can be obtained due to missing or incorrect information in the data source from which information about drug use is obtained. Incorrect classification of exposure status is called 'misclassification' of exposure. The choice of information source will usually depend on the research question. For instance, one may decide that information direct from patients is preferable (e.g. for information about OTC drug use or information about adherence) or that pharmacy data should be used (e.g. if very detailed drug information is needed).

With the development of large computerized databases in the last few decades, pharmacoepidemiology has rapidly evolved. Pharmacies, prescribers, commercial institutions, health insurance companies and other health care institutions started to collect and store their health care data electronically, and this provided many opportunities for pharmacoepidemiological studies. Recently, in the UK, the Clinical Practice Research Datalink has been launched, an online research service incorporating the General Practice Research Database to provide a large computerized database of anonymized longitudinal medical records from primary care, linked with other health care data.

In most databases, the data have been collected in health care systems for purposes other than pharmacoepidemiology research. Research with these databases is relatively inexpensive and studies can be performed relatively quickly after drug alerts arise (e.g. from a spontaneous reporting system). The data are already available on computer, thus little if any extra data collection is required. However, at the same time, it means that not all of the relevant data may be available. In addition, the

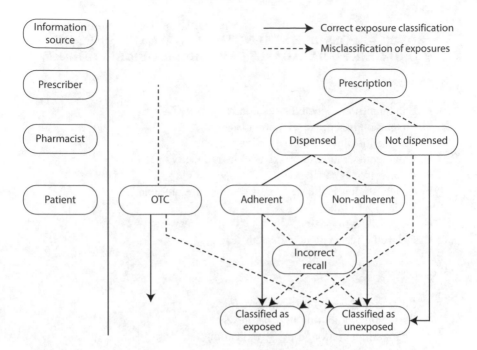

**FIGURE 20.2** Misclassification associated with various information sources of drug exposure. OTC = over the counter.

data may comprise a population that is not representative of the general population, and this may introduce bias into the study. Box 20.3 summarizes the strengths and weaknesses of large computerized databases as sources for pharmacoepidemiology research.

One issue arising with these databases is patient confidentiality. Typically, for clinical research, consent is required from every subject to use their clinical details for research purposes. With these large databases, this is often not feasible because people are followed up for a long time and may be difficult to track down at the time that the study is performed. However, ethical approval is often obtained for this type of study when the confidentiality of subjects is protected, because of the utility of these studies for public health. These issues regarding patient confidentiality in large health care databases have been addressed in the European Data Protection Act.

## MEASURING DISEASE FREQUENCY

If we want to measure whether a drug results in an increased frequency of a disease or other adverse event, we need to compare the frequency of that adverse event in a population that has been exposed to the drug with the frequency in the unexposed population. Two measures of frequency are commonly used in epidemiology: prevalence and incidence (Hennekens and Buring 1987).

Prevalence is the proportion of people in a population that has the disorder (e.g. the number of children with a nut allergy in a school class or the number of people

---

**BOX 20.3   POSSIBLE STRENGTHS AND WEAKNESSES OF RECORD-LINKED DATABASES IN PHARMACOEPIDEMIOLOGY***

Strengths

- Can quantify suspected risks relatively quickly
- Population based: no selection bias
- Can identify increased risks of rare events
- Can identify increased risks with infrequently used drugs
- Relatively inexpensive
- Cohort studies and case–control studies are possible
- Little loss to follow-up
- Long follow-up period
- Delayed effects can be detected

Weaknesses

- Comparator groups difficult to define
- Residual confounding may be present
- Channelling/confounding by indication
- Misclassification of exposure/outcome
- Research is not the primary aim for data collection
- Not always representative of the general population, hence generalizability may be a problem

---

* These vary with databases.

---

with dementia in a nursing home). Specifically, it is the number of existing cases of the disease in a defined population at a given point in time or over a defined time period, divided by the total number of people in that population. It is calculated as 'P', which is the number of existing cases of a disease divided by the total population at a given point in time. For example, if in a nursing home with 500 residents the number of people with dementia is 175, then the prevalence of dementia in that nursing home is 175/500 = 0.35. Typically, the prevalence is a proportion, and it always has a value that lies between 0 and 1. It can give us information about how common a disease is, and in that sense it can be useful in planning or budgeting for health care. However, it does not give us any information about the rate at which new cases of a disease develop.

Incidence provides additional information, and may be defined as the number of new cases of a disease that develops over a defined time period in a defined at-risk population, divided by the number of people in that at-risk population in that same time period. For example, in Tayside, Scotland, 799 new cases of heart failure were identified in 1995. However, the denominator of the population can be defined in two ways, and this leads to two different types of incidence: the cumulative incidence

(CI) and the incidence density. With the CI, the denominator is the number of people in the at-risk population at the beginning of a time period. It is calculated as 'CI', which is the number of new cases of a disease during a given period of time divided by the total population at risk. The CI provides an estimate of the probability – or risk – that an individual will develop a disease during a specified period of time. It assumes that the entire at-risk population at the beginning of the study period has been followed for the specified time interval for the development of the outcome under investigation.

Often, however, people will enter a study population over a period of a year or several years and are then followed to a single study end date or until they leave the study population (e.g. because they move to another country). With the calculation of the incidence density, only new cases are incorporated in the numerator, but now the actual person-time at risk is used in the denominator. Each individual's time at risk is calculated, followed by the sum of each individual's person-time at risk, or the sum of the time that each person remained under observation and free from the disease. The incidence density is the number of new cases of a disease during a given time period, divided by the total person-time of observation. Example calculations for CI and incidence density are presented in Box 20.4.

## MEASURING DRUG USE

The frequency of drug use can be calculated in a similar manner to disease frequency. For example, if 53% of nursing home residents use laxatives for more than 10 months per year, then the prevalence of laxative use is 53%, or 0.53. For longitudinal or temporal comparisons of drug utilization between studies or between countries, a classification system was needed to systematically classify drugs within drug groups. To this end, the WHO has developed a hierarchical drug coding system (the ATC classification system) to facilitate these studies. ATC stands for Anatomical, Therapeutic and Chemical, and this is the hierarchy with which drugs are coded in this system (World Health Organization 1990). An overview of the coding system plus an example is given in Table 20.2.

ATC codes are seven-digit codes, enabling the user to evaluate drug use at various levels (the level of a therapeutic group, such as NSAIDs, or the generic level of individual drugs). The ATC system distinguishes 14 anatomical groups represented as the first letter of the group name. Depending on the indication for which it is used, a drug can have more than one ATC code. For example, acetyl salicylic acid is classified in main group B (blood and blood-forming organs) as an anti-thrombotic agent (B01AC06), but also in main group N (nervous system) as an analgesic (N02BA01). To quantify drug use, the DDD measuring system was developed together with the ATC system. DDD stands for Defined Daily Dose: the recommended daily dose for adults when the drug is used for its main indication. For virtually every ATC code (with the exception of dermatological preparations and vaccines), a DDD value has been established.

An example of calculating DDDs is given in Table 20.3. This example illustrates that the use of several different drugs can be added up and compared (e.g. between people). However, in most cases, the DDD is used to measure drug utilization at the

**BOX 20.4   EXAMPLE CALCULATIONS OF CUMULATIVE INCIDENCE AND INCIDENCE DENSITY**

Consider a study of the incidence of dementia in five nursing homes from 2010 to 2015. At the beginning of the study period, 1,600 elderly people in these nursing homes do not have dementia. Therefore, they are 'at risk' of dementia (they have the possibility of developing it). Suppose that of these 1,600 people, 400 die (of whom no one developed dementia during the study period) and 200 develop dementia. This means that the cumulative incidence is $200/1,600 = 0.125$: the number of people that develop dementia divided by the number of people at risk at the beginning of the study period. Like the prevalence, the cumulative incidence is a proportion: its value always lies between 0 and 1.

The incidence density, however, takes into account the person-time 'at risk' that each individual contributes to the study. We assume that as soon as people in the nursing home die, other elderly people are admitted to the nursing home. Let us assume that of these 400 newly admitted people, 75 suffer from dementia at the time that they are admitted to the nursing home, and these 75 people, therefore, are *not* at risk of developing dementia. Hence, they do *not* contribute person-time at risk. The other 325 newly admitted people do not develop dementia during the study period. We also assume that, on average, people who develop dementia do so at the midpoint of the 5-year study period (some of them will develop dementia before this date, others after, and we assume that this averages out). Similarly, on average, the people who die do so at the midpoint of the study period. The person-time at risk, thus, becomes:

$1,600 \times 5$ person-years (the complete population at risk multiplied by the study period) minus $200 \times 2.5$ (the number of dementia cases multiplied by the time that they contribute to the person-time at risk) minus $75 \times 2.5$ (the deceased elderly people who were replaced by people with dementia, who do not contribute person-time at risk) $= 7,312.5$ person-years. The incidence density, therefore, becomes $200/7,312.5$ person-years. This would be expressed as an incidence density of 27 per 1,000 person-years.

### TABLE 20.2
### The ATC Classification System

| Group | Level | ATC Code | Example |
|---|---|---|---|
| Anatomical main group | 1st level; 1 letter | M | Musculoskeletal group |
| Therapeutic main group | 2nd level; 2 numbers | M01 | Anti-inflammatory and anti-rheumatic products |
| Therapeutic subgroup | 3rd level; 1 letter | M01A | Non-steroids |
| Chemical main group | 4th level; 1 letter | M01AE | Propionic acid derivatives |
| Chemical subgroup | 5th level; 2 numbers | M01AE01 | Ibuprofen |

## TABLE 20.3
### Example of Quantifying Drug Use with Defined Daily Doses

| Drug | Defined Daily Dose Value | Daily Dose | Dose (mg) | Defined Daily Doses/Day |
|------|--------------------------|------------|-----------|-------------------------|
| Nitrazepam | 5 mg | 5 mg at night | 5 | 1 |
| Oxazepam | 50 mg | 3 × 15 mg | 45 | 0.9 |
| Flunitrazepam | 1 mg | 2 mg at night | 2 | 2 |
| Paracetamol | 3 g | 3 × 500 mg | 1,500 | 0.5 |
| *Total* | *4 drugs* | *8 tablets* | *1552 mg* | *4.4 defined daily doses/day* |

population level. Examples of the DDD as a volume measure of drug use on a population level are

- The number of DDDs/1,000/day (e.g. in a country)
- The number of DDDs/100 bed days (e.g. in a hospital department)
- The number of DDDs/day (e.g. in nursing homes, or also in hospitals)
- The cost/DDD of a drug (e.g. to compare costs of this drug with other drugs that are used for the same indication)

The ATC and DDD systems have advantages in the sense that even if drug choice changes over time or differs between countries, drug use can be compared and general trends in use can be identified. In addition, they are international systems, hence it is unequivocal as to which drugs are and which are not included in a study as soon as the ATC codes are published with such a study. However, local prescribing may of course differ from WHO guidelines on the recommended daily dose for an indication. Hence, one DDD does not necessarily indicate one treatment day for an adult. Sometimes, drugs are prescribed for other indications than the main indication for which they are registered. An example would be the use of amitriptyline (an anti-depressant) for neuralgia.

Nevertheless, the systems are useful for providing overviews of drug use on a population basis. In general, the ATC and DDD systems are used in drug utilization studies to monitor drug use and changes over time, to evaluate the effects of market regulations and to plan medical and health policy.

## STUDY DESIGN

In pharmacoepidemiology, several epidemiologic study designs are used:

- Descriptive studies
- Case–control studies
- Cohort studies
- Experimental studies

### DESCRIPTIVE STUDIES

These describe patterns of drug utilization in relation to variables such as disease, gender, place and time. The data that are provided by these studies are essential for health care planning, as well as for epidemiologists. For health care planning, knowledge of specific subgroups of people that are most or least affected by the drugs, or most likely to use the drugs, allows the most efficient allocation of resources and the targeting of specific parts of the population for intervention programmes. For epidemiologists, next to drug alerts from spontaneous reporting systems, drug utilization studies are often the first hypothesis-generating step in the search for determinants or risks of drug use. Usually, these studies can be performed with existing databases and are therefore relatively inexpensive and can be carried out relatively quickly. Typical descriptive studies in pharmacoepidemiology are case reports and cross-sectional studies of populations.

## CASE–CONTROL STUDIES

These are analytical epidemiological investigations in which subjects are selected on the basis of whether they do (cases) or do not (controls) have a particular disease under study. The groups are then compared with respect to the proportion having or not having been exposed to the drug of interest. The advantages of the case–control design are best illustrated using a classic example of a case–control study in pharmacoepidemiology: the discovery that diethylstilboestrol (DES) could cause vaginal cancer in women who had been exposed to DES *in utero*. In the 1960s in Boston, US, this disease was diagnosed in eight women between 15 and 22 years old, whereas this disease usually occurs only very rarely in women younger than 50 years old. Prior to 1967, no one had presented with this disease in the hospital where the physicians worked. One of the women asked her doctor whether the cancer might have been caused by her mother's use of DES during pregnancy. Because they could not find any other apparent cause, the physicians designed a structured study that would systematically compare these women – the 'cases' – with an appropriate comparator group – the 'controls' – to identify factors that might be associated with the disease. For each case, four female controls were found that were matched for age and hospital ward where the cases were born, and the mothers of cases and controls were interviewed. Apart from the use of DES, cases and controls did not differ with respect to the medication taken by the mothers (Herbst et al. 1971).

This study illustrates all of the advantages of the case–control study design. It can be used to explore associations with disorders that are very rare and where there is a long lag time between exposure and outcome. This design can be used relatively quickly and inexpensively, and it can examine multiple aetiological factors for a single disease. Limitations of this study design are that, unless the attributable risk is high, it is inefficient for the evaluation of rare exposures and particularly prone to bias. For example, the selection of controls can lead to bias, and recall bias is often also mentioned in association with this study design. This bias results from cases being more likely to recall prior drug use than controls. Case–control studies have a particular utility in the investigation of both rare diseases and the potential roles of multiple risk factors. Because of their lower costs and relative efficiency, with careful planning and study conduct, this study design is often a useful first step in the identification of possible risk factors.

## Cohort Studies

In these, a group or groups of individuals are identified on the basis of the presence or absence of exposure to a drug as a suspected risk factor for the disease. At the time that exposure status is established, all subjects must be free from the disease under study. Subsequently, they are followed over a period of time to assess the occurrence of the disease. Another name for this design is a 'follow-up study'. Cohort studies are particularly suited for the evaluation of rare exposures, and they can study multiple effects of exposure. In addition, because exposure status is established in disease-free individuals and these are subsequently followed up, the temporal relationship between exposure and subsequent development of the disease is easier to establish. Finally, this study design is less prone to bias in the estimation of exposure than are case–control studies. This is particularly true if the study is prospective, when subjects are recruited and followed up prospectively rather than retrospectively. Limitations of the cohort study design are that such studies can be relatively time-consuming and therefore expensive, especially when they seek to evaluate rare diseases or when they involve the prospective collection of data. If they are carried out retrospectively (e.g. within a multipurpose database), this requires the availability of adequate records. Finally, in cohort studies, people are followed up over time. Inherent in this design is that individuals may be 'lost to follow-up' (i.e. they withdraw from the study). This may be due to factors that are unrelated to the study (e.g. if they move abroad), but it may also be that this loss to follow-up is inherent to the exposure. For example, it may be that people decide to withdraw from the study because they develop serious adverse effects, and therefore refuse to cooperate further in a study of that drug, or it could be that the drug cures an illness so efficiently that subjects think they are no longer needed in this study (because they are cured). If such individuals are simply excluded from the study, this type of loss to follow-up will give biased estimates of the drug's effects, because only a selected population will reach the end of the study period.

## Experimental Studies

A special type of cohort study is the 'randomized controlled trial' (RCT), an experimental study design that is used in the evaluation of new drugs before they can be introduced to the market (see also Chapters 22 and 27). In RCTs, study subjects are randomly allocated to exposed or unexposed status and subsequently followed up over time. In this way, comparability of the exposed and the unexposed populations is ensured, which reduces the chance of obtaining biased risk estimates.

## Risk Estimates

In case–control studies, then, prior exposure to drug use is compared between cases and controls, whereas in cohort studies, cohorts of exposed and unexposed study subjects are followed up for an outcome. From both study types, we can calculate risk estimates of exposure and subsequent outcome (Figure 20.3).

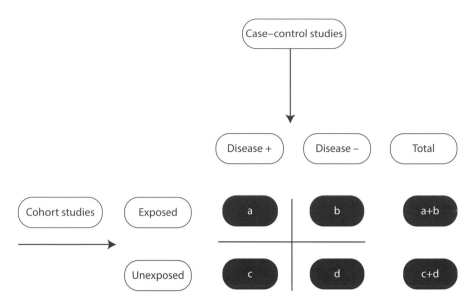

**FIGURE 20.3**   Presentation of data from case–control and cohort studies.

In cohort studies, because we can estimate the true incidence of the outcome studied in the exposed and the unexposed population, a relative risk (RR) can be calculated as the incidence of the outcome in the exposed population divided by the incidence in the unexposed population. This is calculated as follows:

$$RR = I_{exp}/I_{unexp} = CI_{exp}/CI_{unexp}$$

where I is the incidence rate, CI is the cumulative incidence, exp is the exposed population and unexp is the unexposed population.

From this formula, it follows that if $RR = 1$, then the incidence is the same in both populations: there is no association between the exposure and the outcome. If $RR > 1$, however, then exposure is associated with an increased risk of the outcome under study. Finally, if $RR < 1$, then exposure is associated with a decreased risk, or a protective effect, with respect to the outcome under study.

In case–control studies, it is usually not possible to calculate the incidence of the outcome, and therefore the RR cannot be calculated from these studies. However, it can be estimated by calculating the ratio of the odds of exposure among cases to that among controls. Referring to Figure 20.3, this odds ratio (OR) can be calculated from:

$$OR = (a/c)/(b/d) = ad/bc$$

Under certain conditions, the OR approximates the RR (see the 'Further Reading' section).

## BIAS AND CONFOUNDING

When an association between exposure and outcome has been found, we need to evaluate whether this association is valid. In other words, could this association have been found due to chance, systematic bias in the study design or due to confounding? In this section, we shall focus on bias and confounding. Two types of bias are generally considered in epidemiology: selection bias and information bias.

Selection bias may occur in a case–control study if the selection of cases and controls is based on different criteria and these criteria are related to the exposure of interest. A classic example is a case–control study in the 1960s of thromboembolism and prior exposure to oral contraceptives. Because the suspicion of this association existed, physicians were more likely to hospitalize women with symptoms of thromboembolism if these women used oral contraceptives than when they did not. As a consequence, the selection of cases from hospitals gave a case population in which oral contraceptives were over-represented compared to the underlying case population. Therefore, due to selection bias, the OR was overestimated from that study. Similarly, in retrospective cohort studies, selection bias may occur when the selection of exposed and unexposed individuals is based on different criteria that are related to the outcome of interest. In these studies, as in case–control studies, both the disease and the drug exposure have occurred at the time that individuals are selected for the study. Selection bias is unlikely to occur in prospective cohort studies, since in these studies, the outcome is unknown at the time of study subject recruitment (Hennekens and Buring 1987).

Information bias includes any systematic differences between the two study groups (cases and controls or exposed and non-exposed individuals, respectively) in the measurement of information on exposure or outcome. This has already been alluded to in the discussion of Figure 20.2, where misclassification of exposure was discussed. If such misclassification differs between cases and controls (e.g. because cases are interviewed regarding their drug use, while, for controls, general practitioners' records are consulted), this may lead to a biased risk estimate.

Well-known examples of information bias are 'recall bias' and 'interviewer bias'. An example of recall bias would be a case–control study of drug safety during pregnancy and subsequent congenital malformations. It is generally assumed that, when they are interviewed concerning drug use during pregnancy, mothers of malformed babies will be more accurate in recalling this than mothers of a healthy baby. Such recall bias will lead to overestimated ORs. Sometimes, researchers try to avoid this by using 'sick controls' (e.g. mothers of babies with Down's syndrome). This congenital disorder is unlikely to be caused by drug use. Similarly, when interviewers know the health status of cases and controls, especially if they are aware of the exposure that is being studied, it is assumed that their interview techniques may differ between cases and controls, also leading to spurious associations or overestimated ORs.

If the inaccuracy of data collection is the same for both groups, this will lead to a dilution of the effect and the risk estimate will be closer to 1 than it would have been had the data been completely accurate. This is called non-differential misclassification (i.e. the same for both groups).

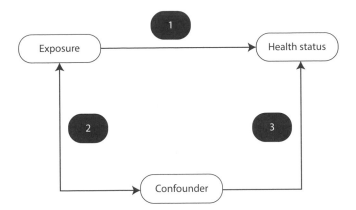

**FIGURE 20.4** Concepts of confounding.

Finally, risk estimates can be over- or under-estimated due to confounding. Confounding involves the possibility that the observed association can, in part or totally, be explained by differences between the study groups other than the exposure under study. These differences could affect the risk of developing the outcome of interest.

The principle of confounding is represented in Figure 20.4. As can be seen from this figure, for a determinant to be a true confounding factor, the following criteria must be met. A confounding factor:

- Is an independent predictor (although not necessarily a cause) of the occurrence of the disease
- Is associated with the exposure of interest
- Must not be an intermediate link in the causal pathway between exposure and outcome

An example of confounding is the association between the use of ulcer-healing drugs and the development of lung cancer. This association is confounded by smoking. If you perform a study of lung cancer and prior exposure to ulcer-healing drugs, you may find an increased risk of lung cancer in the exposed population: there is an association between the drug and the disease (arrow 1 in Figure 20.4). However, people who smoke are more likely to have gastric complaints and, therefore, use ulcer-healing drugs (arrow 2). In addition, we know that smoking is associated with an increased risk of lung cancer, which is independent of exposure to ulcer-healing drugs (arrow 3). Finally, smoking is not an intermediate link in the causal pathway: the use of ulcer-healing drugs does not cause people to take up smoking, which subsequently causes lung cancer.

Unlike bias, which is introduced by the investigators or study participants, confounding is an underlying function of relationships between exposure, disease and other determinants. In addition, unlike bias, as long as the possible confounding factors are known, they can be controlled for in the study design or in the analysis (Hennekens and Buring 1987).

However, in pharmacoepidemiology, one particular kind of confounding is more difficult to control for in the analysis and is usually dealt with at the stage of study design: confounding by the reason for prescription, or 'confounding by indication'. In some cases, it is also referred to as 'channelling'. Treated people differ from people who are not treated (e.g. new drugs are usually prescribed to the sickest patients). There is always a reason for prescribing, and especially with studies of beneficial drug effects, this reason is often associated with the outcome of interest. An example of confounding by indication is the association between the extensive use of beta-agonists, or use of the newest beta-agonists, and asthma mortality. This association is said to be confounded by disease severity – hence, by indication. Another example was the association between selective serotonin re-uptake inhibitors (SSRIs) and suicide rates when the SSRIs were first marketed. Compared to classic anti-depressants, suicide rates were higher among SSRI users, but this was said to be entirely due to confounding by indication. It is difficult to control for this at the analysis stage in a study. People try to avoid this type of bias by measuring and controlling for disease severity or by conducting RCTs (experiments) rather than observational studies.

## CONCLUSION

Pharmacovigilance is used to evaluate the beneficial and adverse effects of medicines and, as such, provides an important information source for the advice that pharmacists give on drug use. This may be required for market approval, the development of prescribing guidelines in general or for the implementation of research findings locally (e.g. in their hospital, community pharmacy, peer-review group or their Drugs and Therapeutics Committee). Pharmacists, with their therapeutic knowledge and ability to critically review the outcomes of spontaneous reporting and pharmacoepidemiology studies, can contribute to the development and implementation of such guidelines. In the long run, this should result in rational drug use, so that, eventually, good pharmacovigilance leads to good medicine. In addition, pharmacovigilance provides the basis for health service research and pharmacoeconomics.

## FURTHER READING

Aronson, J.K. and Ferner, R.E. 2003. Joining the DoTS: New approach to classifying adverse drug reactions. *British Medical Journal*, **327**, 1222–1225.

Hartzema, A.G., Porta, M.S. and Tilson, H.H. 1998. *Pharmacoepidemiology. An Introduction* (3rd Edn.). Cincinnati: Harvey Whitney.

Hennekens, C.H. and Buring, J.E. 1987. *Epidemiology in Medicine*. Boston: Little, Brown.

Hosmer, D.W., Lemeshow, S. and Sturdivant, R.X. 2013. *Applied Logistic Regression*. New York: Wiley-Blackwell.

Rothman, K.J., Lash, T.L. and Greenland, S. (Eds.) 2013. *Modern Epidemiology* (3rd Edn.). Philadelphia: Lippincott Williams and Wilkins.

Schlesselman, J.J. 1982. *Case–Control Studies. Design, Conduct, Analysis*. New York: Oxford University Press.

Strom, B.L. and Kimmel, S.E. (Eds.) 2013. *Textbook of Pharmacoepidemiology* (2nd Edn.). Chichester: Wiley-Blackwell.

Strom, B.L., Kimmel, S.E. and Hennessy, S. (Eds.) 2012. *Pharmacoepidemiology* (5th Edn.). Chichester: Wiley-Blackwell.

Zizam, A., Rosenberg, E., Kleinbaum, D.G. and Kupper, L.L. 2013. *Applied Regression Analysis and Other Multivariable Methods* (5th Edn.). Belmont: Brooks/Cole.

## REFERENCES

Hartzema, A.G., Porta, M.S. and Tilson, H.H. 1998. *Pharmacoepidemiology. An Introduction* (3rd Edn.). Cincinnati: Harvey Whitney.

Hennekens, C.H. and Buring J.E. 1987. *Epidemiology in Medicine.* Boston: Little, Brown.

Herbst, A.L., Ulfelder, H. and Poskanzer, D.C. 1971. Adenocarcinoma of the vagina. Association of maternal stilbestrol therapy with tumor appearance in young women. *New England Journal of Medicine*, **284**, 878–881.

Hill, A.B. 1965. The environment and disease: Association or causation? *Proceedings of the Royal Society of Medicine*, **85**, 295–300.

Inman, W.H.W. (Ed.) 1986. *Monitoring for Drug Safety.* Lancaster: MTP Press.

Strom, B.L., Kimmel, S.E., Hennessy, S. (Eds.) 2012. *Pharmacoepidemiology* (5th Edn.) Chichester: Wiley-Blackwell.

Sukkar, E. 2015. Searching social networks to detect adverse reactions. *Pharmaceutical Journal*, **24**, 75–78.

World Health Organization 1990. *Guidelines for ATC Classification.* Oslo: WHO Collaborating Centre for Drug Statistics Methodology and Nordic Council on Medicines.

World Health Organization 1998. *Safety Monitoring of Medical Drugs. Guidelines for Setting Up and Running of a Pharmacovigilance Centre.* Geneva: World Health Organization.

# 21 Health Economics

*Hakan Brodin*

## CONTENTS

---

### KEY POINTS

- The appropriate application of health economics is crucial for the understanding and comparison of treatment options.
- Health economics involves applying economic theories and methods in order to understand and predict the performance of a health care sector.
- The term 'pharmacoeconomics' may be used to describe health economic studies in the pharmaceutical area.
- The predominant health economic activity is the evaluation of new or existing treatments from a social viewpoint.
- Economic studies focus on the use of resources.

- Across nations, gross national product per capita largely explains how much resource is dedicated to health care.
- The concept of costs and benefits is central to the economic evaluation of pharmaceuticals.
- An important contribution of health economics is estimating the advantages and disadvantages of preventing illnesses or injuries.

## INTRODUCTION

Health economics involves the application of economic theories and methods to understand and predict how the health care sector (including pharmacy) will perform from a policy perspective. It is particularly useful for optimizing the use of pharmaceuticals, to promote appropriate drugs and to identify ineffective or obsolete drugs. It may also be used by health authorities and managers to organize pharmaceutical care in an efficient and resource-minimizing way.

Very often the terms 'health economics' and 'pharmacoeconomics' are used interchangeably. In this chapter, 'health economics' will be used for the academic discipline, theories, methodology and techniques. Health economics uses a few theories and methods, mainly from the medical and psychological disciplines, which are not generally used in conventional economics. The term 'pharmacoeconomics' may be used for health economic studies in the pharmaceutical area. There are no specific theories, methods or concepts, other than those used in general health economics, for the study of pharmaceuticals.

## BASIC HEALTH ECONOMIC CONCEPTS

Economic studies focus on the use of resources. Every clinical decision taken by health care professionals has resource implications. A prescription not only impacts on a patient's health, but also on their purse. If the drug is subsidized, the prescription will also have consequences for how taxpayers' money is used.

In the long term, the choice of one drug over another may have positive or negative consequences for both the patient and the health care system. If a doctor asks for a second opinion from a colleague, a certain amount of time (one kind of resource) is withdrawn from the second doctor's work. If a pharmacist calls the doctor to clarify or confirm an issue on a prescription, his or her resources are spent and cannot be used for other ends. An awareness of the simple economic fact that medical work involves resources and costs is not always fully appreciated by health care organizations or the pharmaceutical profession.

Economics, including health economics, does not simply consist of concepts and definitions which are easily learned. Economics is also a way of thinking. Since the end users of health economics are often physicians and pharmacists, with little time and/or interest to invest in this way of thinking, the consequences are that economic knowledge is often used in a scattered and superficial way. An informed guess would be that a large improvement in medical outcomes (i.e. health improvement) is possible for the same amount of resources consequent upon the application of an economic perspective within health care. Pharmacists may have an important role to play in this respect.

## THE SOCIAL CONTEXT OF HEALTH CARE

Modern health care is remarkably similar in different countries. The major characteristic in most countries is that it is heavily regulated by the political and administrative system. Economic markets play quite a minor part in the doctor/patient interface, although there is 'normal' economic behaviour in the relationship between the health care system and, for instance, the producers of medical equipment and pharmaceuticals. Even in the most market-orientated health care systems, such as in the US, about 40% of health care costs are financed outside of normal markets. Other countries strive to deregulate the medical system, and a common trend is to deregulate the pharmaceutical markets in favour of fewer prescription-only medicines to more pharmacy (or even supermarket)-sold medicines (the 'POM' to 'P' shift).

Across nations, it is also possible to identify a single economic factor which would largely explain ($r^2 > 90\%$) how much resources are devoted to health care. This is the gross national product (GNP) per capita. GNP is the value of the sum total of all produced and sold goods and services in a country in one year. GNP per capita is a measure of the average output per person, and it is also a measure of the average income or purchasing power of the population. Thus, it seems that differences in political systems, private or social insurance, general practitioners or hospital-employed physicians, etc., have less impact on the size of the health care sector than the general income level of the nation. However, public financing limits the costs to a small but significant degree when the influence from other variables is taken into account.

It also appears that health care systems in different countries will increasingly converge with time. There are two possible reasons for this. First, there is a financial need to limit the possibilities for expansion of the system, and to control costs. This is due to an increased competition in society for taxpayers' money as the health care sector expands. Second, the demands for efficiency in the health care sector have led to a global search for new technologies, especially within pharmaceuticals. This, in turn, leads to a common international health care behaviour, in that the same or similar resources will be used and the same or similar results obtained in all countries.

Different nations will encounter different epidemiological conditions. A major cause of death in one country could be of minor importance in another. Planning and monitoring health care from a public health perspective have consequently been major issues in the health care sector, as well as at governmental levels. To this end, a special branch of health economics has been established to estimate what economic consequences are attached to a certain illness: cost-of-illness studies. Two approaches can be identified: first, in the prevalence approach, the (national) total annual cost of a particular illness is estimated. It answers the question 'how much money is devoted to health care of the illness this year?' Second, in the incidence approach, the lifetime cost is estimated (i.e. 'What is the cost of the illness for patient and society?').

Very often, cost-of-illness studies provide figures of large economic burden to society, and the implied logic is that if a given disease has a large economic burden, then more resources should be devoted to it. However, it requires that: (a) there is a technology/method of some kind that alters the situation; and (b) that this technology is worth the invested resources.

A major part of cost-of-illness studies is usually the cost to society of lost production. Some criticisms have been directed towards the estimation of lost production. The most important is probably that it is unethical to use the contribution to GNP as a guiding rule for health care, when the sole purpose of health care should be to prolong life and maintain health-related quality of life.

## HEALTH ECONOMICS THEORY

Kenneth Arrow, a well-known economist, has identified three basic 'peculiarities' or characteristics of health care that have led to massive political and administrative interference in the market structure (Arrow 1963). Arrow's analysis of the market mechanisms led to a deeper understanding of why health care was not sold in small shops or in an unregulated marketplace alongside oven-ready chickens and vegetables. He also explained why regulated health care would work better in meeting its primary goals (i.e. to create and sustain health) than a pure market approach. The basic characteristics of health care are:

- Asymmetric information between doctor and patient
- External effects
- The uncertainty of incidence of disease or injury

### Asymmetric Information

Much of this section is based on the work of Evans (1984). Basic economic theory tells us that, in an ideal world, buyers and sellers meet and voluntarily come to agreements about exchanging goods and services according to the principles of supply and demand. However, a number of activities, especially in health care, are too complex to operate in a free-market environment. They are characterized by a principal/agent relationship. Activity is directed by an agent (the pharmacist) with a special knowledge towards a principal (the patient/customer) who has to rely on the agent since the patient does not possess this knowledge. This is called asymmetric information. Clearly, an agent may benefit by telling the principal of the advantages about a product and conceal the drawbacks. The agent can thus profit from the ignorance of the gullible principal.

Throughout the ages, this has led to a credibility problem, such that by 400 BC, Hippocrates had formulated what is widely known as the Hippocratic Oath to maintain the good standards of doctors. The World Medical Association Declaration of Geneva on the Physician's Oath was adopted in 1948, amended in 1968 and is in use today. It contains most of the same elements in a modern form:

- Regulation of behaviour
- A system for education
- An internal regulatory and punishment system

These provide safeguards that are absent from an unregulated market system. The Geneva Declaration also serves as a model for ethical pharmacy practice in many countries.

## EXTERNAL (INTERPERSONAL) EFFECTS

The second characteristic of health care which contrasts with an unregulated market concerns external effects (i.e. that someone, other than the patient, is potentially affected by the health care delivered [or withdrawn]). The simplest example is the parent–child case. It is not the small child, as a patient, that the doctor attempts to persuade to accept treatment, but rather the child's parents. It is also the parents that the doctor will approach for payment for treatment. This is usually termed the 'altruistic external effect'. Someone is interested, by consideration and love, to pay some or all of the money to ensure that another person receives health care.

An example of selfish external effects is vaccination. If all of the students in a class are vaccinated against polio, then the risk to the teacher of infection is considerably reduced, and he or she will, for perfectly selfish reasons, be willing to pay for the students to be vaccinated.

Another case of external effects is the tendency of governments to protect against hazardous behaviour and to promote healthy behaviour. In most countries, there is extensive taxation of alcohol and tobacco, while health care is subsidized. This is an example of a paternalistic external effect. The government considers citizens, in some instances, not to be adequately responsible for their own health. It therefore attempts to persuade people, by giving them economic incentives, to consume less of some goods and more of others, relative to what they would otherwise choose in an unregulated market.

The consequences of these external effects are that health care, in general, is not only financed by the individuals themselves, but is also financed by a variety of third-party payments, blurring the market structure. It is difficult to separate supply from demand, and some critics of a regulated health care system claim that the health professions exert too much power and influence over governments in setting the health care budget.

## RISK OR UNCERTAINTY

The third characteristic that makes health care a special commodity is the presence of risk and uncertainty about who is going to be ill or injured. Risk and uncertainty is most often addressed by the extensive use of insurance. An insurance system leads to a departure from the simple supply-and-demand model because payment for services is not made at the point of delivery.

# ECONOMIC EVALUATION OF PHARMACEUTICALS

## THE CONCEPTS OF SOCIAL COSTS AND BENEFITS

This section builds largely on the work of Drummond et al. (1989). Thorough evaluation of the costs and effects of health care depends on the quality of available data.

Not only are quality of life issues difficult to measure, but the cost side of the analysis may also present significant problems. The concept of cost (i.e. the value of the resources used) is central to the choice and application of the study methodology. For instance, charges and other 'price-tag' figures are not necessarily an indication of the value of resources. In the pharmaceutical area, as in many other areas of human activities, the 'welfarist' approach should be adopted. Apart from ordinary goods and services like pharmaceutical products and pharmacy services, resources also include energy, water and the time allocated by staff to different activities. The skills of the staff and/or users involved in the activities are another kind of resource – human capital.

Consequently, monetary payment does not represent the real cost. In calculating the real cost, the concepts outlined in the following sections are important.

## Opportunity Cost: The Alternatives

When a certain amount of resources is used deliberately in one health care activity instead of another, a judgement should have been required to ensure that the resources are used in the best possible way. Otherwise, resources will have been wasted. When resources are referred to in this way, they are called opportunity costs. When taxpayers' money is used in hospital care to provide a hip replacement rather than providing chemotherapy treatment, the real operating cost is what is lost in terms of chemotherapy treatment.

Applying the concept of opportunity cost to pharmaceutical technology is sometimes difficult and requires that the marginal cost must be considered, instead of the average cost, when estimating the resources used in a health care programme. The marginal cost quantifies how many extra resources are used when one extra unit of output is produced. This is also an expression of alternative actions and is consequently also one aspect of the opportunity cost principle.

In many cases, the marginal cost can be estimated by short-term operating direct costs only, excluding transferred costs for administration, rents for buildings and the supply of energy and heating. This is because, in most cases, it is only possible to save the direct cost if a programme is not applied (opportunity cost). However, staff costs should not be excluded on the basis that staff will be fired or rendered unemployed should the service be used by fewer patients, since staff not used for one service may be used to deliver another.

## THE DISCOUNT RATE

Another important issue, especially when considering prevention activities, concerns the costs and effects at different points in time. In health care, the costs frequently occur at the commencement of a programme, while the benefits will often accrue some years later. In pharmaceutical care, a momentary investment in a particular activity (i.e. advice-giving to certain persons at risk) may result in a reduced risk of becoming ill or being impaired for the rest of a person's life. To be able to compare costs and benefits, these must be considered as if they are occurring at the same point in time, normally the beginning of the activity. Both costs and benefits accruing sometime in the future will be valued less than if they had occurred today. This is because it is usually advantageous to postpone costs and to advance benefits. This would be the case even in a society with no inflation or bank interest charges. In economics, this is referred to as a consequence of the personal discount rate and varies for different people. Some people are impatient and consequently have a high rate, while others (e.g. those in schools and colleges) postpone their earnings for several years, in favour of waiting for some future better living conditions. They have low discount rates.

All personal discount rates are aggregated to a social discount rate, which is used to transform costs and benefits from different points in time into equivalent costs today. Mathematically, it resembles the interests used by banks. In health care programmes, this discount rate is often around 5%, plus an extra percentage for inflation, if any. The equation for calculating the present value $P$ from a future value $F$, in $t$ years with a discount rate $r$ is:

$$P = F \cdot \frac{1}{(1 + r)^t}$$

An example calculation is shown in Box 21.1.

---

### BOX 21.1  EXAMPLE OF A DISCOUNT RATE CALCULATION

A new drug for preventing osteoporosis is proposed. The consequences of preventing osteoporosis are complex, but to simplify the example, let us say that the sole effect of preventing osteoporosis is to avoid hip fractures in old people. Clinical trials have shown that the new drug can prevent 5,100 extra fractures in the country compared to the existing treatments available. The drug is proposed for use by women at menopause and onwards.

The cost of lifelong treatment is easily calculated. We do not need this for this example. We shall concentrate on the prevention effects, adjusted to the time period of the start of treatment. If we assume that hip fractures, on average, occur at the age of 85, we will 'roughly' need to scale down the 5,100 saved cases by 30 years to 55 years of age. If each fracture treatment costs £19,000, then by using this drug, we can save in terms of future treatment, $F$, of $5,100 \times 19,000 = £96.9$ million. To get the value of this treatment in present terms, we use a discount rate of 5%. Then, from the equation:

$$P = 96.9(1 + 0.05)^{30}$$

compared to the cost today, the result is £22.4 million. Since other preventative measures may have other costs and effects in other time perspectives, the conclusion is that if the health care system can find another way to save hip fractures with lower present costs or a higher present value than £22.4 million (e.g. rebuilding houses for the elderly or reducing prescriptions for sedatives), then they should not adopt the new drug. (See also the 'Economic Aspects of Prevention' section in this chapter.)

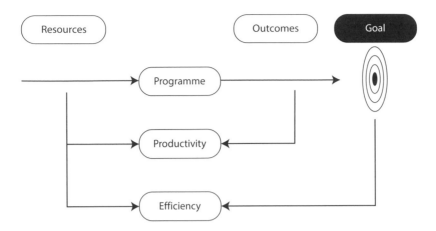

**FIGURE 21.1**   Productivity versus efficiency.

## PRODUCTIVITY VERSUS EFFICIENCY

Economic evaluation usually means evaluation of goal fulfilment. There are other types of evaluation with broader purposes (e.g. process evaluation), but economists tend to regard evaluation as specifying and valuing resources in relation to what can be achieved in terms of the specified purpose. In health care, this is typically prolonged life and increased quality of life. Figure 21.1 illustrates how the inputs/resources are used in some processes (typically unknown and of little interest for the assessment), generating outputs/outcomes of the programme.

A programme has a goal, uses resources and results in outcomes. Inputs and out-puts can be compared, most often in ratios, to measure productivity and efficiency. Efficiency measures the degree of goal fulfilment (health effects) we can achieve with a certain mix and amount of resources. Productivity, on the other hand, only measures how much could be achieved in terms of customers served by the inputs used, regardless of whether health care workers do or do not do a good job in terms of the goal (i.e. increased health among customers). Increased productivity in health care may sometimes even be detrimental to increased efficiency.

## METHODS FOR PHARMACOECONOMIC EVALUATION

Private-sector enterprises have little need for evaluation methods other than to measure net profits (i.e. the return on invested assets). In other words, the goal is to make money. If profit is not sufficiently high, shareholders will transfer their investment to other areas. In health care, there is also a social goal imposed by rep-resentatives of the population to guarantee the provision of health care. If a hospital or pharmacy is not profitable from a business viewpoint, it may still be required to remain in business with government subsidies. In such instances, a different type of evaluation is required.

## Three Techniques of Social Evaluation

### Cost–Benefit Analysis

In cost–benefit analysis, the value of the resources, measured as opportunity costs, is related to the social objective of the programme expressed in monetary terms. All possible effects within the ethical constraints of human behaviour that affect the welfare of individuals are estimated and valued. The most universal value of all is, of course, monetary. The increase in welfare generated by the programme should be measured by willingness to pay; that is, by the sum of money that an individual is prepared to pay to obtain health benefits, or as compensation for the harm inflicted on them. A programme should be undertaken if the social benefits, measured as the sum of all benefits to all individuals, exceed its social costs, measured in the same way (i.e. if the net social benefit is positive).

The expression 'within the ethical constraints of human behaviour' is essential but implicit and sometimes overlooked. In normal activities, economists seldom have reason to discuss the ethical foundations of behaviour. Analysts do not propose illegal actions even if they would be profitable. There are always grey areas, however, between the legal and illegal. When analysing programmes, including personal welfare, utility and quality of life, caution should be exercised about unethical, but not necessarily illegal, actions. One example is the much-discussed inclusion of increased patient work productivity as a measure of the success of a new drug.

Cost–benefit analysis is best suited for limited and well-defined projects. Projects with obscure and/or secondary effects with consequences in many sectors of society are not well suited for cost–benefit analysis. Furthermore, in many cases, market prices or charges made to individuals are inappropriate as measures of the marginal social cost or marginal social value of goods and services. For instance, the charges to users of pharmaceutical services are frequently small. The co-payments made by the consumer may, however, be only a small fraction of the actual costs of those services to the insurance company or health care budget. In such cases, the analyst has to consider more than the market prices, also considering the shadow prices and scrutinizing the accounts to see what the real marginal cost should be.

### Cost–Effectiveness Analysis

As discussed previously, the effects of a social programme are typically not only marketable goods and services, but also savings in time, pain and rehabilitation of lost functioning. In such cases, cost–benefit analysis will become complex and lose its strength as a simple analytical tool. A good alternative may be cost–effectiveness analysis, which only measures the effects in physical units or amounts, instead of monetary values. Cost–effectiveness analysis, on the other hand, loses one of the advantages of cost–benefit analysis: that the net result of the programme only requires it to be positive in money values to determine whether a new treatment programme is to be accepted or not. Since cost–effectiveness measures physical units, it is necessary to present the result of the analysis as a cost–effectiveness ratio (e.g. dollars per saved life, etc.). Therefore, there is no single value that will reveal whether or not the programme is to be undertaken. The cost per unit has to be compared to other

> ### BOX 21.2   THREE POSSIBLE CATEGORIES OF COSTS
>
> - Direct costs are resources that are used to run the programme (e.g. staff costs, costs for drugs, etc.). They also include resources used by the patient or relatives/guardians to access treatment, such as patient charges, travel costs and 'out-of-pocket' drug costs.
> - Indirect costs include the patient's lost income due to illness and treatment, and also the resulting disturbances in their workplace.
> - Intangible costs are difficult or impossible to measure (e.g. anxiety, pain and exhaustion from treatment).

programmes estimated in the same way, and the importance of the different values must then be assessed by political or administrative bodies.

In many cases, the analysis can be so uncertain that it is impossible to achieve a single value representing a 'best guess'. One way of presenting results from this kind of analysis would be to perform a sensitivity analysis; that is, to change the values of critical variables (e.g. the discount rate) and to present the results in terms of maximum and minimum values. The cost could be divided into three categories (Box 21.2).

Another category is often referred to as 'indirect costs'. This category deals with the secondary consequences resulting from a programme. It could be, for instance, an increase in the price of pharmaceuticals as a consequence of new laws requiring economic evaluations before product registration, which increases the development costs. This type of cost should normally not be included in a simple evaluation, since the primary cost has already been included. Likewise, secondary health care effects of increased work, which are a consequence of increased longevity or improved quality of life, should also be excluded from the evaluation to avoid double counting.

## Cost–Utility Analysis

An appealing technique for pharmaceutical activities, which has been developed quite recently, is cost–utility analysis (CUA). The concept of utility has emerged from utilitarian ethics, which were developed during the eighteenth century. Individuals are thought of as 'consistently attempting to achieve maximum satisfaction or well-being or utility, as the concept is variously called' (Parkin et al. 2011). In health care activities, utility often corresponds to 'quality of life', although there are different opinions regarding the relationship between the two concepts. CUA is a complex and still-developing technique. The different psychometric techniques for revealing the quality of life of patients/customers are particularly intriguing. The individual utility cannot be assessed by anyone other than the individual. Therefore, CUA involves extensive use of psychometric questionnaires. Some user-friendly techniques of calculating so-called quality-adjusted life years (QALYs) have been developed. These techniques calculate the product of the changes in length of life between alternative programmes with the quality difference of those extra years. One year of full quality is 1 QALY, as are two years with a halved quality of life (see Chapter 26).

## ECONOMIC ASPECTS OF PREVENTION

One of the most important contributions of health economics is the estimation of the advantages and disadvantages of prohibiting illnesses or injuries. For many people, the prevention of illness appears to be the obvious choice, if possible. However, what is not considered in many instances is the scarcity of resources, and that if resources are used for one purpose, they cannot be used for another. The best use of resources has to be ascertained.

What are the actual alternatives of investing our resources? It would be strange to treat all hypertensive patients at the expense of those needing hip replacements. Instead, we need to ask what can be achieved if the cost of reducing or increasing various activities is varied by a small percentage. In prevention, the appropriate issue is to balance the costs of hypertension screening and subsequent treatment against the costs of the detection and treatment of actual cardiovascular diseases when they appear in the future. When considering alternative uses of resources, a perspective across time must be adopted. It follows from the previous discussion on discount rates that it is always desirable to postpone resource use and to achieve quick treatment results. It is better to save one life today than a life in 10 years (not necessarily the same life, of course). But if we can save two lives in 14 years with the same resources used today to save one life, it is slightly more favourable, if the discount rate is 5%.

If money and other resources are used for hypertension screening, we must compare their values with those of the same resources used for something else, saving further resources for the future when the treatment of cardiovascular disease may be needed. For prevention activities to be favourable, a few rules of thumb may be followed (Box 21.3).

It is obvious that the estimation of the costs and effects of prevention activities often requires more in terms of data and methodology than is available. We need epidemiological data about the incidence and transition probabilities for different phases of the illness. All treatment effects, such as adverse drug effects, should also be known. Additionally, the accounts of hospitals and primary care units do not generally record the resources used per individual. Therefore, the proper modelling

---

**BOX 21.3   FAVOURABLE CONDITIONS FOR COST-EFFECTIVE PREVENTION ACTIVITIES**

- The initial cost of detection of people in the risk groups should not be very high.
- The fraction of people belonging to the risk group should not be very small.
- The probability of prevention success should be very large.
- The probability of future treatment success should be small.
- The timespan from identification to actual illness should not be very long.

of assumptions and consequences in terms of uncertain results are essential elements in economic evaluations.

## MEDICAL ETHICS VERSUS UTILITARIAN ETHICS

Throughout this chapter, ethical issues have been indicated. Even the foundations of health economic theory have ethical underpinnings. Constantly, we touch upon the boundaries between economics and medical ethics, since the Hippocratic basis often interferes with the utilitarian ethics. This section briefly draws attention to some ethical considerations in relation to economics and the consequences of this for health care (for a comprehensive review, see Mooney and McGuire 1988).

The application of medical ethics centres on the individual, requiring the doctor or pharmacist to give full attention to their individual patients or customers. Health professionals are not required to treat only those who would benefit from this attention, but rather those in the greatest need. The need for health care is determined by the professional – not the patient, nor the treatment result.

Utilitarian ethics, on the other hand, takes a broader and more public perspective. It claims that resources should be used as efficiently as possible. The objective of resource allocation is to maximize the greatest benefit for the greatest number of people. The pharmacist has to pay attention not only to the customer in front of him/her, but also to the other customers waiting for service. It then follows that society has to choose between the different possible alternatives in which the resources could be utilized in order to achieve the best possible total results in terms of utility. The concept of choice also implies that the concept of cost has to be treated in a special way. The opportunity cost recognizes the value of the resources used in relation to the benefits missed as a result of not using resources in the best alternative way. This principle underpins what is often referred to as 'evidence-based medicine'.

The two ethical systems place health professionals, including pharmacists, in a dilemma. They traditionally pay full attention to the patient in front of them and use resources for this patient even if the chance of treatment success is low and a waiting patient has greater need for the pharmacist's services than the current one. The painful dilemma arising from the two ethical systems can be reduced to some degree by good leadership and clear professional rules at the pharmacy level, or higher.

## CONCLUSION

Health economics can be an important tool for pharmacists in terms of encompassing the complex and multidimensional nature of high-technology pharmaceutical care. From the health economic perspective, pharmaceuticals are valued in their proper environment, not only in a limited financial sense, but also in a broad social and humanistic framework. They are scrutinized to extract the best available treatments. Their therapeutic effects are related to the costs of the treatment and to other treatment options.

The predominant health economic activity is the evaluation of new or existing treatments from a social viewpoint. The sound application of health economic theory to practical assessment techniques is crucial for the understanding and fair comparison of treatment options. To that end, a small but important number of conventions and guidelines are applied and are increasingly required in the publishing of scientific results. Pharmacists involved in clinical efficiency studies will benefit from recognizing the importance of these.

Finally, this chapter has highlighted the political and ethical implications of health economics in the potential conflict between the professional and the ethical systems. Evaluation techniques are not ethically neutral, and depending on what technique is used, the social implications will differ, and hence, health economic evaluations should not be applied mechanically.

## FURTHER READING

Mooney, G. and McGuire, A. (Eds.) 1988. *Medical Ethics and Economics in Health Care.* Oxford: Oxford Medical Publications.

## REFERENCES

Arrow, K.J. 1963. Uncertainty and the welfare economics of medical care. *American Economic Review*, **53**, 941–973.

Drummond, M.F., O'Brien, B., Stoddart, G.L. and Torrance, G.W. 1989. *Methods for the Economic Evaluation of Health Care Programmes* (2nd Edn.), Oxford: Oxford Medical Publications.

Evans, R.G. 1984. *Strained Mercy*. Toronto: Butterworths.

Mooney, G. and McGuire, A. (Eds.) 1988. *Medical Ethics and Economics in Health Care.* Oxford: Oxford Medical Publications.

Parkin, M., Powell, M. and Matthews, K. 2011. *Economics* (8th Edn.), Harlow: Addison-Wesley.

# Section V

Undertaking Pharmacy Practice and Health Services Research

# 22 Survey Methods

*Jill K. Jesson and Rob Pocock*

## CONTENTS

> ## KEY POINTS
>
> - A social scientific approach is necessary in order to understand the social world.
> - Our social actions have meaning which requires a social scientific interpretation.
> - Social science research methods include surveys, secondary source data analysis, ethnography, observation and interviews.
> - Pharmacy practice research may draw from a range of paradigms with associated methodologies relevant to the research question.

## INTRODUCTION

Along with health care professionals, such as nurses, physiotherapists and other professions allied to medicine, one of the biggest hurdles pharmacists researching pharmacy practice encounter is the introduction of 'alien' thought patterns for which their academic training has often left them ill prepared. The pharmacy degree is based on the 'positivist' philosophical approach to science and the natural world, but to understand the social world, a social scientific approach is necessary. Some social scientists would argue that all knowledge is socially constructed (i.e. scientific procedures and conclusions are in fact not neutral, objective enterprises, but are 'cultural products'). Empirically based scientific 'facts', then, are not simply determined by the nature of the observable physical world – they are also dependent upon socially derived assumptions.

Scientific 'facts' are inseparable from the assumptions, traditions and relations of people at a particular time and place. These assumptions and traditions are motivated by, and in themselves motivate, conceptual modes of thought. Similarly, each professional group develops its own way of knowing. Pharmacists, doctors, lawyers and social scientists are all socialized into the culture, language and methods of their respective disciplines. Consequently, they each make sense of the world in different ways and investigate the world according to their own rules and perspectives.

## PERSPECTIVES ON RESEARCH AND SCIENCE

The social sciences are not constructed on the same principles as the natural sciences. Human actions, unlike the observed effects of molecules when heated, have meaning for both the observer and the observed and involve a process of interpretation. To explore social actions, a different range of methods is used. In the social sciences, it is accepted that there is not one, but several ways of looking at the world. These ways of looking at the world are known as paradigms or perspectives. Each may have its own internally valid 'truths', but accepting the valid existence of several different paradigms means accepting the reality of several possible conflicting truths instead of one single universal truth. 'Paradigm shift' describes the development of new ideas. A classic clinical paradigm shift in beliefs centres on the cause of peptic ulcers. In the past, it was believed genetic factors, a faulty diet or stress caused the condition. Now, with the emergence of bacteriological infection as a primary cause, as Lefanu (1999) observes, '*Helicobacter* has provoked another paradigm shift in changing scientific understanding, not only of the diseases with which it is directly associated, but of all disease'.

## MODELS OF HEALTH, ILLNESS AND DISEASE

In pharmacy practice research and health care research, two paradigms come into conflict: the bio-medical and the social models of illness and disease.

### BIO-MEDICAL MODEL

The dominant model of disease worldwide – the bio-medical model – is based on the Cartesian philosophy (named after the philosopher Descartes) of the body as a machine. Underlying this perspective is the concept that if a body system malfunctions, it can be repaired or replaced. Thus, the bio-medical model is concerned with the treatment of dysfunction. By contrast, illness is the subjective experience of dysfunction. The medical model is based on notions of scientific rationality, with an emphasis on objective, numerical measurement. In this model, health is conceptualized merely as the absence of disease.

The theoretical framework underpinning the bio-medical model is termed 'positivism', an approach to knowledge based on quantitative measurement. This is a view of the world suggesting that phenomena which convey knowledge and meaning are those which are observable and measurable. Positivist researchers are those who believe that, by careful observation, it is possible to identify the relationship between observable and measurable things. It could then be argued that events that cannot be measured cannot be understood. The key relationships of interest are those of 'causality', in which the state of one variable can be said to 'cause' the state of another one – the 'cause and effect' relationship. This is the principle underlying all physical 'laws'.

In the natural sciences, positivists begin with a tentative idea or hypothesis about relationships between variables and then repeatedly test these ideas against the available evidence. This process leads to validation of theory based on the results of observation. Positivism holds that social aspects of human life can be measured objectively and analysed following the principles of the scientific method (i.e. they can be explained in the same way as the natural sciences and other natural phenomena). Such an approach implies that we can predict and explain behaviour. We can produce a set of 'true', 'precise' and 'universal laws', from which we can generalize about the population as a whole.

The gold standard research method for positivists is the randomized controlled trial carried out in a controlled setting, such as the clinical laboratory or hospital, often with a drug therapy or surgical intervention based treatment of the 'subject'. The principle is a simple experiment where the allocation of a remedy to patients is unknown to the physician. Comparing the outcome in patients given a remedy with the outcome of a similar group (the control) that is not provides a test for the efficacy of the remedy. If there is a measurable improvement, it can be presumed that the remedy has had a beneficial effect.

## SOCIAL MODEL

The subject matter in the social model is social action. Social scientists have a range of paradigms that they draw upon in order to understand the world. Pharmacy practice research frequently draws upon a 'realist' paradigm. One way of understanding this is to distinguish between the medical model concept of disease and the subjective feelings and perceptions of disease, usually called illness or sickness by non-health professionals. Illness is not always detectable by biochemical indicators, as a person can be diseased without feeling ill; for example, they may have undiagnosed cancer or feel ill without any obvious biological cause (e.g. myalgic encephalomyelitis). The social model's definition of 'health' can best be described as not merely the absence of disease but a state of complete physical, psychological and social well-being.

The varied range of methods used in social science (Box 22.1) includes surveys, secondary source data analysis, ethnography, observation and interviews. The social science methodologies are often regarded to be a product of the 1960s. However, their origins go back well over a century. For instance, William Henry Duncan, the first Medical Officer of Health in England and Liverpool, conducted a survey

---

### BOX 22.1    THE RANGE OF RESEARCH METHODS

#### QUANTITATIVE METHODS
- Randomized controlled clinical trial.
- Experiments: usually laboratory based.
- Surveys: using postal questionnaires or interview schedules. The method can be self-completion or face-to-face interviewer administered.
- E-mail and faxback offer new choices and samples of respondent.

#### QUALITATIVE METHODS
- Ethnography.
- Participant observation and interview.
- Focus group discussions.

#### OTHER METHODS
- Documentary – secondary data.
- Life history, narratives.
- Diary completion.
- Historical or comparative perspective.
- Nominal group technique.

- Case study.
- Critical incident analysis.

**EVALUATION**

- Uses all methods.

of housing conditions in Liverpool in the 1830s. His findings were used by Edwin Chadwick, a nineteenth century pioneer of the public health movement in the UK, to argue for public health measures to deal with the social causes of the high rate of mortality in Liverpool.

## HISTORICAL DEVELOPMENT OF SURVEY METHODS IN PHARMACY PRACTICE RESEARCH

Pharmacy practice has only recently emerged as an internationally recognized discipline. The range of nations undertaking research is extensive: papers have been published from, for instance, Europe (with the Nordic countries playing a leading role), the US and Canada, Africa, Australia and New Zealand (Wertheimer et al. 1983).

The framework for pharmacy practice research was established in 1997 by the Royal Pharmaceutical Society of Great Britain (RPSGB), with the strategy comprising four key goals, and it is still relevant today (Box 22.2).

---

**BOX 22.2   FOUR KEY GOALS FOR THE DEVELOPMENT OF PHARMACY PRACTICE RESEARCH**

- A clear focus to ensure that the research asks and answers critical questions and produces results that inform not only the progression, but also the wider health and social care policy agenda.
- High quality, to ensure that the research produces scientifically rigorous results that enable it to be a persuasive and effective force for change.
- Raised awareness, to ensure that the results from research are routinely used to improve the effectiveness, efficiency, appropriateness and quality of practice and services provided, as well as to inform professional and policy development in pharmacy.
- Sound funding, to secure the future of pharmacy practice research with adequate investment that is targeted and used to maximum effect.

Adapted from Mays, N. 1997. *A New Age for Pharmacy Practice Research. Promoting Evidence Based Practice in Pharmacy. The Report of the Pharmacy Practice R&D Task Force.* London: Royal Pharmaceutical Society Great Britain.

**TABLE 22.1**

**Key Features of Positivist and Realist Research Paradigms**

| Positivist | Realist |
|---|---|
| Phenomena can only be termed real if their existence can be demonstrated through quantifying empirical evidence. | Studying individuals and organizations is different from studying the physical world. Social reality is the product of social interaction. |
| Positivist research begins with experimental design, based on hypotheses and involves the investigation and discovery of cause-and-effect relationships. | Naturalistic inquiry questions the value of preconceived hypotheses and objectification and emphasizes qualitative research, which describes and explains human behaviour. |
| Positivist research is based on measurement and deductive statistical analysis of large-number data sets. | Small numbers or case studies of examples are valid. Narratives, descriptions and comments can help to give meaning to inductive analysis. |
| Emphasis on treatment and control groups and dependent and independent variables. | |
| Positive researchers are objective, unbiased and apolitical. They remain aloof from the research objects. | Researchers admit to subjective influences and use the practice of reflexivity to discuss the interpretation of results. |

## PARADIGMS AND THE PRACTICALITIES OF CONDUCTING RESEARCH

The description of the medical and social models of health, together with positivist and realist paradigms (Table 22.1), is a polarized view used here to illustrate the conceptual framework that researchers (often unquestioningly) carry with them. However, research often requires a more pragmatic approach. The most effective pharmacy practice research often draws from a range of paradigms with associated methodologies relevant to the research question. Thus, researchers may use three different methods (triangulation) to explore different aspects of the same phenomenon.

## CRITERIA FOR APPRAISING SURVEY RESEARCH

Pharmacy practice research in its infancy was characterized by lack of rigour and inadequate reference to the hallmarks of high-quality survey research, hence the four goals set out (Box 22.2) by the RPSGB (now Royal Pharmaceutical Society [RPS]) (Mays 1997).

### SCIENTIFIC RIGOUR

All research should be conducted rigorously in relation to the scientific paradigm. The essence of science, which applies equally to the social sciences, is the commitment to the 'rules' governing the line of enquiry – the means by which knowledge ('science' as in Latin *scio*, meaning 'I know') is acquired. Positivists emphasize validity and reliability; realists will also look for a statement of context and values in the methodological writing.

## VALIDITY

There are two forms of validity: internal and external validity. Internal validity applies to the study setting and concerns whether or not the empirical evidence properly describes the concepts under investigation. In other words: 'Am I measuring what I think I am measuring?' External validity is the extent to which findings can be generalized beyond the immediate study setting. Replication can confirm findings and may also uncover: 'trimming' – the selection of data which fit hypotheses; 'cooking' – manipulation of the data to make them look better; and 'forging' – a complete fabrication of data. Validation requires one to consider, for example, that if one studies one pharmacy in one area, to what extent can one generalize the findings to all pharmacies and to all areas? In other words, how artificial or atypical is the setting, and has this constrained the findings such that they are particular to one setting and do not represent a valid general model?

## RELIABILITY AND REPLICABILITY

Reliability is extremely important in laboratory-based research. Reliability is less easy to ensure in social scientific studies because we cannot, for both ethical and practical reasons, create precise social conditions and interactions in an experimental setting. Reliability and replicability are often confused with each other. Replicability is about the consistency of results (i.e. the extent to which the research findings are replicable and reproducible using a comparable sample, design and conditions).

## VALUES

The notion that researchers are 'value free' is questionable. In the realist paradigm, we can question the extent to which the researcher imposes their own values on the study. Values, as illustrated by the example in Box 22.3, can be subjective. This subjectivity is expressed through the choice of problem or subject, the theoretical framework underpinning the study, its concepts, indicators and question design, the choice of research methods, the analysis and the report writing.

---

**BOX 22.3   AN EXAMPLE OF SUBJECT VALUE PLACED ON DATA**

A question in a self-completion postal questionnaire to general practitioners (GPs) asked:

Would you support your medical practice funding a GP pharmacist?
❒Yes          ❒No

50% said yes, 50% said no.

The researcher analysed this as a negative, disappointing result and wrote in the report: 'Only 50% of GPs were prepared to pay for a GP pharmacist'. This statement caused some concern at the medical practice because it was perceived to be negative. The report was changed; the word 'only' was removed (Jesson et al. 1998).

## BOX 22.4   ETHICAL ISSUES IN RESEARCH

- Professional integrity, so that other researchers following you are welcomed.
- Relations with, and responsibility towards, the research participants; this raises issues of anonymity, privacy and confidentiality.
- Informed consent, the requirement that participants must be willing and aware of what is involved in participation.
- Relations with, and responsibility towards, sponsors and or funders; this means clarifying obligations, rights and roles at the outset.
- Guarding privileged information and being aware of the political or social impact of your report.

## ETHICS

The first duty of pharmacists is to protect the public. This is particularly relevant when undertaking health research. All higher-education establishments should have their own research ethics committee which will want to approve any proposed study design; their aim is to protect research participants and the institution. There is an additional layer of ethics approval where National Health Service (NHS) patients are involved.

In the UK, all health research involving patients has to be approved by a Local Research Ethics Committee (LREC). Since 2011, the procedure has been led by the NHS Health Research Authority through the National Research Ethics Service. The service streamlined previous regulations to protect and promote the interests of patients and the public. Their website has a decision tool to help researchers determine whether LREC approval is needed (National Health Service and National Research Ethics Service 2015). Every NHS Hospital Trust will also have a formal research ethics procedure which must give approval before commencing a study, whatever the methodology proposed.

Ethical issues to be considered are listed in Box 22.4.

## Stages of Research that Require Ethical Considerations

### Deciding to Do the Survey

Deciding whether a survey can answer the research question is a technical matter, but to undertake a survey which cannot answer the research question is unethical if you are aware of it and incompetent if you are not.

### Sampling

There are no ethical problems regarding the use of public records such as electoral registers or postcode lists, but patient medical records will need ethics committee approval.

### Generation of the Data

This applies equally to all methods of administration. A respondent has the right to know:

- Who you are
- Why the study is being done

- How their name and address was obtained
- How they were chosen
- What is to be done with the information

It is best for the researcher to avoid assuming the dual role of both practitioner and researcher, as the patient may feel compromised and under an obligation to participate. Confidentiality also requires that information is not supplied to anyone outside the research team. Finally, prior to commencing the study, a researcher should plan the action to be taken if a respondent asks for advice or appears to need medical or psychological help.

## Contents of the Questionnaire

Consider whether is it reasonable to ask people about certain subjects which they may find embarrassing or painful. Particular care must be taken for some marginalized groups or where sensitive issues are involved, such as terminal illness or sexual health.

## Data Processing

Ensure that data recorded on a computer cannot be related to individuals without reference to other lists or records correlating names with serial numbers. Researchers should also be aware of any legislation governing the storage of survey data.

## Presentation of the Results

In presenting qualitative data, quotations may be used to illustrate concepts, ideas or other activities. These will usually need an identifier code (e.g. 'Pharm.24' would mean pharmacist interview 24). There is a question as to the extent to which one should camouflage the identity of places, organizations or respondents. Sometimes, it may be difficult if the work has been commissioned. Finally, there may be a dilemma over the suppression of data. Some funding bodies may wish to suppress unfavourable findings, as illustrated in Box 22.5, which is an extract from a review of Local Authority Social Services Departments.

---

**BOX 22.5   AN EXAMPLE OF SENSITIVITY
TO THE SUBJECTS OF RESEARCH**

'Almost by definition, research on complaints procedures is going to involve issues that are sensitive for the authorities concerned. The research has in-built bias. It deals only with situations where something, at some stage, has gone wrong, it does not even begin to look at the things the Department got right. Not surprisingly, they (the Departments) wish to remain anonymous'.

Simons, K. 1995. *I'm Not Complaining But ... Complaints Procedures in Social Services Departments.* York: Joseph Rowntree Foundation.

*Fraud*

It is clearly unethical to fabricate data. Some researchers have been caught out when other researchers have tried to replicate their studies. Many research organizations now have research guidelines or research codes which members are expected to uphold (*British Medical Journal* 1998; Kimmel 1996). The Market Research Society has a code of conduct requiring that a proportion of those interviewed are re-contacted by a supervisor to check that the interview has actually been carried out, as well as checking for conformity with codes of etiquette and courtesy.

## PLANNING AND DESIGNING A SURVEY

### SELECTING APPROPRIATE SURVEY METHODS

Early in an investigation, it is necessary to decide what means of enquiry are best suited to meeting the objectives of the study. There is no single best approach to research methodology, but there is a need to select the approach which is going to be most effective for addressing the research question(s). Before embarking on a survey, researchers should identify what they are seeking to find out, as there might already be a set of someone else's data (secondary data) that will suffice.

### Secondary Data

The research process involves a review of current knowledge. This may vary from a cursory consideration of everyday knowledge to a full-scale systematic literature review. Online computer search bases are a valuable source of information, but they should be supplemented with a manual search of journals and books.

Readily available secondary sources of data include routinely collected census data and government statistics. Before deciding to produce your own survey data, consider whether it has already been collected by another agency. There is a standard format to all research, beginning with a secondary data review and critical analysis, as shown in Box 22.6. Selecting the appropriate method takes place at a much later stage.

---

**BOX 22.6   BASIC STEPS IN CARRYING OUT A RESEARCH PROJECT**

1. Critical review of the literature (secondary data stage)
2. Develop the aims, objectives and hypothesis of the research and specify concepts and theories
3. Clarification of independent and dependent variables
4. Consider research ethics
5. Selection and design of the methods of research and the measurement instruments
6. Data assembly – either secondary sources or through fieldwork and implementation
7. Analysis
8. Report and dissemination of findings

## Referencing

It is important at the commencement of a project to note all of your sources of information systematically as you proceed. Record every source; write the source on photocopies and journal or news articles because you may not find the original again. There are two referencing systems: Harvard and Vancouver. Some studies prescribe the format to be used, but in general, it does not matter which you use, so long as you consistently use one style. Manage your information sources using software-based systems such as EndNote and Reference Manager.

## Surveys

Having decided that a survey is appropriate, it is necessary to work through the associated parts of the process described in the remainder of this section. A survey is a quantitative method (although qualitative data may be obtained through free text using 'open-ended' questions). In the main, however, it deals with quantities of data and relationships between variables, involving the generation and analysis of highly structured data in the positivist tradition. Generally, the technique involves the systematic, structured questioning of a large (statistically valid) sample of people. The structured questioning can be undertaken by self-completion or by interview. Figure 22.1 shows the range of options available within the survey method. An interviewer completes the interviews; they can be face to face in the pharmacy, the surgery, at home or on the street or by telephone. Another increasingly popular option is to distribute questionnaires electronically.

The survey is one method of collecting information from a sample of the population of interest, but not necessarily the whole population. Surveys are suitable in situations where there is sufficient pre-existing knowledge, which can be incorporated into a standard structured 'research instrument', as the questionnaire is often termed. There are many textbooks that describe the survey method in greater detail than is possible here. For a critical review of health service surveys, see Cartwright (1988). A comprehensive review of UK pharmacy practice surveys was undertaken by Smith (1997a,b).

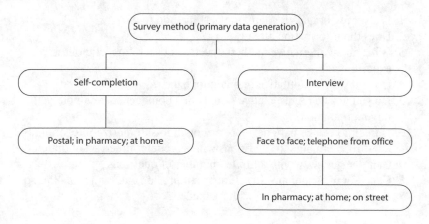

**FIGURE 22.1**   The range of options within the survey method.

## CHOICE OF METHOD

All too often, researchers decide on the method before being clear on the information they need. The availability of resources, time, money, samples of participants or pharmacies often determines options and choices. Although the remainder of this chapter is mainly about quantitative surveys, we look briefly at the full range of options. Box 22.7 illustrates that if you need insight and understanding of rationales for people's beliefs and attitudes, you need a qualitative method, such as a focus group (see also Chapter 24) or depth interview (see also Chapter 23). If you want baseline population data on behaviour patterns (e.g. what percentage of people are loyal to one pharmacy?), a quantitative technique such as a self-completion questionnaire form will be appropriate.

The method by which the survey will be administered is a key early decision. The presentation of the questionnaire or interview schedule and format of the questions is determined by the method of accessing respondents (i.e. is it to be postal, face to face or via telephone, email or the Internet?). At an early stage in learning about research, it is easy to start writing a questionnaire without first thinking about how it will be administered. The words and expressions used will vary considerably, just as written and spoken English are very different.

The design of the research instrument will thus depend on the target audience and the strategy to access them. Before writing the questionnaire, it is important to think through what you want to achieve from your survey. How much time have you got? What research questions do you want to answer? If you are testing a hypothesis, which statistical test will you be using, what size response will you need? Who is going to respond to your survey and how will you identify them?

---

### BOX 22.7   IS A SURVEY APPROPRIATE?

Before you decide that you will undertake a survey, think:

1. Is a survey or questionnaire the best method to use?
2. Does the information already exist?
3. What about alternative methods, such as observation, ethnography or experiments?
4. Do you want quantitative or qualitative data?
5. Do you want a representative sample or a homogeneous sample of the target population?
6. Is the knowledge base developed enough to summarize into straightforward, unambiguous questions with a predetermined set of options?
7. Can you get away with a limited number of questions?
8. Can your questionnaire structure be simply laid out, with few skips so that respondents can deal with it unaided?

## PROJECT PLANNING AND SCHEDULING

Project management is rarely mentioned in research methods textbooks, but it is crucially important. Keep records of everything that you do on the project; set up a systematic filing system; retain a copy of all correspondence; and make a note of all telephone calls and purchase or invoicing orders. There should be a file of all design drafts of research instruments. You can never be sure that computer-held files will not be deleted or lost. This documentation package will be an integral record of the research process and may be important when you write up the methods section of reports or papers. The bigger the survey and the longer the project, the more important a robust data organization system becomes.

The best way to manage day-to-day activities is by using the so-called GANTT project management method. By drawing up a 'GANTT chart' project time plan at the outset, you can see whether the work is feasible within the time allowed and which activities are dependent on another. For more complex or commissioned work, it is the means of identifying resource costs, whether that is for staff, materials or funding.

Figure 22.2 shows a GANTT chart for a survey of pharmacists and their views about services to drug misusers, such as needle exchange schemes and supervised methadone consumption. The project consisted of a number of different methods. The project plan shows a two-tier system of organization – first dividing the project into three stages, and then within each stage, itemizing the activities to be undertaken. Stage and activity are the building blocks of project management. Some activities depend on others having been done first, and these 'dependencies' set demands and constraints on the resulting schedule. Working out the dependencies is vital in helping you decide in what order to do the various tasks.

## SAMPLES AND SAMPLING FRAMES

The type and availability of the sample often determine the choice of survey method. Before you can begin to decide on the choice of research instrument, decide who the respondent sample will be and how you are going to elicit the information you need. What sort of information do you want? If you want to measure 'how many', such a question can easily be answered by a tick box closed option, thus a self-completion postal, telephone or Internet survey could be the desired choice. If you want more in-depth detail and to understand 'why' or 'how', then a face-to-face interview will be needed (see also Chapter 23).

Who will respond to your inquiry? Think through the availability of your respondents. Can you realistically access your sample? Will you need a gatekeeper or can you access them directly? Do pharmaceutical bodies hold an established database, such as their membership lists, or will you need to be more creative in finding respondents?

Surveying customers in a pharmacy might appear easy, but what if you need subjects to meet specific criteria, such as people with coeliac disease, substance misusers or homeless people? If the target audience is small and difficult to access by post or telephone, or you want in-depth information and to understand a social process, then a face-to-face interview will be a more appropriate technique.

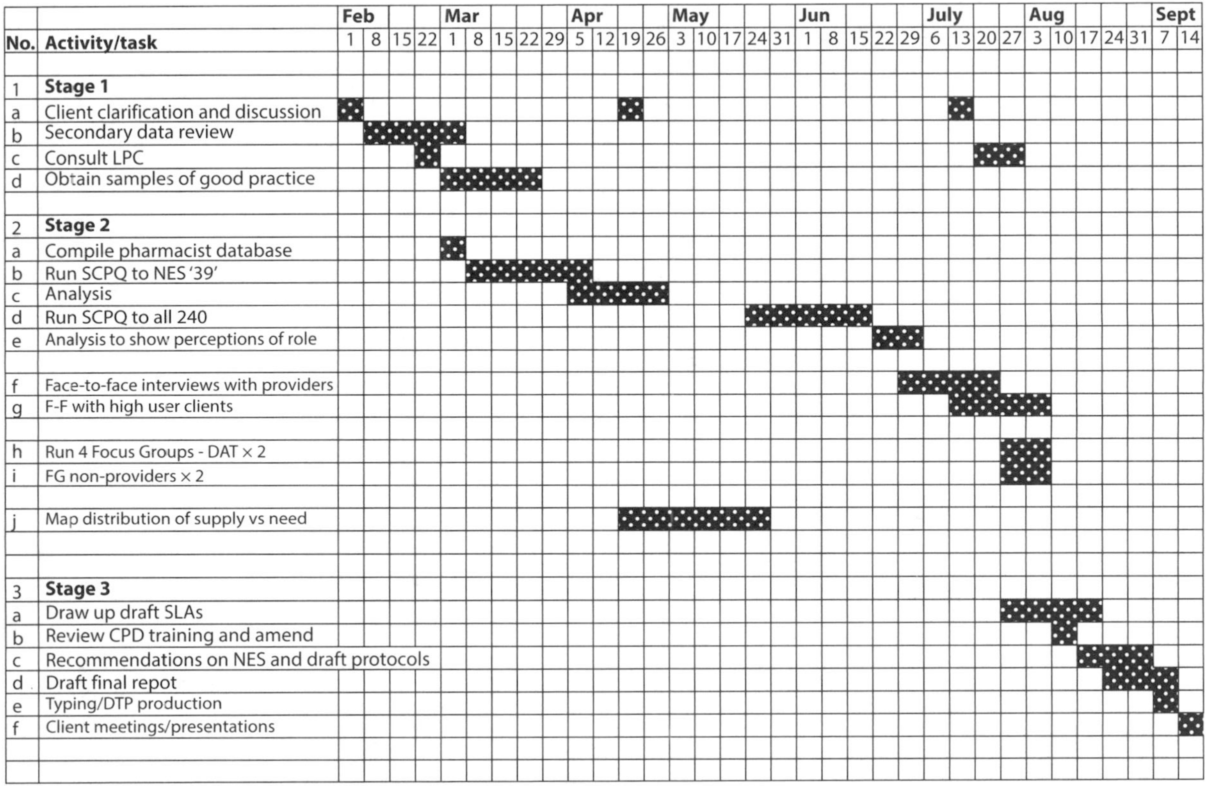

**Stage 1**

1
a  Client clarification and discussion
b  Secondary data review
c  Consult LPC
d  Obtain samples of good practice

**Stage 2**

2
a  Compile pharmacist database
b  Run SCPQ to NES '39'
c  Analysis
d  Run SCPQ to all 240
e  Analysis to show perceptions of role
f  Face-to-face interviews with providers
g  F-F with high user clients
h  Run 4 Focus Groups - DAT × 2
i  FG non-providers × 2
j  Map distribution of supply vs need

**Stage 3**

3
a  Draw up draft SLAs
b  Review CPD training and amend
c  Recommendations on NES and draft protocols
d  Draft final repot
e  Typing/DTP production
f  Client meetings/presentations

Time axis: Feb (1, 8, 15, 22), Mar (1, 8, 15, 22, 29), Apr (5, 12, 19, 26), May (3, 10, 17, 24, 31), Jun (1, 8, 15, 22, 29), July (6, 13, 20, 27), Aug (3, 10, 17, 24, 31), Sept (7, 14)

**FIGURE 22.2** GANTT plan of a community pharmacy and drug misuse study. LPC, Local Pharmaceutical Committee; SCPQ, self completion questionnaire; NES, Needle Exchange Scheme; FF, face to face; DAT, Drug Action Team; FG, Focus Group; SLA, Service Level Agreement; CPD, Continuing Professional Development; DTP, Desk Top Publishing.

## TABLE 22.2
## Key Concepts in Sampling

| Sample | Research Population |
|---|---|
| Sampling frame | List of population from which sample is drawn (contains everyone) |
| Sampling units | Can be pharmacies, general practitioners, Health Authorities, employees in a firm, residents on an electoral register or customers or patients at home, in the street or attending a clinic |
| Types of sampling | Simple random sample; each element has same chance of being selected; makes use of random sample tables |
| Systematic sampling | More even spread of the sample across a list |
| Sampling interval | When total $n$ is known (1 in 10), $n$ = sampling interval |
| Stratified sampling | Identify key characteristics, sex, age and social class |
| Cluster sample | When geographically distributed (e.g. towns in a national survey) |
| Quota sampling | Use census to match proportions in the population (market research) |
| Snowball or network | People recommend someone they know |
| Convenience sampling | Anyone you can get |
| Purposive sampling | A setting chosen for its features |
| Illustrative sample | A small number of case studies which describe concepts or behaviours |

Table 22.2 shows the key terms and the range of sampling options commonly encountered in pharmacy practice research. As you move down the list, the sampling method becomes necessarily more opportunistic in order to access the more difficult-to-reach samples.

## Grouping and Categorizing Samples

Often, pharmacy practice researchers want to survey pharmacies. Surveys can cover a whole health economy, a random sample of registered pharmacy owners, or all pharmacists as the sample frame. Yet if differing types of pharmacy are sought, how are they to be categorized? Traditionally, pharmacies have been categorized by ownership or by location, because that is the easiest variable to identify from existing databases. The competitive nature of pharmacy as a business means that it is extremely difficult to categorize pharmacies by physical size, prescription level or income, yet these may be much more meaningful criteria for understanding the contribution of pharmacy to health care.

There is another important consideration in surveying pharmacies. Researchers often make the mistake of not defining clearly whether it is the pharmacy or the pharmacist they are trying to study. These two entities are intrinsically intertwined, but from the research perspective, they should be distinguished. Surveying practising pharmacists is in one sense a simple task because the individual is the single entity under study. Pharmacies as businesses are much more complex. Business data such as prescription volumes, financial returns from prescriptions and over-the-counter and non-medical sales may be seen as highly sensitive and confidential. Then there is the problem of 'chains'. A small chain is often seen in business terms as a single entity or sample. Financial and operational data (such as counter staff employment) may only be held in aggregate form for the chain. The large multiples often have corporate protocols prohibiting individual pharmacists from responding as individuals, with the chain providing a single group response.

In such cases, questions need to be phrased and expressed with regard to the 'corporate' respondent. Similarly, research concepts such as the 'response rate' are less meaningful and expectations should be geared to the 'norms' of business surveys (where responses of over 15% are acceptable), rather than for surveys of individuals or professionals, where such a response would be seen as unacceptable.

## QUESTIONNAIRE DESIGN, ADMINISTRATION AND RESPONSE

### SELF-COMPLETION QUESTIONNAIRE SURVEY CONSTRUCTION AND LAYOUT

The questionnaire format and question construction are two separate issues, but there are a few key rules that can be quickly used for reference purposes. Box 22.8 shows the complete instrument design for the postal self-completion survey process. Most self-completion questionnaires are sent by post or email, but this is not always the case. It is standard procedure now in pharmacy to invite customers to fill in a satisfaction questionnaire while waiting for the prescriptions to be dispensed. The same happens at the other primary care settings, or at relevant locations for target groups, such as young parents at play groups, older people at day care centres and so on.

With all self-completion questionnaires, the layout and design should encourage the recipient to respond. The first thing is to have a title and an introductory sentence explaining the reason you are asking for the information, then number each question Q1, Q2, Q3, etc., and provide instructions for each question (e.g. 'Please tick box or write in your own words', or 'Rate on a scale of 1 to 5, where 1 is low and 5 is high', and so on). Questions should be written in a clear typeface that looks attractive. The use of arrows, boxes and italics, bold and underlining can draw attention to key words or instructions.

---

**BOX 22.8   STANDARD POSTAL SURVEY DESIGN PROCESS**

1. Think about what you want to ask and what your aims and objectives are.
2. Begin design.
3. Check for clear unambiguous questions.
4. Check layout and visual aspects.
5. Beware of the length.
6. Order freepost envelopes.
7. Set up a database of the sample for logging replies and follow up.
8. Design letter.
9. Pilot or pre-test redesign, and pilot again if necessary.
10. Print.
11. Stuff envelopes and post (select Thursday or Friday and check time of year and holidays).

The visual impact of the instrument is important. Use A4 size paper and a strong staple to hold pages together. An alternative might be A3 paper folded into a booklet form; this makes it easier to turn the pages and it is less likely that the back page will be lost. Questions should not be split across two pages. You do not have to say 'please' in every question. Aim for no more than 50 questions, or 10 pages, printed back to back. In a lengthy paper questionnaire, it is important to print on both sides of the page, as this has a positive psychological effect on the recipient who may not reply to a thick document.

Finally, don't forget to include a reminder telling the respondent how to return the completed questionnaire and, if relevant, enclose a pre-paid envelope. In order to track replies, it is usual to stamp a code or ID number on the back page. This is important when following up non-responders.

Remember, self-completion and postal survey questionnaires are limited in the range of information that can be obtained. In a self-completion questionnaire, you can only measure attitudes, beliefs, behaviour, knowledge, attributes or demographics.

## Question Design

The way in which questions are designed depends on the survey technique. Do not formulate specific questions until you have thought through the research question. Keep asking yourself: 'Why do I want to know this? What will I do with the answer?' – the 'so what?' question. Box 22.9 has some tips on question design that are applicable to all survey types, not just self-completion surveys.

## Piloting

Every survey instrument should be piloted before it is ready to be printed. Test it on colleagues, edit and revise; test on other people of the same respondent group by post and by sitting down with them and asking what they are thinking as they read each question.

Check that the instructions are clear, the design is professional and looks acceptable to the recipient, that the language is easy to understand and that the questions

---

### BOX 22.9   TIPS FOR GOOD QUESTION DESIGN

1. Aim for no more than 20 words in one question.
2. Avoid asking two or more questions at the same time.
3. Avoid using qualifying clauses, phrases and instructions.
4. Avoid hidden questions.
5. Do not use double negatives (e.g. in attitude scales).
6. Avoid hypothetical questions.
7. Do not ask questions everyone can agree with, as this is bias.
8. Beware of meaningless words (e.g. 'regularly' and 'ever').
9. Do not start with a soft phrase (e.g. 'Would you mind saying…?').
10. Do not use questions including 'either', 'if any' or 'if at all'.
11. Do not mix tenses in questions.

are clear and unambiguous. Are the pre-coded options comprehensive, are the skips (instructions to complete only appropriate questions) correct and question number sequence accurate, is there sufficient space to write an answer to open-ended questions? Finally, check how long it takes to complete. It is then ready for printing.

## Administration of the Postal Survey

Ideally, a self-completion questionnaire is limited to 50 questions that take about 10 minutes to complete. It should be printed on attractive paper, with a balance of words and space, easy to complete and handle and well stapled. From the research management side, it needs to be easy to record responses in an appropriate manner for statistical analysis (coding) and for identification. A survey needs a covering letter to motivate completion. It is important to get the letter right in order to maximize the number of completed questionnaires returned (the response rate). The covering letter must answer all the recipients' questions – the who, what, why and when explanations. It should look attractive, be no longer than a page and each sentence should be short and purposeful. Even the heading on the letter can influence completion.

## Letter Content
- Explain the purpose of the study.
- Attempt to convince the reader that they are being useful and have valued information/opinions.
- Ensure confidentiality and anonymity if relevant.
- Do not forget to mention a contact name and number and the freepost or stamped addressed envelope.

The advantage of a postal survey is usually cost. Postal surveys can cost only a third as much as interviews because there are lower organizational costs per respondent (e.g. stamps are cheaper than the equivalent interviewer fees). It is also easier to have a random geographical sample in a postal survey than in an interview model. You can reach working people, those who are rarely at home at 'normal' times and sparsely populated country areas or 'unsafe' housing estates. Self-completion helps to eliminate interviewer bias and personal or embarrassing questions may be answered more frankly. The respondent has more control of the instrument and has time to reflect on their answers before posting at their convenience. Finally, there is a degree of anonymity, which may encourage completion.

The disadvantages of a postal survey are linked to the limitations of the instrument and the completion process. In this method, it is not possible to use lead questions to get at a subset of issues; questions have to be simple, short and straightforward. Thus, they lack qualitative depth and are inflexible.

Once the instrument has been posted, there is no control over the sequence of reading or completing and answers cannot be probed or checked. Loss of control over the process means that it is not always possible to determine who is a nonresponder or reasons for non-response. Returned forms may be incomplete or inaccurate because the person misunderstood or did not read the instructions. One can never be sure who filled the questionnaire in – whether it was the target person or a group effort. There is only the letter to motivate response. Thus, the main disadvantage is the risk of poor response rates and a biased skew to the sample.

## Self-Completion, Non-Postal Surveys

Some self-completion surveys are completed by the respondent in the pharmacy or a general practitioner surgery. The non-postal instrument lacks a target respondent unless someone agrees to hand questionnaires out on your behalf. Quite often, they are left lying around, or on the counter, waiting to be noticed.

In one survey, self-completion questionnaires were to be handed out to all patients attending a surgery over 2 weeks, and the anticipated target had been calculated on attendance numbers as being 500. The reality was that since no one took responsibility for the distribution, it actually took 6 weeks to achieve 289 replies. The following year, a repeat survey was managed differently and that produced a return of 257 replies after 2 weeks (Jesson et al. 1998).

## Electronic Online Surveys

The use of electronic surveys via the Internet is increasingly common these days. For example, everyone who goes shopping will have received a till receipt asking the purchaser to go online and complete a satisfaction survey. The electronic survey is basically a structured questionnaire delivered via the Internet.

There are two approaches:

- Those administered by email, where the questionnaire is embedded in an e-mail to the respondent
- Web-based surveys, where the respondent is directed to a website in order to complete a questionnaire

In the embedded email option, there will be a short introduction; responses are made by use of a simple 'X', or 'delete alternatives that do not apply'. With open-ended questions, the answer is typed in. The advantage of this simple approach is that it is easier for the respondent to return and requires less computer expertise on their part. With this approach, where the target respondent is known, it is easier to follow-up non-responders and measure the response rate.

In a web-based survey, the questionnaire arrives as an attachment. To complete the survey, the respondent can either answer by clicking on a circle in which a dot appears or select an item from a pull-down menu of options. Open-ended questions require a typed-in answer.

## Sample

As with all surveys, the sampling frame and sample depends on who the target respondent is. Few sampling frames exist of the general public online, or of patients, and, generally speaking, Internet users are a biased sample of the population. They tend to be better educated, wealthier and younger (a third of over 65-year-olds have no access to computers) and are not representative in terms of ethnicity. Ideally, access to the email addresses of corporate intranets helps (e.g. university staff or students, pharmacists in a hospital trust or interest groups). The online web-based survey method used to survey pre-registration trainee pharmacists by the General Pharmaceutical Council (GPhC) used their own internal email database (General Pharmaceutical Council 2013). However, the downside of access to a named list may be loss of anonymity; this is less likely with a web-based attachment.

## Design

The design and implementation of e-surveys involves a level of expertise which the new researcher may not have. Web-based surveys need a high level of design skills. There are a growing number of software packages available for survey design, but if the start-up cost is too expensive, there are commercial companies who will, for a fee, carry out the survey for you (Bryman and Bell 2003).

## Response Rate

Online surveys typically generate lower response rates than postal surveys (e.g. the GPhC pre-registration trainees' survey achieved a 35% response rate). There may be a growing antipathy towards uninvited emails. As with other self-completion surveys, it may be difficult to measure the representativeness of those who reply. Online responses tend to come in quicker than postal surveys and the whole survey could be completed in 2 or 3 weeks. There are fewer unanswered questions and fewer missing data because the software controls the progress and does not allow the missing out of items.

### Processing Replies

Once you are ready for distribution, here are some tips that could help. With postal surveys, you should print 2.5-times the number in the sample to allow for two follow-up reminders. Buy self-sealing envelopes to make the 'stuffing' process quicker. Post towards the end of the week to arrive for completion at the weekend. The whole mailing process can take up to 9 weeks.

You can expect:

- 30% returned from the first mailing after 3 weeks
- 20% returned from the second mailing after 3 weeks
- 10% returned from the third mailing after 2 weeks

If the sample is small, an alternative option is to telephone and ask whether the respondent has returned the survey instrument. In this way, you can find out something about the non-responders' attitudes. Sometimes, subjects will be prepared to respond over the phone (i.e. you fill in a spare copy of the survey form while they give you their answers).

Each questionnaire needs a code number before distribution so that you can tag the replies as they come in ready for the follow-up mailings. Set up the questionnaire database and code the replies for entering into a database.

## Face-to-Face Interviews

Face-to-face interviews can be held with patients in their own home or on the street. It is important to remember in face-to-face interviews that this is a social interaction between an interviewer and respondent, so the dynamics of information exchange are different from those obtained in self-completion surveys. There are two types of interview: the structured interview, which produces quantitative data, and the exploratory depth interview, which produces qualitative data (see also Chapter 23). The choice of interview model depends on the purpose of the research, the stage of the research (development or testing), the time available for interview and the skill of the interviewer.

In a structured face-to-face interview, as in a self-completion survey, the questions are standardized. This method is most commonly used in market research surveys, for public opinion polls and in government surveys. The interviewer uses a standard technique, following the format rigorously so that every interview should be the same. In quantitative, structured interviews, the questions are fixed by the designer before the interview, the exact wording is prescribed for each respondent and the sequence is always the same. The interviewer should attempt to be unbiased and objective. However, there is a debate about the extent to which this is possible and whether there should be matched interviewers and respondents in terms of age, sex and ethnicity. The large sample size means that the data should be valid, replicable and reliable, and drawn from a representative sample, which then allows generalization.

The advantage of structured, quantitative interviews is that these interviewers can reach a large proportion of the sample. Standardization of the instrument makes comparison and statistical analysis easier. The quantitative interview allows more scope for creativity through the use of prompts and show or shuffle cards, especially when it takes place indoors. House interviews can take up to an hour, or longer, and have the advantage of building up a rapport with the respondent. Quicker, on-street surveys take about five minutes.

A disadvantage of this method can be the unavailability of respondents. It can be a frustrating experience standing outside a pharmacy in the cold trying to catch the attention of customers, and it may take some time to reach the desired sample size. If you want to interview a pharmacist, this method is problematic for interviewing them in the pharmacy. In addition to the demands of dispensing, there is rarely a suitable place to sit. You may also have to offer to pay a locum fee to cover lost work time. Recruiting and training good interviewers can also be time consuming and expensive.

Time and the cost of interviewers will influence the sampling strategy. Every pharmacy is different. Sometimes, quotas are used, but more often than not, it is likely that an interviewer will approach every other pharmacy customer. Problems arise when the pharmacy is a very busy one, because it is difficult for one person to approach every other customer. Conversely, in quiet pharmacies, there may be a lot of 'down time' because of the lack of customers.

## Telephone Interviews

Telephone interviews are increasingly used in survey work and may be more suitable for interviewing pharmacists. A telephone interview needs to be fairly short, taking about 10 minutes at most. It will need a different construction and format from a face-to-face interview schedule, with more attention needed for spoken explanations.

The main advantages are convenience, the capability of rapid data collection, the lower cost than face-to-face interviews, better access and adaptability and greater interviewer control, plus lower costs in terms of time, effort and money. Telephone interviews share many of the advantages of a face-to-face interview: a high response rate, the potential for the correction of obvious misunderstandings and the potential for using probes and prompts. They are also safer for interviewers, who do not have to enter unknown homes. A disadvantage is the limitation on the scope and complexity of the questions that can be asked. A typical call will last up to 10 minutes. The lack of visual cues may cause some problems in the interpretation of answers.

The sampling frame is usually telephone and business directories. This can also have a bias based on gender and social class. Furthermore, new subscribers are not listed; more and more people are now ex-directory, use a mobile phone or subscribe to one of a range of telecommunication companies. Similarly, the telephone numbers of pharmacies may not be held centrally by the profession's registering body. For more random sample surveys, the technique of random digit dialling is used, which involves the local part of a telephone number being generated randomly using a table or a computer.

The response rate to a telephone survey can be higher than the postal method because the immediacy of the approach gives respondents less time to refuse, or they have the option of calling back at a convenient time. Telephoning pharmacies may not produce the anticipated response rate, especially if it has a busy dispensary and the pharmacist is constantly interrupted or called away from the telephone. Halfpenny et al. (1998) describe the experience of a telephone survey of small companies with a 33% refusal rate. The companies in question had developed resistance to telemarketing because they were deluged with telephone calls that were unproductive for them, because the callers wanted something other than the goods or services sold by the companies. It wastes their time and prevents customers getting through.

In a face-to-face or telephone interview, the time scale can be much shorter than in postal surveys, depending on the size of the sample. You print exactly the sample number of schedules; no reminders are needed. There are no envelopes, freepost inserts or postage costs. Instead, you will need to set up interviewer claim forms, travel cost payments and so on.

## Response Rates

Response rates to survey questionnaires vary tremendously according to the sample, the method (postal, Internet, interview or telephone), design, topic of interest and time of year when they are sent out. Smith (1997a) describes a range of methods for increasing survey response rates. Her review of surveys involving community pharmacists found a range of rates from 30% to 90%; with patients, the range was 34%–88%. The best results for postal surveys can be obtained by sending at least three mailings. The response rate should be described in the report, so that readers are able to understand the scientific validity of the results.

There is no consensus on acceptable response rates. Many research textbooks base their estimates on clinical or medical studies and assert that anything less than a 70% response is not good enough, because there is a potential bias in the data. Bowling (1997) mentions a 40% response rate as common in postal surveys.

In addition to the usual reluctance to answer survey questionnaires, the response rate for pharmacy surveys in the UK is associated with competition and competitive advantage. This is because, as stated previously, a pharmacy survey is often analogous to a 'business survey'. Although the pattern of pharmacy ownership varies with every health economy, competitive advantage limits the amount and type of information that can be obtained. When undertaking a survey that includes the multiples, the superintendent pharmacist should be contacted in advance of posting the questionnaire. The instrument may require amendment, but if support is given, the response rate will be higher.

## CONCLUSION

Surveys are a popular way of generating data in pharmacy practice research. They can be easy to do or extremely difficult. The complexity varies with the study. In this chapter, we have not set out to review the work of published surveys. Instead, we have described the philosophical basis of survey methods as applied to pharmacy practice research and shown the need to bring into pharmacy practice the social or 'realist' paradigms of social survey research. This chapter has demonstrated four basic model options within the survey approach and has described in practical detail the key stages in undertaking a survey using these methods.

It should be borne in mind that survey research is, in itself, a learning process and has to adapt to a dynamic social and technological environment (people are increasingly reluctant to take part in surveys, but on the other hand, technology is opening up new ways of accessing people). There is no definitive text on the subject, nor have we attempted to provide one, because the state of the art is still rapidly developing. Rather, we hope to have stimulated reflective thinking on the subject in order to raise the overall standards of survey research.

## FURTHER READING

Edwards, A. and Talbot, R. 1999. *Hard Pressed Researcher* (2nd Edn.). London: Longman.
Fielding, N., Lee, R.M. and Blank, G. 2008. *The Sage Handbook of Online Research Methods*. London: Sage.
Shipman, M. 1997. *The Limitations of Social Research* (4th Edn.). London: Longman.

## REFERENCES

Bowling, A. 1997. *Research Methods in Health*. Buckingham: Open University Press.
British Medical Journal 1998. The randomised control trial at 50. *British Medical Journal*, **317**, 1217–1246.
Bryman, A. and Bell, E. 2003. *Business Research Methods*. Oxford: Oxford University Press.
Cartwright, A. 1988. *Health Surveys in Practice and Potential: A Review of Scope and Method*. London: The King's Fund.
General Pharmaceutical Council 2013. General Pharmaceutical Council Survey of 2012/13 Pre-Registration Trainees. Available at: www.pharmacyregulation.org.
Halfpenny, P., Hudson, S. and Jones, J. 1998. Researching small companies' charitable giving through telephone interviews. *International Journal of Social Research Methodology*, **1**, 65–74.

Jesson, J., Lacey, F. and Wilson, K.A. 1998. *Second Year Evaluation of the North Birmingham Total Purchasing Pilot Pharmacy Project. A Report to the TPP.* Birmingham: Aston University.

Kimmel, A.J. 1996. *Ethical Issues in Behavioural Research.* Oxford: Blackwell.

Lefanu, J. 1999. *The Rise and Fall of Modern Medicine.* London: Little Brown.

Mays, N. 1997. *A New Age for Pharmacy Practice Research. Promoting Evidence Based Practice in Pharmacy. The Report of the Pharmacy Practice R&D Task Force.* London: Royal Pharmaceutical Society Great Britain.

National Health Service and National Research Ethics Service 2015. Health Research Authority National Research Ethics Service. Available at: www.hra.nhs.uk.

Simons, K. 1995. *I'm Not Complaining But … Complaints Procedures in Social Services Departments.* York: Joseph Rowntree Foundation.

Smith, F. 1997a. Survey research: (1) Design, samples and response. *International Journal of Pharmacy Practice,* **5**, 152–166.

Smith, F. 1997b. Survey research: (2) Survey instrument, reliability and validity. *International Journal of Pharmacy Practice,* **5**, 216–226.

Wertheimer, A., Claesson, C. and Londen, H.H. 1983. The development of the discipline of social pharmacy. *Journal of Social and Administrative Pharmacy,* **1**, 113–115.

# 23 Interviews

*Madeleine Gantley*

## CONTENTS

---

### KEY POINTS

- Structured interviews often centre around the administration of a questionnaire while semi-structured interviews are designed to collect detailed qualitative data from a relatively small number of respondents with experience of the topic under investigation.
- Qualitative interviews are distinct from normal conversations in that they are purposively guided to extract 'rich' data.
- Key considerations when undertaking qualitative research include sampling, designing a topic guide, consideration of ethics, interviewing, data recording and data analysis.

## INTRODUCTION

This chapter addresses interviewing as one means of collecting research data. In some ways, pharmacists use informal, brief interviews as an integral part of their work. However, the shift to research interviewing requires an acknowledgement of the distinction between routine conversations with the aim of extracting information in order to make a particular decision and the semi-structured interview designed to encourage research respondents to talk at some length about a particular phenomenon.

The choice of data collection methods is made within the broader choice of research methods appropriate to answer a particular research question (see Chapter 22). Interviews may be formal or informal, structured or unstructured. The formal, structured interview, often centred around the administration of a questionnaire, falls within the quantitative framework in which researchers focus on the collection of large structured data sets. The informal, semi-structured interview, in contrast, is one of the key methods of data collection within qualitative research, which is designed to produce detailed data from a relatively small number of research respondents with experience of a particular phenomenon.

## APPROPRIATE RESEARCH QUESTIONS

Qualitative research is essentially exploratory, and the choice of qualitative methods is made in order to maximize the amount of data generated. If the research question focuses on how many people at risk of heart disease take aspirin regularly, the appropriate method is a large survey, using a standard data collection tool. If, on the other hand, the question is why people with heart disease do not take aspirin regularly, then a relatively small number of in-depth interviews will provide appropriately detailed information to help the researcher understand their concerns. An example of a qualitative study is illustrated in Box 23.1.

## SAMPLING STRATEGIES IN QUALITATIVE RESEARCH

Bearing in mind the nature of qualitative research, sampling concentrates on maximizing either the range or depth of explanations and reasoning. Sampling is described as purposive and is subdivided into a number of different strategies. The most frequent include maximum variety, intensity, typical and dissonant case. These are summarized in Box 23.2.

Sampling strategy is of more importance than sample size, but qualitative studies tend to draw on 30–40 hours of data collection. For a review of sample sizes in qualitative research, see Denzin and Lincoln (1994).

## INTERVIEWS VERSUS FOCUS GROUPS VERSUS OBSERVATION

Face-to-face interviews are not the only way of collecting data for qualitative research. Many qualitative studies use a mixture of interviews and focus groups, and some also draw on observation. It is important to be clear about the strengths

---

**BOX 23.1   A QUALITATIVE STUDY OF
IDEAS ABOUT MEDICINES**

Recognizing that little attention had been paid to patients' ideas about medicines and their potential relevance for understanding non-adherence to medication, Britten (1994) set out to research patients' ideas about medicines and adherence. She conducted 30 semi-structured interviews with patients in two socially contrasting general practices and identified a number of different themes:

- Perceived properties of medicines
- Orientation/general preferences for taking or not taking medicines
- Actual use of medications

She found that while much medicine taking was taken for granted, patients had many fears and powerful negative images of medicines.
On the one hand:

Something like penicillin, it's sort of reached the status of, like an aspirin, it's something people accept, it's been around for a long time, it's proven if you like.

And on the other hand:

I have a belief whether I am right or wrong that all medicines to an extent are carcinogenic. It's like everything else, if you take enough of it and overdose over a long period of time, you are always prone to perhaps advancing the nature of things like cancer.

---

and weaknesses of each method (Table 23.1) and to choose the most appropriate approach. Each method is a balance between gathering appropriately detailed data and ensuring that such data are relevant for the research question. Interviews have the maximum potential for obtaining such data, allowing the interviewer to follow the respondents' own priorities and to encourage discussions at some depth. Focus groups (see Chapter 24) are a relatively rapid method for generating a range of topics, but may be more difficult for the facilitator to control. Thus, the data may lack both relevance and depth. Observation may be either direct or participant, depending on the nature and relevance of the researcher's involvement in the research site, and entails prolonged exposure to the research setting. It may be used to supplement information collected by interviews or may comprise the principal method of data collection, as with ethnographic studies. Observation is very time consuming, but has the advantage that the observer sees what people do, rather than collecting data on what they say they do. However, there is no guarantee that data are relevant and the researcher has minimal control over the research setting. Bear in mind that for each method, the researcher has an impact on the research setting.

**BOX 23.2   SAMPLING STRATEGIES (PATTON 1990)**

Maximum variety: purposefully picking a wide range of variation on dimensions of interest. Documents unique or diverse variations that have emerged in adapting to different conditions. Identifies important common patterns that cut across variations.

Intensity: information-rich cases that manifest the phenomenon intensely, but not extremely, such as pro-medication/anti-medication.

Typical case: illustrates or highlights what is typical, normal or average.

Deviant case: learning from highly unusual manifestations of the phenomenon of interest.

Snowball: identifies cases of interest from 'people who know people who know people', who know what cases are information rich or good examples for study. May be used when respondents are hard to reach (e.g. injecting drug misusers).

Theoretical sampling: finding manifestations of a theoretical construct of interest so as to elaborate and examine the construct. Often used within the context of grounded theory.

Perhaps the most important type of sampling is combination or mixed purposeful sampling, which allows triangulation of data and ensures sufficient flexibility to meet multiple interests and needs.

---

**TABLE 23.1**

## Advantages and Disadvantages of Qualitative Methods

| Advantages | Disadvantages |
| --- | --- |
| **Interviews** | |
| Depth | Skilled interviewer essential |
| Opportunity to explore ideas | Sampling strategy essential |
| Context rich | Expensive |
| Data collected in 'natural setting' | |
| **Focus Groups** | |
| Generate breadth of ideas | Skilled facilitator essential |
| Document development of ideas | Audio recording more difficult |
| Spin off among participants | May be too hard to control |
| Relatively rapid data generation | May be dominated by |
| |   vociferous participants |
| | Expensive |
| | May tend to consensus |
| **Observation** | |
| Seeing people in 'natural setting' | Skilled observer essential |
| Observing process | No control over setting |
| Context rich | Time consuming |
| Can be used to complement interviews | Lack of focus |
| Sensitizing researcher to research setting | |

## PREPARATIONS

The first step in conducting a qualitative study is the preparation of a topic guide. This involves a critical assessment of the relevant literature and reflection on your own beliefs and assumptions about the research question. In conducting the literature review, ensure that you search across different disciplinary fields, including sociology, anthropology and psychology, as well as pharmacy and other relevant fields, such as primary care. Reflecting on your own assumptions is rather more difficult. This is sometimes known as 'bracketing'. Ahern has provided 10 'tips for reflexive bracketing' (Box 23.3).

## MAKING THE FAMILIAR STRANGE

Another technique for promoting reflection on your own assumptions is that of 'making the familiar strange'.

Imagine you are on holiday in France. Your companion twists a knee and needs to buy painkillers and a knee bandage. You go into the local pharmacy. Here is my brief account of what happened on a visit to a small town east of Paris!

> My immediate impression was that I had entered a clinical environment. White coats, bright lights, a slightly antiseptic smell. The assistant was immediately at hand, behind a glass-topped counter. She offered anti-inflammatories and insisted on my companion sitting down while she measured the painful knee in order to fit a support bandage. She then offered an array of walking sticks of varying heights and strengths. Two other people entered the pharmacy while we were being attended to, and joined in the provision of advice and help.

This kind of observation is useful in encouraging us to reflect on what is familiar to us in our own cultures. It is what anthropologists call 'making the familiar strange', or recognizing what we take for granted in our own cultures. The short account above identifies the notion of the clinical environment, the focus on serving the customer rather than self-service and a consultation involving the inspection and tailoring of care to the individual concerned. I remember each of these aspects precisely because of the contrast with my own perceptions of visiting a community pharmacy in the UK.

Beware, however, of the apparently simple observation: 'Don't they do things differently here!' This has been characterized as 'the trap of tourism' by David Silverman (2015), and carries the inherent danger of focusing on what is different while ignoring those features that are common to both settings.

## PREPARING AN INTERVIEW TOPIC GUIDE

The next step is the preparation of the interview topic guide. This is a list of topics to be covered in each interview (see also Chapter 24). Topics may be addressed in any order, and the list may be added to throughout the research collection period. An example of a topic guide for use in a pharmacy setting is shown in Box 23.4.

The topic guide may then be developed into a semi-structured interview guide, with specific open questions, followed by more exploratory, probing questions. An

## BOX 23.3   TEN TIPS FOR REFLEXIVE BRACKETING

1. Identify some of the interests that you, as a researcher, might take for granted in undertaking this research (e.g. the assumption that you will be able to gain access to your professional peers to conduct research, or broader assumptions associated with power, gender, skin colour, socioeconomic status and so on).

2. Clarify your personal value systems and acknowledge areas in which you know you are subjective. This is important in recognizing the assumptions that you bring to the analysis of the data and developing a critical perspective throughout the research process.

3. Identify possible areas of role conflict and your responses to particular types of situations. How would you respond, for instance, to being interviewed about your own professional practice? How is this likely to influence recruitment of research respondents and the data collection process?

4. 'Gatekeepers' are people with whom you need to negotiate in order to recruit research respondents. For instance, the pharmacist may be the gatekeeper to his or her customers, or the Superintendent Pharmacist may be the gatekeeper to pharmacists employed by a particular multiple. Try to identify gatekeepers' interests and consider their enthusiasm, or lack of it, towards your research.

5. Identify and recognize feelings that could indicate a lack of neutrality on your part. This could include, for instance, your feelings towards injecting drug users, or female colleagues combining professional practice with parenthood. How will you deal with these feelings in conducting the research?

6. Is anything new emerging from the data collection or analysis? This may be an indication of 'saturation' or a lack of critical reflection. This is the time to talk to colleagues, ideally drawn from a variety of academic and professional backgrounds, to increase your capacity for reflection.

7. Learn to recognize 'blocks' in the research process and to reframe them. Think laterally and review the methodology; is additional data collection needed, or an alternative method?

8. As you complete the analysis, reflect on the presentation of the data. Are you citing one person more than another, and if so, why? Are you citing the articulate professional, rather than the quiet layperson?

9. Review the literature that you have cited. Does it too bring a critical perspective to the findings of the research, or have you selected the literature in order to reinforce your own research question or findings?

10. Become aware of potential 'analytical blindness', which is ignoring data that do not support your conclusions. Again, draw on multidisciplinary discussions of data analysis to reflect on your own assumptions about the data.

Adapted from Ahern, K.A. 1999. *Qualitative Health Research*, **9**, 407–411.

> ## BOX 23.4 EXAMPLE OF AN INTERVIEW TOPIC GUIDE
>
> - Role of the pharmacist: advice giver, counsellor, expert on medication, entrepreneur, primary care team member, advisor on minor illnesses or instant-access substitute general practitioner.
> - Customers' expectations: dispensing prescriptions, giving advice, selling common medicines, health promotion or selling cosmetics.
> - The place of pharmacies: in the high street, in supermarkets or in out-of-town shopping mall.
> - How do pharmacists describe those who use their services: clients, customers, patients or users?

> ## BOX 23.5 EXAMPLE OF A SEMI-STRUCTURED INTERVIEW GUIDE
>
> - Could you describe to me how you see your role as a pharmacist? (Probes: advice giving, expert on medication, etc.)
> - Where do you think pharmacies should be situated? (Let respondents describe the range of situations; probe for potential strengths and weaknesses of each if necessary.)
> - How do you see the people who use your shop? (Try not to use the terms 'customer' or 'client', leave it to the respondent to decide what language is most appropriate to describe the users of their service.)
> - How do you see the future of pharmacists and pharmacy? (Open question designed to encourage respondents to look to the future.)

example is shown in Box 23.5. Some researchers find it easier to work with a topic guide, and some with a semi-structured interview guide. It may also be that at an early stage of the research process a topic guide is appropriate, and as the research develops, a semi-structured interview guide becomes more useful.

## TYPES OF INTERVIEW QUESTION

As can be seen from the interview guide in Box 23.5, there are a number of different types of questions that can be used. Box 23.6 summarizes the range of approaches that may be helpful.

## GETTING IN: NEGOTIATING ACCESS AND RECRUITMENT

Having identified your sampling strategy, the next step is recruitment. How will you identify and reach appropriate respondents? How will you present the research to potential participants? How will you ensure that respondents' confidentiality is maintained and that they understand the nature and potential use of the research data?

## BOX 23.6  INTERVIEW QUESTIONS
## (BRINKMANN AND KVALE 2013)

Introducing questions: opening questions designed to yield spontaneous, rich descriptions where respondents provide what they experience as the main dimensions of the phenomena under investigation. May include 'Can you tell me about...?' or, 'Do you remember an occasion when...?'.

Follow-up questions: the interviewer adopts a curious attitude, inviting the respondent to explain through a further question, a nod, non-vocal encouragement or repeating significant words.

Probing questions: asking the respondent to explain or provide an example of a particular phenomenon. This involves recognizing areas of concern to the respondent and finding alternative ways of addressing such areas.

Specifying questions: invite the respondent to provide more detail that is often specific to their own experience, rather than general beliefs: 'What did you do then?' or, 'How did you react?'.

Direct questions: used only later in the interview, after the opening exploratory questions.

Indirect questions: invite the respondent to comment on how other people might feel or react; useful in conjunction with direct and specifying questions.

Structuring questions: sometimes called 'signposts' and used to indicate to the respondent the sequence of questions to be used or the stage of the interview that has been reached.

Interpreting questions: a variety of follow-up questions, allowing the interviewer to check that their understanding or interpretation matches that of the respondent.

Silence: don't be afraid to pause in order to leave the respondent to break a silence. Sometimes people need time to think, and some respondents speak less or more slowly than others. Allow the respondents to pace the interview and to use (short) silences for reflection.

## INTRODUCING YOURSELF

Make sure people know who you are, what role you will play (this is particularly important if respondents know you either as a professional colleague or as a local pharmacist), the purpose of the research, what will happen to their interview (e.g. transcribed anonymously, data analysed and extracts may be used in a final research report and in publications for academic journals) and offer to let them see a copy and to comment on it. Assure them that they may withdraw from the research at any time, and that this would have no impact on their care/service. Offer a prepared information sheet, to be left with respondents, to provide information to them, to reassure them of your own identity and to allow them to contact you if they have comments to add.

> **BOX 23.7 ETHICAL QUESTIONS WHICH SHOULD BE ASKED AT THE START OF AN INTERVIEW STUDY**
>
> - What are the beneficial consequences of the study?
>   How can the study contribute to enhancing the human condition? Will potential contributions be primarily for the research participants, for their group or for humanity more generally?
> - How can the informed consent of the respondents be obtained?
>   Should informed consent be agreed orally or should there be a written contract? Who should give this consent? How much information should be provided in advance? How can informed consent be handled in exploratory studies where investigators themselves have little advanced knowledge of how the interviews will proceed?
> - How can the confidentiality of the respondents be protected?
>   How important is it that respondents remain anonymous? Who will have access to the interview transcripts? Are there potential legal problems concerning protection of the respondents' anonymity?
> - What are the consequences of the study for participants?
>   Will the interviews touch on therapeutic issues, and if so, what precautions can be taken? When publishing the study, what consequences can be anticipated for the research participants?
> - How will the researcher's role affect the study?
>   How can the researcher ensure the scientific quality of the study and protect the independence of the research, including his/her own critical perspective?
>
> Adapted from Brinkmann, S. and Kvale, S. 2013. *Interviews: Learning the Craft of Qualitative Research Interviewing (3rd Edn.)*. Thousand Oaks, CA: Sage.

## ETHICAL ISSUES

What sort of ethical issues are raised? If your respondents are also pharmacists or other health professionals, are specific professional or ethical issues raised? If your respondents are clients, what sort of professional and ethical dilemmas might be raised?

Brinkmann and Kvale (2013) have suggested a number of ethical questions that should be addressed at the start of an interview study (Box 23.7).

## GETTING ALONG

Having prepared a topic guide, managed the recruitment of research participants and negotiated access, you are now in a position to start talking. The aim of the interview is to be respondent centred, to establish the respondent as the expert and to place them in a position to explain to you their views of a particular topic. It is the researcher's role to guide, to establish an atmosphere in which the respondent feels comfortable to talk in depth and to ask questions that allow the respondent to think and reflect on their particular experiences. Thus, it is important to emphasize that there are no 'right' answers. The point of the exercise is a 'guided conversation', rather than a series of questions and answers. It is important to recognize that, particularly in research of this kind, the knowledge generated is a social product; that is to say, it is the result of the interaction between you as interviewer and the interviewee.

As a research interviewer, you will be expected to strike a balance between the needs of the research and creating a guided conversation using the topic guide or interview guide that makes sense to your respondent. For this reason, the sequencing of questions is important, from the general to the specific, and from the relatively easy to the more complex topics. One strategy is to start with the 'grand tour' question, to ask respondents an initial open question that allows them to talk at some length. To return to the example of aspirin, an opening grand tour could be: 'Could you start by telling me about your general feelings about taking medicines?'.

Another useful strategy is to use 'signposts' to let your respondent know the broad direction of the interview, when you are changing topics or focus and when you are getting close to the end of the interview. Phrases such as: 'I'd like to start by asking you to tell me about...' and, 'I'd like to move on now' can be used. A signpost such as: 'The final thing I would like to ask you about is...' tells your respondent that the end is in sight, and may prompt them to relax and speak more discursively. It is always worth finishing with: 'Any other comments you would like to make about this?'.

## INTERVIEWING COLLEAGUES

There are particular issues in interviewing colleagues, sometimes encapsulated as the 'you know what it's like' syndrome. If this happens, have probe questions at your disposal to encourage respondents to make their views explicit; these may be phrases such as: 'If you were describing this to a new colleague, how would you do so?' or, 'Imagine you were explaining this to a colleague from abroad, how would you start?'.

There are both advantages and disadvantages to interviewing colleagues. On the one hand, it is likely to be relatively easy to gain access to professional peers, and on the other hand, you may simply reinforce each other's beliefs and not create an environment in which respondents can think critically and question their own professional beliefs and assumptions. It may be that it is less easy to give a glib, publicly acceptable answer to an outsider than to a pharmacist colleague. For instance, if you were asked to be interviewed for a study of the role of community pharmacists within primary health care, you may say very different things to a pharmacist than to a non-pharmacist, and as an interviewer in this particular scenario, you are well placed to ask the probing follow-up question.

## KEEPING ON TRACK

While it is important to encourage respondents to be discursive, it is equally important to keep them on track. Strategies such as: 'Could I bring you back to...?', 'You mentioned...' or, 'Some people have mentioned...' are subtle ways of steering an interview while remaining informant centred and working with your own agenda as a researcher.

# RECORDING THE DATA

There are two important aspects to recording data: note taking and audio recording.

## TAKING NOTES

Taking brief notes during each interview and expanding upon them immediately afterwards allows you to record your own observations of the interview, to note wording that either did or did not work well, to identify new topics or opinions that were generated during the interview and to identify additional topics for future interviews. In short, it is the beginning of the work of data analysis, of generating an analytical framework from the data.

## AUDIO RECORDING

The second way of recording data is through the use of a digital recorder. Make sure you have spare batteries; make sure that 'pause' is not on and don't use 'voice activation'. In short, take every care to avoid losing data and to allow you to concentrate on the interview, not on problems with recording. Audio files then need to be passed to a transcriber. Files should be encrypted, anonymized and numbered before being passed to the transcriber. In costing for research of this kind, ensure you budget for an audio recorder, transcriber and a transcribing time of approximately 5 hours for each hour of interview time.

Remember that if the transcription is not going to be undertaken by the researcher, it may take several weeks for transcripts to be produced. During this time, you will be carrying on with data collection. Again, notes taken after each interview allow you to keep track of the data collection process, of new topics emerging from interviews and of ways of addressing particular topics. Ensure that notes are numbered in sequence in the same way as interviews in order to allow you to link the notes with their original interview and to establish their place in the sequence of data collection.

# DATA ANALYSIS

Much contemporary health services research adopts an approach to knowledge that could be described as 'common sense', accepting a physical world that is both knowable and researchable. Such an approach relies on a positivist definition of the world (see Chapter 22), in which what is being researched may be reduced to its constituent parts, understood and reassembled, either physically or metaphorically. Such an approach is appropriate in certain circumstances (e.g. the assessment of the physical properties of a particular drug). However, in addressing more complex questions which relate to the social world or to the ways in which we attempt to explain or make sense of particular phenomena, a more complex consideration of knowledge allows the development of a more subtle and complex analysis. Qualitative research is appropriately used in little-understood areas, and its methods are embedded in disciplines such as anthropology and sociology, which provide the scope for a more theoretical analysis (see Chapter 25). The choice of the depth of analysis lies in the nature of the research question.

There are a number of methods that are used in qualitative research, from 'framework' analysis (at the most empiricist end of the spectrum), through thematic analysis, conversation, discourse and narrative analysis, to grounded theory. The general principle of qualitative analysis is that the analytical framework is generated from the data, rather than being predetermined by the researcher. Data analysis commences at the same time as data collection, and new data are used by the researchers to review their sampling strategies and data collection methods. The analytical framework is developed throughout the data collection period, with new data being used to question or refine the analysis.

## VALIDITY AND RELIABILITY IN QUALITATIVE RESEARCH

The *British Medical Journal* criteria for assessing the rigour of qualitative research are largely methodological, but emphasize that the methods need to be discussed within their theoretical framework. This is particularly important given that the

---

**BOX 23.8   QUESTIONS TO ASK OF A QUALITATIVE STUDY**

- Overall, did the researcher make explicit in the account the theoretical framework and methods used at every stage of the research?
- Was the context clearly described?
- Was the sampling strategy clearly described and justified?
- Was the sampling strategy theoretically comprehensive to ensure the generalizability of the conceptual analysis?
- How was the fieldwork undertaken? Was it described in detail?
- Could the evidence be inspected independently, and could the process of transcription be independently inspected?
- Were the procedures for data analysis clearly described and theoretically justified? Did they relate to the original research questions? How were themes and concepts identified in the data?
- Was the analysis repeated by more than one researcher to ensure reliability?
- Did the investigator make use of quantitative evidence to test qualitative conclusions where appropriate?
- Did the investigator give evidence of seeking out observations that might have contradicted or modified the analysis?
- Was sufficient use of the original evidence presented systematically to satisfy the sceptical reader of the relationship between the interpretation and the evidence?

Adapted from Mays, N. and Pope, C. 1995. *British Medical Journal*, **311**, 182–184.

research process is essentially inductive, which is to say that the analytical framework is derived directly from the data, and therefore reflects both the theoretical and practical concerns of the researcher and the researched. It is therefore essential to make explicit your own theoretical and practical starting points as outlined above in the discussion of bracketing and reflexivity. There is no absolute expectation that any two researchers will analyse data in precisely the same way; the question to be asked is why conflicting analyses are different. Is it a feature of the researcher's theoretical background in a particular discipline or a result of assumptions based on experience and beliefs? Consequently, there are a number of pertinent questions one should ask when presented with a qualitative study (Box 23.8).

## CONCLUSION

The research interview is a powerful method for the collection of qualitative data. Choosing both to conduct a qualitative study and to use interviews within the study has a number of specific implications for the conduct of the research. While all qualitative studies entail careful sampling strategies and the collection and management of detailed data, interview studies require particular reflection on the ways in which the interviewer affects the data that are collected and the data analysis. When the interviewer is also known in a professional capacity and is interviewing either fellow professionals or clients, a number of specific strategies need to be adopted in order to protect the confidentiality of research informants and the integrity of the data.

## FURTHER READING

Britten, N. 1995. Qualitative interviews in medical research. *British Medical Journal*, **311**, 251–253.

Crabtree, B. and Miller, W. 1999. *Doing Qualitative Research*. Newbury Park: Sage.

Gantley, M., Harding, G., Kumar, S. and Tissier, J. 1999. *An Introduction to Qualitative Methods for Health Professionals*. London: Royal College of General Practitioners.

Glaser, B.G. 2006. *Doing Formal Grounded Theory*. Mill Valley: Sociology Press.

Glaser, B.G. and Strauss, A.L. 1995. *The Discovery of Grounded Theory*. Piscataway: Transaction Publishers.

Hoddinott, P. and Pill, R. 1997. A review of recently published qualitative research in general practice. More methodological questions than answers? *Family Practice*, **14**, 313–319.

Kirk, J. and Miller, M. 1986. *Reliability and Validity in Qualitative Research*. London: Sage.

Kitzinger, J. 1995. Introducing focus groups. *British Medical Journal*, **311**, 299–302.

Mays, N. and Pope, C. 1995. Observational methods in health care settings. *British Medical Journal*, **311**, 182–184.

Mays, N. and Pope, C. 1995. Rigour and qualitative research. *British Medical Journal*, **311**, 109–112.

Murphy, E. and Mattson, B. 1992. Qualitative research and family practice: A marriage made in heaven? *Family Practice*, **9**, 85–91.

Patton, M.Q. 2014. *Qualitative Evaluation and Research Methods* (4th Edn.). Newbury Park: Sage.

Riessman, C. 2008. *Narrative Methods for the Human Sciences*. London: Sage.

Ritchie, J. and Spencer, L. 1994. Qualitative data analysis for applied policy research. In: A. Bryman and R. Burgess (Eds.), *Analyzing Qualitative Data*, London: Routledge, pp. 173–193.

Silverman, D. 2013. *Doing Qualitative Research: A Practical Handbook* (4th Edn.). London: Sage.

Spencer, L., Ritchie, J., Lewis, L. and Dillion, L. 2003. *Quality in Qualitative Evaluation: A Framework for Assessing Research Evidence.* London: Government Chief Social Researcher's Office.

Strauss, A. and Corbin, J. 1990. *Basics of Qualitative Research.* London, New Dehli and Thousand Oaks: Sage.

Strauss, A. and Corbin, J. 2015. *Basics of Qualitative Research* (4th Edn.). London: Sage.

Tesch, R. 1991. *Qualitative Research: Analysis Types and Software Tools.* London and Philadelphia: Falmer Press.

## REFERENCES

Ahern, K.A. 1999. Ten tips for reflexive bracketing. *Qualitative Health Research*, **9**, 407–411.

Brinkmann, S. and Kvale, S. 2013. *Interviews: Learning the Craft of Qualitative Research Interviewing* (3rd Edn.). Thousand Oaks: Sage.

Britten, N. 1994. Patients' ideas about medicines: A qualitative study in a general practice population. *British Journal of General Practice*, **44**, 465–468.

Denzin, N. and Lincoln, Y. 1994. *Handbook of Qualitative Research.* Thousand Oaks, London and New Delhi: Sage.

Mays, N. and Pope, C. 1995. Rigour and qualitative research. *British Medical Journal*, **311**, 109–112.

Patton, M.Q. 1990. *Qualitative Evaluation and Research Methods.* Newbury Park: Sage.

Ritchie, J. and Spencer, L. 1994. Qualitative data analysis for applied policy research. In: A. Bryman and R. Burgess (Eds.), *Analyzing Qualitative Data.* London: Routledge.

Silverman, D. 2015. *Interpreting Qualitative Data* (5th Edn.). London: Sage.

# 24 Focus Groups

## *Felicity Smith*

## CONTENTS

---

### KEY POINTS

- Focus groups are a qualitative method used to explore a topic from the perspective of a particular population group.
- Focus groups are the research method of choice where interactions between group members may stimulate more wide-ranging thoughts, ideas and experiences of participants.
- Group discussion often has the effect of strengthening the average or dominant view within the group, rather than stimulating a discussion on a range of views.
- Focus groups are particularly useful in helping to develop hypotheses for testing using quantitative methods.

---

## INTRODUCTION

Focus groups (group interviews) are a popular method of data collection in health services and pharmacy practice research and their value as a research tool is now widely acknowledged. There are many examples of focus groups as a sole method in research studies or in combination with other methods of data collection to address specific objectives at a particular stage of research.

Focus groups are a qualitative method used to explore a topic from the perspective of a particular population group. In line with processes of qualitative enquiry, data are gathered and analysed in the context of the experiences, views, priorities and concerns of the participants.

Focus groups are often seen as an alternative means of data collection to face-to-face interviews, with interaction between group members being the essential feature that distinguishes focus groups from one-to-one interviews (see Chapter 23). Researchers generally opt to conduct a group rather than individual interviews when they believe that the group interaction will have a positive effect on the data collection process for achieving the study objectives. Group interviews may, for instance, uncover more wide-ranging thoughts, ideas and experiences as the participants may stimulate each other. Listening to the views and arguments of other group members may assist individuals in recalling experiences or feelings, or in developing and clarifying their own thoughts. Should differences of opinion be expressed, the researcher has the opportunity to explore the reasoning behind them. This enables 'how?' and 'why?' questions to be addressed, in addition to providing descriptions of events or experiences.

## ABOUT THE NATURE OF GROUPS

Interaction between people is part of everyday life. Thus, in some respects, focus group research simulates a natural interactive process in which people express and modify their views and opinions. As with all qualitative research, the aim of the researcher is to explore issues from the perspective of people's lives, experiences and concerns, and is thus context specific.

When individuals come together in a group, each brings their own personal history, views and perspectives, which contribute to the character of the group. Consequently, all groups will be unique and the members share the experience of being part of the group and the production of data.

Many researchers, in particular in sociology and psychology, have examined and reviewed aspects of group behaviour. For example, group polarization is widely acknowledged. This is defined as 'a group-produced enhancement of members' pre-existing tendencies' (Myers 1993). Researchers have observed that group discussion often has the effect of strengthening the average or dominant view within the group, rather than resulting in a split within it. Thus, a group of people with a tendency to take risks, following a group discussion, would be expected to assert enhanced risk-taking tendencies, while a group of people naturally more prudent would tend to have more cautious views. A number of explanations are given for this. For example, in a group discussion, a high proportion of contributions from the group would favour the dominant view, while minority viewpoints, if expressed, may not receive the corresponding attention. Participants may be unaware of the extent to which alternative or competing views are considered. People are also more likely to be persuaded by the arguments of individuals with whom they identify. In the context of focus group research, the participants in a group will generally share some background and/or experiences.

In focus group research, interaction between group participants is seen as an important feature (often the reason that the approach is selected). In the analysis and interpretation of the data, it is important to remember that the data are a product of the group interaction process (Kitzinger 1994).

## APPROPRIATE RESEARCH OBJECTIVES FOR FOCUS GROUPS

As in other qualitative research, the aim of the researcher is to explore issues from the perspective of the research participants (group members). This may be to gain insights into people's understanding and perceptions of issues, and to explore how these relate to people's experiences, priorities and concerns. In general, qualitative methods are used to explore the research questions 'how?' and 'why?', rather than to quantify the frequency of events and statistical relationships between variables. Qualitative approaches are used to generate hypotheses and facilitate the development of theories to explain phenomena, rather than to provide conclusions based on quantitative assessments. A common aim of focus groups is also to scope wide-ranging experiences and perceptions on a topic.

Focus groups are employed in different ways and at varying stages in research projects. When conducted in the early stages of a research project, they can be helpful in developing research objectives. For example, they may be used to inform the development of a quantitative study (e.g. a survey instrument). Focus groups will enable exploration of the issues of importance to the population of interest on any topic so that the researcher, in building their instrument, can check that all relevant data are collected (i.e. that content validity is achieved). Focus groups have also been used by researchers subsequent to quantitative work to explore, in greater depth, topics of interest arising from previous work. For phenomena uncovered in a survey, focus group discussions may provide the opportunity to explore responses in more detail. For example, 'why?' and 'how?' questions can be addressed, which will enable contexts and reasons for respondents' views or experiences to be examined.

Increasingly, focus groups (often in combinations with other qualitative approaches) are employed to examine feasibility and acceptability aspects in intervention studies. Service evaluations, intervention studies and clinical trials will have quantitative outcome measures. Commonly in these studies, researchers will be looking for a difference between groups (e.g. intervention and control) in performance on primary outcomes. However, many such studies are complex and may impact on different stakeholders in diverse ways, which will not be reflected in the primary outcome measures. For example, factors such as the acceptability and workability of an intervention in practice will be important to wider implementation, but not captured in a formal quantitative evaluation. Focus groups with study participants can provide additional contextual data on how, when and why the intervention may or may not be acceptable or feasible. They can also be used to explore perceived benefits and reasons for positive or negative outcomes.

Focus groups are sometimes adapted in a format to achieve specific research objectives. For example, the nominal group technique is employed to develop consensus between group members. It is a structured procedure that includes group discussion as well as individual appraisal of material at different stages. Group discussions may also include 'workshop' activities (e.g. pairing of participants to reflect on particular scenarios), which may then be shared with the group. Some structuring of group activities and open discussion of selected hypothetical and 'real-life' case studies can promote more in-depth consideration of issues of interest.

Depending on the research objectives, either group or one-to-one interviews may be more effective. The generation of a comprehensive range of issues, which is seen as a strength of focus groups, may be at the expense of detailed discussion of issues of particular concern to individual participants. In the light of the objectives of the study and preliminary fieldwork, the researcher must decide the most effective method of gathering the data required.

Feasibility is also a consideration in the decision to gather data in focus groups versus one-to-one interviews. For many research studies, either method may be effective. The choice of approach may be determined by practical considerations (e.g. finding a time slot and venue that is convenient for a number of people).

## SAMPLING: SELECTION OF GROUPS AND/OR PARTICIPANTS

Focus group research has been conducted in both established community groups and those convened by the research team for the purpose. Each approach has its own advantages and disadvantages.

Research among established community groups enables the researcher to gather data in the context of a 'real-life' situation. Qualitative studies, in particular ethnographic work, aim to examine people's views, priorities and concerns in the context of their daily lives and experiences. The groups people join are natural settings in which they will discuss issues, hear views and form and modify their thoughts and ideas. Thus, research among these pre-existing groups enables the researcher to follow some principles of ethnographic research, collecting data in a naturally occurring social context rather than in an artificially created research environment. Group interviews with established community groups will often be conducted as part of a regular meeting of the group. If people are interested in the research, then willingness to participate may be high. The meeting may be held at a group's usual venue, which minimizes both the costs (e.g. room hire) and the administrative tasks associated with organizing the meeting.

However, there may be important disadvantages. In attending the meetings of established community groups, the researcher has only limited control over who attends and the suitability of the venue. The quality of the data and the extent to which research objectives are met may be severely compromised if, for instance, the number of participants is too large, or the room is unsuitable. In arranging the meeting, the researcher must ensure that their minimal requirements (determined in advance) can be met. As focus group research has become more popular alongside an increased emphasis on health services research in ensuring users' views are solicited, some community groups may find it difficult to respond to all requests for involvement. Some groups may be reluctant (and should not be expected) to devote too much of their meeting time that is intended for a different purpose.

Convening groups specifically for the purpose of the research generally involves more administration than arranging to meet with established groups and attending one of their regular meetings. The costs may also be greater (e.g. financial incentives may be required to elicit cooperation from individuals). However, subject to response rates, the researcher retains control over the group size, who is invited to the group and can ensure the suitability of the venue.

Inevitably, interactions and relationships between group members will have an impact on the data collected. This applies to both established community groups and those specially convened for the study. Participants in established groups will often know each other well, are likely to be friends and may be more likely to be supportive of each other, rather than unfriendly or antagonistic. They may also be less shy and more willing to participate in discussion, and natural 'leaders' may have emerged. Groups which are convened for the purpose of the study may or may not include individuals known to each other. Members of the group are generally selected on the basis of sharing some experience or characteristics. They may include health professionals from a particular geographical area or people who have been involved in a particular initiative. It is not usually necessary or desirable to aim for group members who are unknown to each other.

Decisions regarding sampling procedures relate to both the groups and the individual members of the groups. Common strategies employed are purposive, maximum diversity sampling and representative sampling. There will usually be an element of self-selection, in that participants will have chosen to take part. The researcher will often have limited control over the individuals attending established community groups. However, they do make decisions regarding the selection of the groups themselves, and similar considerations will apply.

Appropriate procedures will depend on the objectives of the study. In the selection of individuals into groups convened for a study, the researcher may wish to ensure that group members are broadly representative of the population of interest. Where a sampling frame (a list of all members of a population) is available (e.g. of community pharmacies, pharmacy students, people attending a surgery or clinic, etc.), the researcher can randomly select individuals and invite them to participate. In many cases, a sampling frame may not be available and the researcher may have to resort to less rigorous methods of achieving some degree of representativeness in the groups. Quota sampling involves the selection of individuals with particular characteristics (e.g. ensuring representation from people in particular age groups). Although not randomly selected, the group will include representatives of people with particular characteristics. In preliminary fieldwork, convenience samples (individuals accessible and willing to participate) may be acceptable to the researcher.

Some studies require the participation of individuals who share some common experience, have taken part in particular programmes or possess other characteristics. Individuals may be 'purposively' selected for these studies.

The researcher makes an informed decision and purposely selects individual participants (e.g. individuals who have taken part in a particular programme or have experienced certain adverse events). Thus, the focus group may include a group of experts on any topic who can share their similar and differing perspectives.

Maximum diversity sampling is employed when the researcher wants to explore the extremes of view or experience. For example, an effort may be made to include participants who have had positive and negative experiences, who work in a range of health care settings or who are from diverse socio-economic backgrounds. Maximum diversity may also be applied to the groups themselves (e.g. contrasting locations).

In discussion, groups in which the individuals are from varied backgrounds may raise a wider range of issues than groups of like-minded individuals. However, groups in which the individuals share background characteristics and experiences may provide the researcher with an opportunity to explore, in some depth, issues that may be of shared concern. Thus, there may be some trade-off between the variety of issues raised for discussion and the depth of discussion achieved around each of these issues.

In selecting or convening groups, the researcher must decide the extent to which their study objectives are best served by either groups whose members share many common features or those that are more heterogeneous in nature. The number of groups required will be determined by the objectives of the study. If the aim of the researcher is to include issues important to individuals in order to inform a more structured instrument, sufficient groups should be consulted so that the researcher is confident that all important perspectives are identified. A technique that can be employed is to meet with successive groups until no new issues emerge. This is referred to as 'sampling to saturation'. In some studies with a very specific focus or among a limited population group, all major issues may emerge from just one or two meetings.

## DETERMINING GROUP SIZE

The groups should be small enough to allow all participants to contribute to the discussion. Too large a group may potentially undermine the efficacy of this method (Box 24.1).

In a large group, the task of the facilitator in maintaining a single 'floor' for the discussion and participation of all individuals is more difficult. A wide range of viewpoints may be shared, but this may be at the expense of more detailed exploration of specific issues. It is worth realizing that in a 90-minute meeting with nine participants, each would have an average of less than 10 minutes to contribute their views. This could be viewed as an inefficient use of their time. Five or six participants may be more worthwhile from all perspectives.

Bales et al. (1951) found that as group size increased, larger proportions of participants contributed less than their fair share, there was greater differentiation between the most active people and others and the involvement of the group leader increased.

---

### BOX 24.1   POTENTIAL ISSUES OF TOO LARGE A FOCUS GROUP

- The group may fragment.
- Comments made to neighbours may be inaudible (and lost to the data set).
- Several people may attempt to speak at once.
- Contributions of some individuals relevant to the discussion may not be voiced.
- Insufficient time may be available to explore everyone's perspectives on any question.

Participation in relation to group size was also analysed in a series of focus groups held with community groups to discuss experiences of medicines (Smith 1999). Group size ranged from four to ten. Irrespective of group size, the duration of contributions from the most active members was similar. Increasing the group size beyond about six participants had the effect of increasing the number of participants who made a minimal contribution. The optimal number of participants for most focus group discussions is considered to be five to seven participants. Larger numbers may be preferred in some studies when more structured formats or break-out groups may be employed.

## VENUE AND ENVIRONMENT

The venue and environment must be conducive to a group discussion. The surroundings should be comfortable and the layout of the room such that all participants feel equally part of the group and able to take part in the discussion with similar ease. Prior to the start of the meeting, the researchers should prepare the room to ensure that these needs are met.

The usual procedure (as in all qualitative interviews) is for the meeting to be audio recorded. Audio-recording equipment should be situated centrally where contributions from all group members will be captured.

## ROLE OF FACILITATOR AND CO-FACILITATOR

Focus groups are conducted by a facilitator and co-facilitator. The facilitator has responsibility for steering the group discussion. He or she will endeavour to encourage participation by all members of the group. In welcoming people to the group, all participants should be asked to introduce themselves. The facilitator should explain the purpose and operation or agenda for the event. It should be emphasized that individual group members may have different perspectives, experiences and concerns regarding the issues to be discussed and that all views are important. The facilitator should encourage participants to express differences in opinion and experiences. When these arise, this provides the facilitator with an opportunity to probe into the reasons and contexts of differences and similarities. Then, in the subsequent analysis, both the range of views and rationale (how and why questions) behind them can be examined.

In accordance with an interview guide (see below), the facilitator will introduce topics for discussion and follow-up responses and contributions from group members to obtain further details or contextual information, rationales for particular viewpoints, alternative perspectives and the reasoning behind them. The facilitator will aim to encourage all participants to engage in the discussion.

The co-facilitator's role is to ensure the smooth organization of the group meeting, operating the audio-recording equipment so that a high-quality recording is obtained and noting contextual information to aid the interpretation of the transcript (e.g. interruptions or late arrivals, etc.). The co-facilitator should be able to see all participants and identify who is speaking. As the discussion proceeds, the co-facilitator should maintain a record so that contributions of different group members can be identified and attributed in the transcript. A diagram of the seating plan should be made, including the position of the facilitator, co-facilitator, all group members, the microphone and any other relevant features that may be useful.

Meetings are generally followed by a 'debriefing' session between the facilitator and co-facilitator in which relevant observations or thoughts can be noted (e.g. features of the interactions between group members that may be important and not apparent from the audio recording).

## THE INTERVIEW TOPIC GUIDE

Following an introduction to the meeting, the group discussion will be based around an interview topic guide (see also Chapter 23). This will generally comprise a series of predominantly open questions on topics relevant to the subject area of the research. Open questions allow group members to respond with issues which are important to them. They give participants an opportunity to express their views, experiences and concerns in their own words.

The interview guide may also include a range of prompts and probing questions to assist the facilitator in achieving an in-depth discussion of the issues raised in response to the open questions. For example:

Would you say more about…?
Why do you think…?
What do you think are the reasons for…?
Has anyone else had a similar experience?
Does anyone have a different view?
What others issues are important regarding…?

As is common in all qualitative interviews, the issues raised and discussed are determined by the respondents, rather than following the agenda and perspectives of the researcher.

## DATA MANAGEMENT AND ANALYSIS

In the analysis of focus group data, the principles of one-to-one qualitative interviews are generally followed (see Chapter 23). The first step will be verbatim transcription of the focus group discussion. Then, commonly, a coding frame will be developed. This may be informed by the interview guide, but may also employ qualitative procedures involving the identification of emergent themes as in a more 'grounded' approach. Depending on the objectives of the research, a descriptive approach scoping the range of issues may be important. If a more in-depth discussion was achieved, a further stage of coding and analysis may enable some analysis in relation to the context and reasoning behind participants' experiences and views. The data from focus group discussions have the added complexity in that the group process will have an impact on the data obtained. For example, it may be pertinent to examine whether all positive or negative comments on any topic came from a small number of participants, or were more widely shared. In addition, if several participants expressed similar views, were there subtle differences in their reasoning or experience?

## ETHICAL CONSIDERATIONS

All research raises ethical issues. Informing potential participants of the purpose of the study, what it will involve, ensuring there is time to ask questions and to consider whether they wish to take part, maintaining confidentiality of data, appropriate arrangements for storage, obtaining consent, etc., are important for all research.

Particular methodologies may present their own ethical issues. Researchers frequently choose to conduct focus group interviews rather than individual interviews because they believe that they will be more effective in identifying a wide range of issues, considering alternative viewpoints and securing an in-depth discussion. This will be the case only if group members are willing to share their thoughts and experiences with others. If relevant issues are not raised in the discussion, this will impact on the validity of the data. In groups that include people who know each other, individuals may have had experiences that they have shared with another group member, but that they would not wish to be raised for open discussion in the context of the research study. Circumstances could arise in the course of the discussion that leave individuals feeling vulnerable and uncomfortable.

Focus group discussions are generally audio recorded. Verbatim transcripts are seen as important to ensuring that the detailed and comprehensive data required for qualitative analytical procedures are obtained. In individual interviews, respondents will be informed of the researcher's wish to audio record the interview and their consent will be requested. A similar procedure is adopted when working with groups. An objection by any member of the group must be respected. If the reasons for the need to audio record are stated (i.e. that it is important that everyone's views and thoughts are documented), permission is generally granted. During transcription, data are anonymized, with all identifiers being removed.

## CONCLUSION

With careful planning and preparation, focus groups are a valuable tool that have been widely used in health services and pharmacy practice research. They are no longer viewed as a novel approach, but are nowadays employed widely and flexibly to meet the needs of many different types of research study.

## FURTHER READING

Krueger, R.A. 1994. *Focus Groups: A Practical Guide to Applied Research*. London: Sage Publications.

Morgan, D.L. 1996. *Focus Groups as Qualitative Research* (2nd Edn.). London: Sage.

Silverman, D. (Ed.) 2011. Part IV: Interviews and focus groups. In: *Qualitative Research* (3rd Edn.). London: Sage Publications, pp. 129–184.

## REFERENCES

Bales, R.F, Strodtbeck, F.L, Mills, T.M and Roseborough, M.E. 1951. Distribution of participation as function of group size. *American Sociological Review*, **16**, 461–468.
Kitzinger, J. 1994. The methodology of focus groups: The importance of interaction between
research participants. *Sociology of Health and Illness*, **16**, 103–121.
Myers, D.G. 1993. *Social Psychology* (4th Edn.). London: McGraw-Hill.
Smith, F.J. 1999. Analysis of data from focus groups: Group interaction – The added dimension. *International Journal of Pharmacy Practice*, **7**, 192–196.

# 25 Analysing Qualitative Data

*Geoffrey Harding, Madeleine Gantley and Kevin Taylor*

## CONTENTS

---

### KEY POINTS

- The scope of problem-based qualitative research is limited.
- Applying a theoretical perspective to qualitative pharmacy practice research can generate an enhanced perspective.
- Findings from qualitative syntheses are able to generate findings that contribute to the evidence base.

---

## INTRODUCTION

Qualitative methods, such as depth interviews (Chapter 23) and group interviews (Chapter 24), are increasingly popular as investigators explore the broader context of pharmacy services (e.g. the behaviours and attitudes of users and providers of pharmaceutical services). The use of qualitative methods in pharmacy practice research, as in much health services research, produces analytical insights from recounted experiences, beliefs and views.

Using qualitative methods in pharmacy practice research without an understanding of the theory that informs the types of questions asked and the data generated from these methods can result in their being used merely as a technique for collecting or organizing data. Qualitative research is frequently a 'catch-all' term used variously to describe the type of data to be collected (e.g. documents or transcripts of interviews), the method of data collection (e.g. participant observation), methods of data analysis or the particular theoretical perspective adopted (e.g. interpretative).

## THEORY-ORIENTATED VERSUS PROBLEM-ORIENTATED QUALITATIVE RESEARCH

The 'theory-orientated' and 'problem-orientated' distinction in research reflects researchers' contrasting epistemological stances; that is to say, differing assumptions about what constitutes legitimate knowledge. Theory-orientated research is essentially exploratory and theory generating. Thus, the nature and significance of empirical inquiry are fully meaningful only within the context of social science theories. On the other hand, problem-orientated research is embedded within an epistemology in which 'facts' do not require theoretical interpretation, but are readily observable and describable.

Published qualitative studies in pharmacy practice, based on depth interviews, are often characterized by a similar presentational format, with raw data (i.e. selected quotes) grouped together and listed along identified themes to generate an account of individuals' actions. Such qualitative studies are then little more than a reiteration of what subjects reported when interviewed. Typically, publications from these studies comprise little more than a stream of selected quotes whose significance is assumed to be self-evident in relation to the conclusion of the research.

'Applied' research, as exemplified by health services research and pharmacy practice research, is generally less theoretically driven than 'pure' social science research, which has many theoretical assumptions. Pharmacy practice research has a clear end objective defined in terms of outcomes, centred on the efficient and effective delivery of pharmaceutical services. However, without an appreciation of the theoretical framework that underpins such research methodologies, investigators run the risk of conducting 'shallow' analyses, yielding apparent insights which differ little from common sense or are invalidated by the misapplication of a particular method.

Qualitative methods in the theoretical disciplines comprising the social sciences require interpretation of data from a theoretical perspective. At the core of such interpretation lies the assumption that what people say and do can be analysed as a particular form of behaviour; that is, social action. Behaviour is therefore not self-evident, but requires interpreting within a wider social and cultural environment. The interplay with this environment both shapes and is shaped by social action. Thus, principles of social theory (e.g. ethnomethodology or symbolic interactionism, which regard social interaction as comprising meaningful communicative activity between people) essentially define the nature of a social scientific research problem, how it is to be explored and the interpretation of the qualitative data collected (Atkinson 1995). In contrast to 'theory-orientated' social science research, however, pharmacy practice research has often utilized 'common sense' rather than 'theory', derived from a discipline as a basis for analysis. Theory in qualitative analysis becomes secondary to assembling 'facts' and descriptions in order to answer predefined research questions, such as how to contain prescribing costs or how to identify the constituent

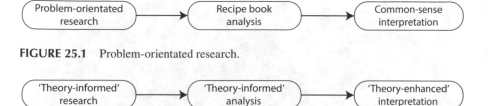

**FIGURE 25.1** Problem-orientated research.

**FIGURE 25.2** Theory-informed research.

elements of 'best practice'. The scope of problem-orientated qualitative research questions and the chosen method of analysis becomes defined, then, by practical rather than theoretical considerations. Transcripts and notes recounting experiences, views and beliefs are taken at face value. Problem-orientated qualitative research thus becomes little more than a set of simple techniques or practices as in 'content analysis', which involves identifying and cataloguing themes from transcripts.

It is arguable whether pharmacy practice researchers should (and equally importantly could) adopt the social scientist's approach to qualitative analysis. In short, is qualitative data interpreted within say a sociological epistemology valid and relevant to the objectives of pharmacy practice research? Correspondingly, should qualitative methods in pharmacy practice research be informed by and interpreted within a social theory frame of reference? When used as a managerial tool for planning and rationing services, where the role of problem-orientated research is to provide information to bring about organizational change, pharmacy practice research which draws on social theory is neither tenable nor necessary. However, to avoid too simplistic an application of qualitative methods and to enhance the quality and value of qualitative analysis in pharmacy practice research, a theoretically-informed approach is vital. Qualitative pharmacy practice research should develop beyond a 'cookbook approach' (i.e. simply following a recipe for data collection and interpretation) (Figure 25.1). Rather, the potential contribution of theoretical frameworks from within the social sciences, particularly sociology, social psychology and social anthropology, should be considered in framing research questions and informing subsequent analysis (Figure 25.2).

## AN EMERGENT COMMON GROUND

The problem-orientated approach of pharmacy practice research and health services research and the pre-eminence of theory in social scientific research might seem irreconcilable. However, common ground is emerging, as funding for theoretically-orientated research is diminishing relative to the funding available for health services research. This has led social scientists increasingly to temper their emphasis on analytical or exploratory research with pragmatism, researching social rather than sociological concerns. Likewise, pharmacy practice and health services researchers can develop a theoretical foundation by framing research questions within a broad theoretical perspective (Figure 25.3). Thus, the theory-orientated/problem-orientated dichotomy is less defensible and less relevant in the current economic climate.

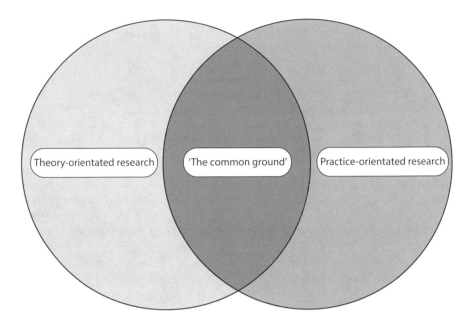

**FIGURE 25.3** The common ground.

However, while arguing against pharmacy practice research simply applying qualitative methods divorced from a theoretical context, it should nevertheless draw on social theory only to the extent of building up its own theoretical foundation, which in turn would be subject to a continual process of refinement through hypothesis testing. A first step would be for practice researchers to eschew qualitative analyses founded on the principles of what has been termed 'abstracted empiricism' (i.e. treating what people say and do as self-evident, leading in turn to the discrete accumulation of empirical data, thus stultifying the development of theoretical insights, however limited). Qualitative analysis should extend beyond ordering the content of individuals' responses along identified themes. The question becomes not simply what pattern can be discerned from people's responses, but also why this pattern and not others? A central assumption of a theoretically-informed qualitative analysis in pharmacy practice research may be that the authenticity of people's experiences is not necessarily to be taken at face value.

## TREATING 'COMMON SENSE' AS A TOPIC FOR ANALYSIS

In the absence of theory, it is not possible for pharmacy practice researchers to produce a detailed analysis of the processes whereby meanings are attached to behaviour. Theoretical structures are needed in which to analyse the common-sense assumptions of both the researcher and the subjects of research to lend meaning to behaviour. A leading figure in sociological qualitative analysis, David Silverman (1993), notes the philosopher Wittgenstein's observation that 'The aspects of things that are most important for us are hidden because of their simplicity and familiarity'. Silverman suggests that this applies equally to the social sciences as to philosophy. Introducing a theoretical perspective from the social sciences thus seeks to make common-sense knowledge of the way in which the world (and indeed pharmacy) is organized as the topic of analysis, because once perspectives enter the category of 'common sense', they cease to be examined or questioned.

## INTRODUCING A THEORETICAL PERSPECTIVE: AN EXAMPLE

A pharmacy-based example of theory-informed practice research might be a study of the relationships between pharmacists and other health professionals. Typical questions to pharmacists and general practitioners might include: 'How would you describe your relationship with your colleagues? Do you participate in joint decision making? How would you describe good inter-professional communication?'. In the absence of a theoretical underpinning, responses to such questions would not inform the researcher about the broader social processes which have formed that response. A research methodology and an analysis of the data informed by social theory (e.g. the application of the theoretical concepts of the 'proletarianization' and 'bureaucratisation' of professions) would, however, enable searching questions to be posed in order to explore the extent to which inter-professional collaboration is influenced by the various professions' susceptibility to these processes and their impact on collaboration. Such questions might include: 'How do you make professional judgements? To what extent can your judgements be challenged by other professions?' The answers to such questions will then provide insights into the dynamics of the relationship between the occupational groups that each stake claims to making professional judgements in health care.

## META-ETHNOGRAPHY

Qualitative research continues to be a popular methodology within pharmacy practice research, and a considerable repository of findings covering a wide spectrum of pharmacy practice activities have accrued over recent years. By their nature, research findings using qualitative methods are applicable only to the population from which the results are derived – they are not generalizable and therefore, in themselves, collectively do not contribute to an evidence base for pharmacy practice. However, by synthesizing selected research findings, it is possible to contribute to an evidence base. One technique for synthesizing qualitative analyses – meta-ethnography – was developed by Noblit and Hare (1988). This approach involves seven sequential steps (Box 25.1).

Meta-ethnography is one of a number of methods for synthesizing qualitative research findings and may potentially contribute to the evidence base of pharmacy practice. There are a number of published worked examples of this method, though none have focused on pharmacy issues *per se* (e.g. see Britten 2002). There are also commentaries on methodological issues arising from its use (e.g. see Atkins et al. 2008), which provide a useful starting point for researchers who are not familiar with this method.

**BOX 25.1   SEVEN SEQUENTIAL STEPS
OF META-ETHNOGRAPHY**

Step 1 – getting started: in order to undertake a meta-ethnography study, the initial task is to determine a research question appropriate to qualitative methods and which provides the focus of the synthesis.

Step 2 – deciding what is relevant to the initial interest: having established the research question, the next task is to identify research findings of potential relevance by a systematic search of electronic bibliographic databases. This process involves determining inclusion/exclusion criteria, together with a critical appraisal of relevant studies, in order to determine their quality and robustness.

Step 3 – reading the studies: studies identified as being of potential interest to the synthesis are interrogated and their emergent themes and categories are extracted.

Step 4 – determining how the studies are related: themes and categories identified from the studies are listed or displayed onto a grid or table to allow relationships between these to be explored, revised and merged as appropriate.

Step 5 – translating the studies into one another: compare the themes and concepts from the first study with the second, which are then synthesized. This synthesis of themes and concepts is then compared with the themes and concepts from the third study to create a synthesis of the three studies, and so forth with the remaining studies.

Step 6 – synthesizing translations: the next step involves moving from describing the relationships between the concepts and themes derived from translating the studies into one another towards an explanatory analysis in which the composite themes and concepts form the basis for what is termed a 'line of argument' underpinning the development of an overarching model.

Step 7 – expressing the synthesis: the resultant line of argument derived from what is a series of complex processes, together with emergent hypotheses generated from the synthesis, may be expressed diagrammatically in order to illuminate the research question. This is particularly important if the findings are to contribute towards an evidence base.

Adapted from Noblit, G.W. and Hare R.D. 1988. *Meta-Ethnography: Synthesizing Qualitative Studies*. Newbury Park: Sage.

## CONCLUSION

By paying attention to the unremarkable and to seemingly uneventful descriptions and events – as well as the strikingly different – qualitative pharmacy practice research, informed by social scientific theories, has the potential to contribute to our understanding both of social processes and of how they may be modified in the pursuit of desired ends. While using a recipe book approach to research methods may produce practical solutions to specific problems, it does not provide researchers with the broader concepts in which to place contemporary and/or immediate problems. Theory is 'good to think with...' (Levi-Strauss 1964) and provides researchers with new insights and a broader context for the development of a theoretical foundation for pharmacy practice research. Moreover, the increasing emphasis on evidence-based practice within health care provides opportunities to capitalize on the increasing volume of qualitative pharmacy research.

## ACKNOWLEDGEMENT

This chapter is adapted from a paper published in *Family Practice* (1997) **15**, 76–79, with permission of Oxford University Press.

## FURTHER READING

Britten, N. 1995. Qualitative interviews in medical research. *British Medical Journal*, **311**, 251–253.

Bryman, A. and Burgess, R. 1994. *Analysing Qualitative Data*. London: Routledge.

Fitzpatrick, R. and Boulton, M. 1994. Qualitative methods for assessing health care. *Quality in Health Care*, **3**, 107–113.

Harding, G. and Gantley, M. 1998. Qualitative methods: Beyond the cookbook. *Family Practice*, **15**, 76–79.

Kitzinger, J. 1995. Introducing focus groups. *British Medical Journal*, **311**, 299–302.

Mays, N. and Pope, C. 1995. Observational methods in health care settings. *British Medical Journal*, **311**, 182–184.

Mays, N. and Pope, C. 1995. Rigour and qualitative research. *British Medical Journal*, **311**, 109–112.

Silverman, D. 2013. *Doing Qualitative Research: A Practical Handbook* (4th Edn.). London: Sage.

## REFERENCES

Atkins, S., Lewin, S., Smith, H., Engel, M., Fretheim, A. and Volmink, J. 2008. *BMC Medical Research Methodology*, **8**, 2. Available at: http://www.biomedcentral/1471-2288/8/21.

Atkinson, P. 1995. Some perils of paradigms. *Qualitative Health Research*, **5**, 117–124.

Britten, N., Campbell, R., Pope, C., Donovan J., Morgan, M. and Pill, R. 2002. Using meta ethnography to synthesise qualitative research: A worked example. *Journal of Health Services Research and Policy*, **7**(4), 209–215.

Levi-Strauss, C. 1964. *Totemism*. London: Merlin Press.

Noblit, G.W. and Hare R.D. 1988. *Meta-Ethnography: Synthesizing Qualitative Studies*. Newbury Park: Sage.

Silverman, D. 1993. *Interpreting Qualitative Data: Methods for Analysing Talk, Text and Interaction*. London: Sage.

# 26 Measuring Health and Illness

*Sally-Anne Francis*

## CONTENTS

> **KEY POINTS**
>
> - Health and health outcome measures have an important role in allo-cating resources, informing clinical decision making and facilitating patients' autonomy.
> - The choice of approach to measuring health is determined by the con-ceptual model and the purpose for which health is being measured.
> - Traditional approaches to measuring health include mortality data, morbidity patterns and service-use data.
> - Broader, subjective measures of health, such as functional ability, self-reported health status and health-related quality of life, focus on the impact of disease and treatment on the lives of individuals.
> - Rigorous scientific methods should be adopted to measure subjective indicators of health in a reproducible and valid way.

## INTRODUCTION

Health services must continually change to ensure that a population's needs and expectations are met. The World Health Organization (WHO) identified the follow-ing aims for an evolving health service (World Health Organization 2010):

- To improve the health status of individuals, families and communities
- To defend the population against what threatens its health
- To protect people against the financial consequences of ill health
- To provide equitable access to people-centred care
- To make it possible for people to participate in decisions affecting their health and health system

The consequences of any health service development must be evaluated in terms of the impact on the health of the population (i.e. the health outcome).

Traditionally, health care practitioners have used objective criteria, such as signs of disease, laboratory data and radiological examination, to inform the diagnosis of disease and its management. Measures of mortality and morbidity have been used to evaluate the consequences of medical treatment. There are also broader measures of health outcomes that include both objective and subjective indicators, such as functional ability, self-reported health status and positive concepts of health, such as health-related quality of life. Often, social and economic approaches to measuring health outcomes are employed alongside traditional methods, and the patient's view-point has become central to monitoring and evaluating of health care interventions.

This chapter will review approaches to the measurement of health and illness. Traditional approaches such as mortality data, morbidity patterns and service-use data will be described, followed by broader measures, such as subjective health indi-cators and health-related quality of life. The choice of approach is dependent on the definition of health adopted (i.e. the conceptual model) and the purpose for which health is being measured. Therefore, the chapter begins with a brief discussion of the concept of health.

## THE DEFINITION AND CONCEPT OF HEALTH

Disease may be defined as 'an abnormal condition of the body with a complex of physical signs, symptoms and effects that can be attributed to a cause (known or unknown)' (Youngson 1992). By contrast, illness is often referred to as a subjective state resulting from a perceived change in functioning where disease may or may not be present. Sickness is endorsed behaviour that signifies illness, despite the presence of disease or illness. However, these definitions can be influenced by factors such as the cultural context of the individual, class, gender, ethnic group and other factors, such as availability of support from family members (Scully 2004). Furthermore, definitions of disease will change over time according to evolving diagnostic criteria and social and economic factors.

Health is also difficult to define. For example, the health of a population may be said to have improved if the life expectancy of that population has increased. Similarly, if a person who is diagnosed with schizophrenia receives a drug therapy that is effective at reducing the symptoms of illness and has an improved side-effect profile compared with previous drug therapy, then it may be said that the health of that individual has improved. Each of these examples may represent a different aspect of health.

Health may be defined in negative terms, such as the absence of disease, illness and sickness. However, the widely acknowledged WHO definition of health went beyond the absence of disease, to include 'a state of complete physical, mental and social well-being' (World Health Organization 1948). A number of limitations have been identified with this definition (e.g. its lack of clarity, its exclusion of physiological states, its lack of guidance on which health states are preferable to others and the boundaries of social well-being in relation to health) (Patrick and Erickson 1993). Ware's definition (1995) compounds the criticism that health is often unrealistically represented as an ideal state: 'Health also connotes completeness – nothing is missing from the person – and proper function – all is working efficiently'.

Absolute definitions such as these are often unhelpful in providing a conceptual base to guide the measurement of the concept (i.e. to serve as an operational definition). By developing measures without a firm conceptual base, confusion arises when interpreting the results of studies and making comparisons between studies. In response to these limitations, different concepts of health have been proposed, such as focusing on the ability to adapt and self-manage according to the three domains of health: physical, mental and social (Huber et al. 2011).

The lack of consensus on the definition or concept of health has resulted in the development of health indicators. For example, the number of times a person consults with their doctor may be considered a health indicator. However, it is unlikely that one indicator alone, such as doctor consultation rates, could reliably measure the multidimensional concept of health; more frequently, a number of indicators are employed. For example, the health status of a patient after a hip-replacement operation may be determined by the results of radiological examination, range of movement compared with the pre-operative state, experience of pain and the use of analgesia and functional ability (e.g. ability to carry out activities of daily living, such as climbing stairs).

## WHY MEASURE HEALTH?

Current health systems are concerned with the most effective treatment strategies, while considering the best use of their finite resources for a given population. In clinical settings, health status measurement may be concerned with determining the choice and effectiveness of interventions for an individual patient or comparing the outcomes of different treatment approaches between patient groups.

Population-based health outcome measurement can provide a baseline against which to measure future medical and public health practices, and any consequent social and economic legislation. For example, what would be the health outcomes associated with incorporating pharmacists more fully in the delivery of urgent and emergency care in England? In addition, examination of the relationships between health status and the environment provides evidence for the aetiology and transmission of disease, and informs the control of infectious diseases.

Life expectancy continues to improve worldwide. In the developed world, this has been largely due to preventative care and health-promotion strategies, in conjunction with effective treatments for major causes of mortality. Consequently, demands on health care services continue to grow due to the increased prevalence and presentation of chronic, non-communicable disease. Therefore, the objective of many treatments is to reduce morbidity rather than curing or prolonging life. In addition, advances in health technology have raised society's expectations of health care interventions. Patients' experiences are now central to the decisions concerning the risks and benefits of different treatment options. Therefore, the measurement of health outcomes has an important role in allocating scarce resources, informing clinical decision making and facilitating patients' autonomy.

## APPROACHES TO MEASURING HEALTH AND ILLNESS

### TYPES OF MEASURE

Mortality and morbidity patterns and service-use data have traditionally been used as measures of health outcome. Epidemiology (the study of the occurrence of conditions that affect health in a given population) has two main measures that it employs to represent disease frequency: incidence and prevalence. The incidence of a disease is the rate at which new cases of a specified condition presents in a particular population during a given period; prevalence is a measure of the proportion of people experiencing a particular condition in a given population at any one point of time. Mortality may therefore be termed as the incidence of death from a disease (Coggon et al. 2003).

### Mortality Data

Mortality data provide population-based information on the patterns of disease and causes of death. The crude death rate is calculated by dividing the number of deaths in a given population by the total number of people in that population. This permits the comparison of death rates between populations and over time. However, the composition of a population can influence its death rate (e.g. the proportion of elderly people or the proportion of men or women). Therefore, 'standardized' values are often calculated to take into account factors such as the age and gender structure of a given population. Expressed as standardized rates, mortality data are important indicators of public health and may be used to estimate the size and distribution of health problems. For diseases where treatment is likely to have an impact on length of life, survival time is frequently used as a primary endpoint in the evaluation of new drug therapies.

The application of mortality statistics as a global indicator of health status has limitations. For example, patterns of mortality in the developed world have changed (i.e. death from disease is now more commonly age related). In addition, it is an insensitive health outcome measure for assessing the impact of most health care interventions. It is essential that health outcome measures can identify the impact and consequences of alternative treatment options, even if there is no effect on survival.

The advantages of using mortality data as a measure of health, then, are twofold:

- Mortality data are often routinely collected by age, gender, cause of death and geographical area.
- Data are inherently reliable indicators, since death is definitive.

However, there are also two notes of caution:

- The extreme nature of the endpoint makes mortality data insensitive to identifying important changes within people's continuum of health and illness experiences.
- Cause of death information has limited value regarding patterns of disease over time due to the continued refinements made to the classification systems of disease.

## Morbidity and Service-Use Data

Morbidity data aim to capture information about the experience of disease and illness. In health care evaluation, frequently used morbidity data include biological endpoints such as blood pressure, condition-specific markers such as symptom lists or performance-related indicators such as number of days absent from work through illness. However, external factors such as environmental conditions and advances in diagnostic criteria can influence patterns of disease. In particular, performance-related indicators have a number of limitations. For example, changes in employment patterns and society's attitude to work and sickness suggest that 'days absent from work through illness' has severe disadvantages as an indicator of health. It may represent information on a range of other factors such as age, economic and social opportunities and the provision of health care resources. In addition, it only provides information on the proportion of the population that is in the workforce, thereby excluding children, full-time students, the unemployed, the retired, those looking after a home and full-time carers.

Service-use data (e.g. the number of people discharged from hospitals over a given period of time, hospital readmission statistics and doctor consultation rates)

are frequently used as indicators of health status, but they can obscure the true picture of health or disease in society. Access and availability of services and the illness
behaviour patterns of a population will affect the use of health services.

Morbidity and service-use data are often collected through service-based audits and
surveys. For example, since 1993, the Health and Social Care Information Centre has
been carrying out The National Study of Health and Well-Being (also known as the
Adult Psychiatric Morbidity Survey) (McManus et al. 2009). This is a series of household surveys (which has been repeated at seven-year intervals) which provide information on the prevalence of both treated and untreated psychiatric disorders in the adult
population in England, and is used to inform the planning of health and support services.

The main limitation associated with morbidity and service-use data is whether
patterns of change can be attributed to a change in health status or whether it is identifying change in some external factor. Other limitations include the lack of information about the impact of treatment on the patient's life and the difficulties associated
with making comparisons across different groups or populations. Comparisons
between international data can often reflect the influence of different cultural values
and health care systems, as well as identifying differences in the health of the populations being studied.

## Disability-Adjusted Life Years

A summary measure of population health is the disability-adjusted life year (DALY).
It is a principal measure used by the WHO in its Global Burden of Disease project
and can be used to represent and enable a comparison of the burden of disease suffered by different populations. It is a measure that combines mortality and morbidity
into a single number.

> …the disability-adjusted life year (DALY) [is] a time-based measure that combines
> years of life lost due to premature mortality and years of life lost due to time lived
> in states of less than full health, or years of healthy life lost due to disability. (World
> Health Organization 2014)

Therefore, those diseases associated with a higher number of DALYs are considered to have a greater impact than those associated with fewer DALYs. In terms of
evaluating interventions, it is considered that those interventions that have the greatest impact on reducing DALYs will bring most benefit.

## Subjective Health Measures

Mortality, morbidity and service-use data focus on disease, illness and access to
health care services. However, determinants of the effects of treatment go beyond
symptom alleviation and biological and physiological functioning to include patients'
outcome criteria such as role performance (e.g. the ability to go to work and the ability to fulfil household duties), levels of interest and energy and the ability to enjoy
oneself (Hunt and McKenna 1993). Therefore, subjective measures of health, such
as functional ability, self-reported health status and health-related quality of life, are
broader outcome measures that focus on the impact of disease and treatment on the
lives of individuals.

Subjective health measures are important approaches to health outcome measurement since they reflect a comprehensive range of factors known to influence a patient's health outcome, such as motivation, psychological well-being, adherence to treatment, social support networks and an individual's value system (Bowling 2004). In addition, directly involving patients in the assessment of health outcomes has been identified as the best approach to determining whether a treatment or medical intervention facilitates a patient to meet their needs or expectations (Ware 1995). For disease states where future drug therapies and surgical procedures are likely to have marginal effects on quantity of life, there is a need to incorporate broader, patient-led measures, such as functional status, health status and quality of life, into the assessment of health outcomes.

Functional measures focus on the impact of the disease and its treatment on activities of daily functioning. Interruptions of usual activities and roles are often important outcome indicators for the individual. This approach also permits comparison of the burden of disease between different disease states. One of the oldest measures of functioning is the index of activities of daily living (Katz et al. 1963; 1970). This was developed for use with elderly people where an observer rates the degree of independence/dependence associated with the completion of activities such as bathing, dressing, mobility, continence and feeding. As with any standardized instrument, the judgement is limited to functioning in those areas included within the content of the instrument. Therefore, functioning in relation to other activities that may be important to individuals is not considered.

Health status measurement can encompass functional status, physiological measures (e.g. signs, symptoms and clinical data) and measures of subjective well-being, thereby permitting the identification of differences in the clinical condition and functional capacity of people with the same 'disease'. There are two approaches to measuring health status: the first focuses on an individual's subjective perception of their health, and the second comprises symptom checklists (Bowling 2004). Health status measures can provide valid assessments of the health of individuals or populations and the positive and negative outcomes of health care interventions. Health status measurement may be presented as a single global index or a profile. These approaches to measurement are discussed later.

Health-related quality of life has multiple components and considers the impact of disease and its treatment on aspects of life such as functional ability, health status and life satisfaction. It should be noted that health-related quality of life is a narrower concept than quality of life *per se*. The concept of quality of life is more than those aspects of life affected by disease and its treatment, and includes life areas such as the environment, standard of living and financial status. While the WHO's definition of health (World Health Organization 1948) may be criticized for its idealistic stance, its commitment to a positive concept of health and related concepts such as quality of life must be acknowledged.

Quality of life is defined as an individual's perception of their position in life in the context of culture and value systems in which they live and in relation to their goals, expectations, standards and concerns. It is a broad ranging concept affected in a complex way by the person's physical health, psychological state, level of independence,

**BOX 26.1   REASONS PHARMACISTS NEED TO
UNDERSTAND THE CONCEPT AND MEASUREMENT
OF HEALTH-RELATED QUALITY OF LIFE**

- Pharmacists need to be able to critically analyse studies that incorporate health-related quality of life as an outcome measure. Such information may be used as evidence to support therapeutic decisions at a clinical, formulary or policy level. Patient-centred outcome assessments, such as health-related quality of life, are an important component of health care evaluation.
- Providers of health care (including pharmacists) are monitored for performance in terms of their contribution to both the clinical and health outcomes of patients. Patient-centred data, such as health-related quality of life, provide evidence of the consequences of health care services and interventions.
- Drug therapy is the most common form of treatment for chronic disease and illness. Pharmacists have a role in monitoring both the positive and negative effects of drug treatment on the health-related quality of life of patients in order to minimize distress and non-compliance. Information concerning the impact of drug treatment on health-related quality of life may be used to improve the health care practitioners' understanding of the outcomes of care for individual patients (e.g. patient monitoring and patient preferences and satisfaction).

Adapted from MacKeigan, L.D. and Pathak, D.S. 1992.
*American Journal of Hospital Pharmacy,* **49**, 2236–2245.

social relationships, and their relationships to salient features of their environment. (World Health Organization Quality of Life Group 1993)

## Health-Related Quality of Life

Health-related quality of life is an important endpoint for those diseases where treatment is likely to have a limited impact on survival. The importance of including measures of health-related quality of life is of particular significance where the benefits of treatment are weighed against potential impaired functioning due to disabling adverse effects. With the increased prevalence of chronic disease due to increased life expectancy in the developed world, the primary outcome measure must focus on the well-being of those being treated.

The importance of pharmacists' understanding of the concepts and measurement of health-related quality of life is shown in Box 26.1.

## THE SCIENCE OF HEALTH STATUS MEASUREMENT

With increasing emphasis placed on measuring the outcomes associated with health care interventions, it is essential that scientific methods be adopted to measure subjective indicators of health in a reproducible and valid way. Superior data are collected when using a standardized, well-tested instrument with robust psychometric properties (Bowling 2001).

## CHOICE OF AN INSTRUMENT: GENERIC, CONDITION SPECIFIC OR PATIENT SPECIFIC?

Standardized instruments have been developed for use as generic or condition-specific measures. Generic health measures focus on functional status and well-being. They assess health concepts that are relevant to basic human values. Generic measures have a limited number of core health concepts that are sensitive to the impact of a wide range of diseases (e.g. physical and social functioning, role performance and mental health). As such, they should be administered in studies where one wishes to draw conclusions about general health outcomes. The advantage of generic methods is that the breadth of areas of life (domains) covered by the instrument maximizes the opportunity for detecting unexpected or iatrogenic effects. However, the disadvantage is that by including such a wide range of domains, responsiveness to the measurement of outcomes of health care can diminish. Generic measures are more suited to measurements across populations for estimating the burden of disease and can provide useful information for comparing alternative treatments.

The choice of generic measure is extremely important when comparing the outcomes of different diseases or alternative treatment programmes in order to avoid confounding (see Chapter 20). Preferably, one must ensure that the items included in the measure do not favour the symptoms of a particular disease or the adverse effects of a particular treatment (Ware 1995).

Condition-specific measures are developed with a detailed knowledge of the disease, the treatments and interventions used in the management of that disease (e.g. cancers, respiratory conditions and cardiovascular diseases) (see Bowling 2001 for a comprehensive review of condition-specific measures). Therefore, condition-specific measures are more likely to detect subtle changes resulting from treatment within a particular patient group. Administering both generic and condition-specific instruments concomitantly can capture the burden of disease and treatment effects in specific terms, as well as according to general health outcome indicators.

Using standardized instruments has been criticized for reducing the individual to Mr and Mrs Average (Hunt 1997). Alternative patient-specific measures have been developed in response to the question of the relevance of standardized instruments when an external value system is imposed on respondents (e.g. the Schedule for the Evaluation of Individual Quality of Life [SEIQoL]) (O'Boyle 1994). This approach to outcome assessment permits the respondent to nominate the areas of life that determine their quality of life and the relative importance of each of these life areas.

Some authors have recommended the use of a patient-specific approach in clinical trials, since the measurement of items nominated by respondents has an increased sensitivity to change that allows a smaller sample size to be employed compared with standardized instruments (Chambers 1993; Tugwell et al. 1990). Similarly, a risk–benefit analysis of treatment, weighing the positive effects of the medication (in terms of treating the disease) against the toxicity of the treatment, is an individual judgement and levels of acceptable toxicity are likely to vary between individuals

(Fayers 1992). Individuals have different coping abilities and will make different adjustments to their lives in response to various health states (Hunt 1997).

By adopting a patient-specific approach, cross-sectional data will vary between individuals, but the responsiveness of individual measurement is likely to be greater when considering the effects of different interventions and detecting unexpected or iatrogenic effects. A disadvantage of the patient-specific approach is that items reported at a follow-up interview may not be related to those items reported at the baseline. On such occasions, respondents could also be asked to re-prioritize baseline items.

The argument against the use of individual measurements of quality of life and condition-specific measurements is that such measurements cannot inform resource allocation decisions because there is limited potential for comparison between individuals, groups or societies with different diseases (Cairns 1996).

## CHARACTERISTICS OF INSTRUMENTS

### Administration Method

The most common method of collecting subjective data is by questionnaire, either self-administered or administered by an interviewer. The measurement strategy depends on the purpose of the study, financial resources and the characteristics of the respondents.

Self-report instruments are the most popular methods since they access subjective assessments of health and its related domains, such as functional status and well-being. Self-report measures may be single-item measures, a battery or a scale. The usefulness of a single-item method is limited, since it is unlikely to provide comprehensive information about a given concept. Scales are the preferred method of measurement because they contain a large number of items, and the summed and weighted scores are more able to withstand statistical analysis.

Interviewer-administered instruments introduce the potential of rater bias into the assessment process. However, depending on the target population, interviewers may be essential in studies of patients with reading or cognitive difficulties that preclude the use of some self-administered instruments. Bowling (2001) advises the use of trained interviewers to reduce bias in health-related quality of life studies. Interviewers must be as objective as possible and it is preferred that they are not staff responsible for the health or social care of the respondents. This can help guard against respondents wishing to give desirable answers. Interviewer-administered instruments also have the potential advantages of boosting response numbers, giving participants the opportunity to clarify issues or ambiguous questions, helping motivate respondents to complete the interview and, if sufficient rapport is developed, can lead to increased reliability in the reporting.

The length of an instrument is another important factor in the choice of administration method. Shorter instruments are more akin to self-completion, although they are likely to be less sensitive. Longer instruments may be preferable. However, they are more expensive to administer (especially if interviewer administered) and more time consuming to analyse (see also Chapter 23). Given that respondents may perceive health-related quality of life as an abstract concept, another issue of importance is the perceived need by respondents to answer such questions. One study that has considered these issues concluded that patients enjoyed completing the question-naires and thought that the information was relevant for their doctor to know (Nelson and Berwick 1989).

## Scoring Method

Three alternative methods used for scoring measurement instruments are the health profile, health battery and the health index (Box 26.2).

Health profiles and health batteries provide comprehensive information pertain-ing to impairments in those dimensions of life measured (e.g. physical functioning, role performance and psychological well-being). However, limited information can be achieved with these methods in comparative studies unless measurement is higher in all dimensions for one comparator. Some health indexes provide dimensions scores, as well as an overall score, which are useful for their descriptive detail. Other health indexes simply provide the summary score, which cannot be disaggregated and is therefore less sensitive. Health indexes have the advantage of being easier to analyse and better for informing decisions, particularly for economic analyses.

Weighting reflects the preferences and priorities of certain items/domains within a given scale. Values (which may be represented by the number of items proportional to significance) are often assigned to constructs during the testing of the instrument. However, Joyce (1994) questioned the likelihood that the weightings developed dur-ing testing would be identical to those an individual may set with whom the scale may be used. Najman and Levine (1981) also drew attention to the arbitrary nature with which weightings and priorities are given to any life area. They believe that the values and perceptions of the respondents should be understood in order to be able

---

### BOX 26.2   THREE METHODS FOR SCORING MEASUREMENT INSTRUMENTS

- The health profile is derived from a single instrument that scores a number of individual dimensions separately (e.g. physical function-ing, psychological well-being and social functioning). This method does not attempt to aggregate the component scores into a single sum-mary score.
- The health battery comprises a series of questions, or independent instruments, which each measure a separate dimension of the same concept. Each dimension is scored separately.
- The health index is a single instrument whose dimension scores are aggregated to form one summary score. It is not usually recom-mended to simply sum the components; each dimension should be weighted before totalling.

Adapted from MacKeigan, L.D. and Pathak, D.S. 1992.
*American Journal of Hospital Pharmacy,* **49**, 2236–2245.

to interpret the ratings. Critics may want to consider the year and place of testing of the instrument, the sample characteristics used to derive the weightings and whether these reflect the sample and study conditions for which the instrument is to be employed. Joyce (1994) recommended that, ideally, in order to assess an individual's quality of life, weights should be allocated to each item (or at least the dimension) for each individual on each test occasion. Two examples of patient-specific measures where authors have adopted this method successfully are the McMaster Health Index Questionnaire (Chambers 1993) and the SEIQoL (O'Boyle 1994).

Other approaches do not examine the preferences of the respondents, but assume equal weighting among items. Häyry (1991) suggested that it is contrary to common sense to suppose that all items in a given scale have equal importance, and that it is equally unrealistic to assume that all individuals would have the same preferences and priorities. Methods where the values comprise a single score and then groups of patients are aggregated to form a single mean score have been criticized since they lose any aspect of an individual's preferences and values (Hunt 1997; Rosenberg 1995).

## PSYCHOMETRIC PROPERTIES OF STANDARDIZED INSTRUMENTS

The selection of an instrument to measure health or illness should be influenced by its psychometric properties. The Medical Outcomes Trust (1997) recommended eight attributes by which to evaluate an instrument (Box 26.3). The relative importance of each criterion depends on the instrument's intended use and application. For example, if the instrument is intended for discriminative or evaluative purposes between individuals or populations, or if the instrument is intended for research or clinical practice settings, the criteria should be assessed accordingly. The context of use is an essential factor that influences the properties of an instrument, and therefore, evidence should be presented for each of the instrument's intended applications. A clear description of the sample size, characteristics of the sample, testing

---

**BOX 26.3   CRITERIA BY WHICH TO EVALUATE A
MEASURE'S STRENGTHS AND WEAKNESSES**

- Conceptual and measurement model
- Reliability
- Validity
- Responsiveness
- Interpretation
- Alternative forms
- Burden
- Conceptual and linguistic equivalence

Adapted from Medical Outcomes Trust 1997. *A Resource Directory for the Health Outcomes Field.* Boston: Medical Outcomes Trust.

conditions and study design methods should be detailed for any work undertaken to test or adapt a new instrument. Bowling (2001) has also listed a review of the important criteria to consider when generally selecting and administering a scale.

## Conceptual and Measurement Models

A conceptual model is the justification for, and description of, the concept(s) that the instrument claims to measure and the relationship between those concepts. A measurement model represents the structure and scoring methods of the instrument's scale and sub-scales. The scale should also demonstrate adequate variability in domain scores relative to its intended use (i.e. the avoidance of 'floor' or 'ceiling' effects). The level of measurement (e.g. ordinal, interval or ratio scales) and the rationale for the chosen scoring methods (e.g. use of raw scores, standardization or weighting) should be stated.

## Reliability

The reliability of an instrument is a measure of the degree of freedom from random error and may be judged using a number of methods: test–retest reliability, inter-rater reliability or intra-rater reliability. Reliability can be expressed as 'a ratio of the variability between individuals to the total variability in the scores' and is represented by a number between zero (indicative of no reliability) and one (perfect reliability) (Streiner and Norman 1989).

For instruments used on two or more occasions with the same group of participants, a test–retest reliability (also known as reproducibility or external reliability) attribute may be tested (i.e. on repeated administrations of the same instrument, this assesses the extent to which similar results are obtained when conditions have remained stable). However, the influence of the first administration may affect the responses collected on the second administration, causing reliability to be overestimated. This is known as a repeat effect. Conversely, reliability may be underestimated due to the detection of true variations. Careful consideration should be given to the time permitted between measurements and the nature of the underlying concept (i.e. whether the concept is likely to change in given circumstances).

If more than one interviewer is involved in administering an interview and coding the data, inter-rater reliability may be measured (i.e. the degree of agreement between two interviewers). The reliability of measurements made by the same interviewer on two separate occasions may also be determined: the intra-rater reliability.

The internal consistency of an instrument considers the relationship between multiple items of a scale. It is an estimate of the reliability based on all possible correlations between two sets of items within the test on a single administration of the instrument. It assesses whether the group of items is consistently measuring different aspects of the same underlying construct. One of the most frequently used statistics for estimating internal consistency is Cronbach's alpha (Cronbach 1951).

An explicit decision must be made concerning the acceptable level of variation in measurement. Acceptable levels of the reliability coefficients differ according to whether comparisons are being made between groups (0.70) or between individuals where the standard is much higher (0.90 or above) (Nunnally 1978). Cronbach (1951) reported that a value greater than 0.50 was an acceptable level of good internal consistency, as well as test–retest reliability. Other authors are more conservative and expect values of greater than 0.8 for internal consistency and greater than 0.5 for external reliability (Bryman and Cramer 1997; Streiner and Norman 1989).

## Validity

While reliability data indicate the random error associated with the measurement of an attribute, it does not mean that the correct attribute is being measured. The validity of an instrument is concerned with the extent to which a measure assesses the underlying attribute. Evidence of validity may be gained through observation, expert and lay judgement and empirical enquiry.

Face validity is a measure of whether the items included in the scale make sense, are unambiguous and could reasonably measure the underlying concept. Face validity is an estimate of the meaning and relevance of the items (Bowling 2004).

Content validity is a judgement of the standard of clarity, comprehensiveness and redundancy of items and scales of an instrument, relative to its intended use and name. A definition or conceptual framework is required as a standard against which content validity may be evaluated. All items should be relevant to the content areas (domains) of the instrument. Items should be reviewed for their relevance to the instrument's objectives, and similarly, the instrument's objectives should be reviewed for comprehensiveness. The number of items per domain should reflect the relative importance of that domain to the instrument construct. Lay groups have been suggested as the best source for determining the content validity of measures of subjective health status (Hunt et al. 1986). It is important that due consideration is given to the items and domains of instruments in light of the specific condition under study. This is of particular significance when the data from the questionnaire are reduced to a single index and so mask the items and domains tested by the instrument.

Construct validity is concerned with hypothetical instrument attributes that cannot be directly measured. Testing of the instrument involves developing theories about the relationship between the instrument attribute and other measures. Testing is undertaken to confirm or dispel these theories. Problems arise when the hypothesis is disproved since it is not clear whether the hypothesized theory was wrong or whether there was a problem with the instrument. Construct validity may be subdivided into convergent and discriminant validity. Assessment of the relationships between the new instrument and other variables, as well as other constructs to which it should be related, are tested. Correlations provide evidence of the extent of these relationships. If the correlation coefficient is too high, the new instrument may be measuring the same concept. Convergent validity requires the new instrument to correlate moderately with measures of the same construct (0.4–0.8) (Streiner and Norman 1989). Discriminant validity requires the instrument to have no associations with dissimilar variables. It has been suggested that a low or zero correlation is more informative, since it clearly shows that instruments are measuring different concepts.

Criterion validity refers to the ability of an instrument to correlate with other widely accepted and validated measures of the construct under test. It is difficult to perform tests of criterion validity with health outcome measures due to the lack of widely accepted measures of health and related concepts, such as quality of life. Criterion validity may be subdivided into concurrent and predictive validity.

Concurrent validity involves administering the new instrument and the criterion instrument simultaneously to establish whether the new measure may be a suitable substitute for the criterion measure. Predictive validity considers the ability of the new instrument to predict future differences. For this test, the criterion is available at a future endpoint.

## Responsiveness

Responsiveness (i.e. the extent to which scores change when the concept under study improves or deteriorates) is a particularly important criterion for studies that occur over a period of time. Sufficient sample sizes and variability of scores are required to detect a real change. When evaluating the impact of a health care intervention, it is vital that instruments can detect change, both clinically and that which is important to patients.

## Interpretation

The degree to which qualitative meaning may be assigned to the quantitative scores of an instrument is an important aspect of interpreting the scores of that instrument. For example, if the instrument is scored so that it provides a summary score, it is important that this number has meaning.

## Burden

During the administration of an instrument, demands may be placed on those participating in the study and those conducting the study. Consideration must be given to the abilities of the participants and the feasibility of the study. Missing data (questions not answered by participants) and refusal rates should be made explicit as measures of acceptability of the instrument to the target population.

## Alternative Forms of Instrument

The above properties should be reported during the development of any instrument in combination with the form of the instrument (e.g. telephone-administered, interviewer-administered, self-administered, observer-rated, proxy reports, etc.). All instrument criteria and information relating to its use must be demonstrated with the alternative forms of the instrument. It is unacceptable practice to use an interviewer-administered instrument for a postal survey by assuming that the psychometric properties of the instrument will be stable.

## Cultural and Language Adaptations

Of concern to many health providers and researchers is the need to include the views of participants that are representative of local populations. However, this can cause problems when using standardized instruments for measuring health and illness with respondents who have a variety of cultural backgrounds and speak different languages. The reliability and validity properties of instruments developed in a particular language or culture must be reassessed if translated into a different language or adapted for use in a new culture.

The main concerns are of conceptual equivalence (i.e. what are the relevance and meaning of concepts across different languages and cultures?) and linguistic equivalence (i.e. are the wording and meaning of questions in all aspects of the instrument shared across different languages?). Conceptual and linguistic equivalence equally apply to the use of American measures in the UK and other European settings, and vice versa.

## CONCLUSION

From the range of approaches to measuring health, it is evident that there is not a single best method. The choice of approach is determined by the conceptual model and the purpose for which health is being measured. Multiple approaches offer the most comprehensive method for measuring health. All health care professionals should be interested in determining the impact of disease and treatment from the patient's perspective and using this information alongside clinical variables to optimize the health care of their patients.

It is essential that considerable thought is given to the choice of instrument for measuring health and illness. Uncritical use of instruments can influence decision making in an inappropriate manner. The relative strengths and weaknesses of instruments influence their appropriateness for measuring change in certain illnesses, and consequently data can give inaccurate pictures of the impact of interventions.

## FURTHER READING

MacKeigan, L.D. and Pathak, D.S. 1992. Overview of health-related quality of life measures. *American Journal of Hospital Pharmacy*, **49**, 2236–2245.

## REFERENCES

Bowling, A. 2001. *Measuring Disease: A Review of Disease-Specific Quality of Life Measurement Scales* (2nd Edn.). Milton Keynes: Open University Press.

Bowling, A. 2004. *Measuring Health: A Review of Quality of Life Measurement Scales* (3rd Edn.). Milton Keynes: Open University Press.

Bryman, A. and Cramer, D. 1997. *Quantitative Data Analysis with SPSS for Windows. A Guide for Social Scientists*. London and New York: Routledge.

Cairns, J. 1996. Measuring health outcomes. Condition specific and patient specific measures are of limited use when allocating resources. *British Medical Journal*, **313**, 6.

Chambers, L.W. 1993. The McMaster health index questionnaire: An update. In: S.R. Walker and R. Rosser (Eds.), *Quality of Life Assessment: Key Issues in the 1990s*. London, Kluwer Academic, 131–149.

Coggon, D., Rose, G. and Barker, D.J.P. 2003. *Epidemiology for the Uninitiated* (5th Edn.). London: British Medical Journal Publishing Group.

Cronbach, L.J. 1951. Coefficient alpha and the internal structure of tests. *Psychometrika*, **22**, 293–296.

Fayers, P. 1992. Untitled contribution to the discussion on Cox D. et al. Quality-of-life assessment: Can we keep it simple? *Journal of the Royal Statistical Society*, **155**, 382.

Häyry, M. 1991. Measuring the quality of life: Why, how and what? *Theoretical Medicine*, **12**, 97–116.

Huber, M., Knottnerus, J.A., Green, L. et al. 2011. How should we define health? *British Medical Journal*, **343**, d4163.

Hunt, S.M. 1997. The problem of quality of life. *Quality of Life Research*, **6**, 205–212.

Hunt, S., McEwan, P. and McKenna, S. 1986. *Measuring Health Status*. London: Croom Helm.

Hunt, S.M. and McKenna, S.P. 1993. Measuring quality of life in psychiatry. In: S.R. Walker and R.M. Rosser (Eds.), *Quality of Life Assessment. Key Issues in the 1990s*. London: Kluwer Academic, pp. 343–354.

Joyce, C.R.B. 1994. Requirements for the assessment of individual quality of life. In: H.M. McGee and C. Bradley (Eds.), *Quality of Life Following Renal Failure. Psychosocial Challenges Accompanying High Technology Medicine*, Switzerland: Harwood Academic, 43–54.

Katz, S., Downs, T.D., Cash, H.R. and Grotz, R.C. 1970. Progress in development of the index of ADL. *Gerontologist*, **10**, 20–30.

Katz, S., Ford, A.B., Moskowitz, R.W., Jackson, B.A. and Jaffe, M.W. 1963. Studies of illness in the aged. The index of ADL: A standardized measure of biological and psychosocial function. *Journal of the American Medical Association*, **185**, 914–919.

McManus, S., Meltzer, H., Brugha, T., Bebbington, P., Jenkins, R. (Eds.) 2009. *Adult Psychiatric Morbidity Survey 2007*. Colchester: Health and Social Care Information Centre.

Medical Outcomes Trust 1997. *A Resource Directory for the Health Outcomes Field*. Boston: Medical Outcomes Trust.

Najman, J.M. and Levine, S. 1981. Evaluating the impact of medical care and technologies on the quality of life: A review and critique. *Social Science and Medicine*, **15F**, 107–115.

Nelson, E.C. and Berwick, D.M. 1989. The measurement of health status in clinical practice. *Medical Care*, **27**(Suppl. 3), S77–S90.

Nunnally, J.C. 1978. *Psychometric Theory* (2nd Edn.). New York: McGraw-Hill.

O'Boyle, C.A. 1994. The schedule for the evaluation of individual quality of life (SEIQoL). *International Journal of Mental Health*, **23**, 3–23.

Patrick, D.L. and Erickson, P. 1993. *Health Status and Health Policy. Quality of Life in Health Care Evaluation and Resource Allocation*, New York: Oxford University Press.

Rosenberg, R. 1995. Health-related quality of life between naturalism and hermeneutics. *Social Science and Medicine*, **41**, 1411–1415.

Scully, J.L. 2004. What is a disease? *EMBO Reports*, **5**(7), 650–653.

Streiner, D.L. and Norman, G.R. 1989. *Health Measurement Scales. A Practical Guide to Their Development and Use*. Oxford: Oxford University Press.

Tugwell, P., Bombardier, C., Buchanan, W. et al. 1990. Methotrexate in rheumatoid arthritis: Impact on quality of life assessed by traditional standard item and individualised patient preference health status questionnaires. *Archives of Internal Medicine*, **150**, 59–62.

Ware, J.E. 1995. The status of health assessment 1994. *Annual Review of Public Health*, **16**, 327–354.

World Health Organization 1948. *Official Records of the World Health Organization, No. 2*. Geneva: World Health Organization, 100.

World Health Organization 2010. *Key Components of a Well Functioning Health System*. Geneva: World Health Organization.

World Health Organization 2014. Global Burden of Disease. Available at: http://www.who.int/healthinfo/global_burden_disease/gbd/en/.

World Health Organization Quality of Life Group 1993. *Measuring Quality of Life: The Development of the World Health Organization Quality of Life Instrument (WHOQOL)*. Geneva: World Health Organization.

Youngson, R.M. 1992. *Collins Dictionary of Medicine*. Glasgow: HarperCollins.

# 27 Evaluating Pharmacy Services

*Felicity Smith*

## CONTENTS

---

### KEY POINTS

- Resources for health care are constrained; to justify funding, evidence is required to demonstrate the value of services and potential developments in service provision.
- Evaluation is the systematic and scientific process of determining the extent to which an action or a set of actions was successful in the achievement of predetermined objectives.

- Evaluation provides the pharmacy profession, governments and funding bodies with a picture of the value, strengths and weaknesses of existing services and potential service developments.
- Evaluation can be considered in terms of efficacy, effectiveness and efficiency, which relate to the extent to which the objectives of a pharmacy intervention are met.
- Appropriate study design, relevant and reliable outcome measures, systematic data collection and correct analytical procedures are essential for a robust evaluation of any health care technology or intervention.
- Evaluations require scientific rigour combined with an element of pragmatism to ensure that findings are relevant to real-life and diverse pharmacy settings.

## INTRODUCTION

In response to the changing health needs of populations and the priorities of governments, the health care professions are continually reappraising the services they offer. Pharmacy services are no exception. In many parts of the world, pharmacy services are viewed by professional bodies and governments as an underutilized resource (see Chapter 2). Their presence in local communities and accessibility to the public are commonly highlighted unique strengths. Pharmacists are seen as having the potential to contribute more effectively to public health goals and supporting the optimal use of medicines by patients. However, the evidence base for these services remains limited. Resources for health care are similarly constrained, so to justify funding, there needs to be evidence of the value of services and potential developments in provision. Robust evaluation is central to this evidence base. For successful service development, it is essential that initiatives are demonstrated to be:

- Effective in achieving their objectives, especially health outcomes
- Deliverable in a wide range of pharmacy settings
- Appropriate to the needs and expectations of clients
- Cost effective

Evaluation provides the pharmacy profession, governments and funding bodies with an invaluable picture of the value, strengths and weaknesses of existing services and potential developments. This information is vital to decisions regarding the commissioning of services.

The methodological principles of service evaluation are transferable across the different branches of the health services. However, the application of different designs and methods in various settings will present a unique set of considerations and challenges. In addition, because of the diversity within pharmacies, procedures which are feasible and acceptable in one setting may be unworkable in another.

# WHAT IS EVALUATION?

The World Health Organization has defined evaluation as 'the systematic and scientific process of determining the extent to which an action or a set of actions was successful in the achievement of predetermined objectives' (Shaw 1980). Within this definition, a number of components can be distinguished that must be addressed when evaluating health (including pharmacy) services. In particular, a scientific approach requires the use of an appropriate study design, relevant and reliable outcome measures, systematic data collection and the correct analytical procedures.

Researchers generally make a distinction between evaluation and audit. Audit consists of reviewing and monitoring current practice against agreed standards. As a cyclical process, it includes evaluative procedures. It is often undertaken as an integral part of the normal provision and delivery of health services as a means of maintaining and improving standards of care.

## EFFICACY, EFFECTIVENESS AND EFFICIENCY

Evaluation may be considered in terms of efficacy, effectiveness and efficiency, which all relate to the extent that the objectives of a pharmacy intervention are met:

- Efficacy – can it work?
- Effectiveness – does it work?
- Efficiency – is it cost effective?

### Efficacy

Innovations in pharmacy frequently begin with individual practitioners who perceive a need in the population they serve. They may develop a service in response to this need and then evaluate it in terms of the extent to which specific objectives are achieved. Many potential service developments, prior to widespread implementation, are evaluated as pilot projects and may involve small numbers of pharmacies and pharmacists who are keen to participate.

It may be expected that, in these special conditions (of self-selected settings and personnel), an innovative service may be more likely to succeed than in a wide range of more representative environments. Thus, the study may be seen as an 'efficacy study', with the question being, 'Can this work?' If the service is unsuccessful in 'ideal' conditions, then it is unlikely to work in a more diverse range of settings.

To examine operational aspects and the workability of an intervention in practice, a 'feasibility study' is often conducted. This will provide an assessment of specific features or circumstances that would be deemed essential for success, prior to recommendations for more extensive implementation or evaluation.

### Effectiveness

Having demonstrated that an intervention can work, in terms of achieving specific objectives in selected settings, the next question may be 'does it work?' when implemented more extensively. That an innovation *can* work in a particular setting does not necessarily mean that it *will* work when delivered more widely. The effectiveness of any new intervention should be assessed in a range of environments and conditions that reflect the diversity of the settings in which it will ultimately be delivered. Thus, when assessing the effectiveness of a service, researchers may need to gather data on a wider range of variables that allows the researcher to take into account the different types of setting, conditions, workforce and individual characteristics of practitioners and patients/public.

## Efficiency

Demonstrating that an intervention achieves worthy objectives may not be sufficient. Researchers may also wish to demonstrate that the programme is a cost-effective method of achieving these objectives, and is thus an appropriate use of limited health care resources. Therefore, many researchers will include some assessments of costs and cost implications as part of a service evaluation.

Assessing the costs of a health care programme requires decisions by the researcher regarding which costs to include (e.g. direct and indirect, average or marginal) and who incurs these costs. Cost savings that accrue to a health authority may be offset by consequential costs to service users or their relatives and friends. Many new programmes will confer advantages and disadvantages that cannot readily be converted into monetary costs. Thus, the comparison of different programmes in terms of costs may be difficult.

A number of methodologies have been developed and employed by health economists, including cost–minimization analysis, cost–effectiveness analysis, cost–benefit analysis and cost–utility analysis (see Chapter 21). These techniques are commonly incorporated in evaluations of health interventions, including pharmacy services.

## EVALUATION: STUDY DESIGN AND METHODOLOGY

Appropriate study design, relevant and reliable outcome measures, systematic data collection and the correct analytical procedures are all vital in a robust evaluation of any health care technology or intervention. To ensure a robust approach, researchers commonly refer to CONSORT guidelines. CONSORT stands for Consolidated Standards of Reporting Trials, and the CONSORT group has produced statements and guidelines in response to inadequate reporting in randomized clinical trials (CONSORT 2010). CONSORT guidelines provide a framework for researchers to ensure a scientific approach to design and methodology.

### STUDY DESIGN

#### Randomized Controlled Trials

In the evaluation of health care interventions and technologies, randomized controlled trials (RCTs) are seen as the 'gold standard'. Employing an experimental design (with adherence to the principles of a RCT) enables an evaluation in which the impact can be confidently attributed to the intervention, rather than known or unknown extraneous factors. Key features in the design of a RCT are shown in Box 27.1.

## BOX 27.1   KEY FEATURES IN THE DESIGN OF A RANDOMIZED CONTROLLED TRIAL

- Intervention and control arms, so differences in treatment outcomes can be assessed
- Randomization of participants to avoid any systematic differences between individuals in the two arms
- Blinding of the research team to the allocation of participants to control or intervention arms to avoid any possible bias in data collection or analysis
- Blinding of participants and health professionals, if possible, to avoid a placebo or nocebo effect
- Control of experimental conditions and assurance of fidelity to protocol regarding delivery of the intervention
- Identification of relevant and robust outcome measures
- A systematic approach to the collection of all data

While seen as a gold standard, RCT design is not always possible or practicable, and RCTs have a number of inherent limitations. RCTs may be confined to a limited range of settings, according to pre-specified eligibility criteria. Evaluation of an intervention across widely dispersed locations is expensive. A smaller number of sites assists the researcher in controlling experimental conditions and ensuring the reliability of the results. However, a more localized study may compromise the generalizability of the findings to wider or more representative settings.

Blinding is not always possible. In a clinical trial of medicines, control-arm participants can take a placebo, so that they are blinded as to whether they are in the intervention or control arm, but if the intervention is, for example, an educational intervention, participants will necessarily be aware of which arm they are in.

## Other Study Designs

A 'quasi-experimental design' is sometimes employed when randomization is not possible for practical or ethical reasons. For example, in comparing the impact of an intervention in two different types of setting, the features of the settings (e.g. with and without counselling areas) may be fixed. A control group is still employed, and this should be selected so that the intervention and control arms are equivalent in all respects other than the intervention under evaluation. This is generally achieved by 'matching'. For each individual in the intervention arm, an individual similar in all important respects is selected for the control arm. If systematic differences between the two groups are present, it may be these confounding factors to which differences in study outcomes could be attributed. Every attempt should be made to identify potential confounding factors and to ensure that the control group is similar (matched) in these respects to the intervention group.

'Before-and-after' studies are sometimes employed in the evaluation of pharmacy services. These are more powerful if a control group is also included; they may then also be described as a RCT or a quasi-experimental study, depending on whether allocation to study and control groups is by randomization or a matching procedure.

## Process Evaluation

Many service evaluations will include an integral process evaluation. This assesses the implementation and operation of the intervention, its workability in settings and secondary or perceived impacts. Data are often collected by a variety of methods. The process evaluation enables an assessment of the feasibility of an intervention in practice; it examines the types of settings, situations or circumstances in which an intervention is more or less likely to be effective. If the intervention is not demonstrated to have a significant impact, the process evaluation may be helpful in establishing why it was not successful (e.g. if it is due to difficulties in implementation, rather than its inherent inefficacy).

## SAMPLING STRATEGY

The sampling strategy, sampling procedures and sample size will all depend on the objectives, design and operation of the study. Researchers aim for representative samples, so they can make inferences regarding the wider relevance of the research findings. Random procedures, in both the selection of participants and in allocation to intervention and control arms, are required for the application of probability statistics.

Sampling strategy is part of study design. Probability samples (random selection procedures) are preferable. There are a number of approaches to this. A simple random sample is the most straightforward. The sample is drawn from the entire population of interest, with each individual having an equal chance of being selected. However, this is often not practicable, and an alternative study design may have to be adopted. For example, many studies will be undertaken in limited geographical areas or selected locations, but random procedures may be applied to the selection of these locations or sites within them. A further stage may involve individual participants being (randomly) selected from each of the selected sites. Samples which are drawn from (clustered within) particular locations are termed cluster samples. Clustering is often necessary for practical reasons. For example, if recruiting clients from pharmacies or clinics, there will necessarily be a limited number of sites involved. But, even if random selection procedures are employed, because of clustering, less diversity on some important features is expected. This is referred to as intra-cluster correlation.

The sample size will depend on the degree of variability in the population and the precision required in the results. If clustering is adopted as a sampling strategy, this has to be taken into account, and larger numbers of participants are generally required. This is because clustering will reduce the overall variability in the sample.

Many intervention studies are undertaken in one or a few self-selecting locations. For instance, the evaluation of a new service in a community pharmacy environment may, in the first instance, include only one or a small number of pharmacies. While providing a useful indication of the feasibility or problems of a service, caution must be exercised in generalizing the findings to other settings.

In studies in which the researcher wishes to compare structures, processes or outcomes among population subgroups, the sample must include sufficient numbers from each of these subgroups.

## RECRUITMENT PROCEDURES

Recruitment of participants is commonly one of the most challenging stages of any study. The time and resources required are often underestimated. Recruitment procedures need to be designed so that no bias is introduced. This can often require the presence of a member of the research team at each site for extended periods. In some studies, researchers have depended on pharmacy or other health care staff to identify and recruit participants. The immediate advantage is that a researcher does not have to be present in every site during the recruitment stages of a study. However, in charging others with this responsibility, the researcher may no longer be assured of the extent to which protocols are adhered to, the reliability with which eligible participants are approached or the comprehensiveness of records of non-responders. Thus, the representativeness of the sample can be in doubt. In addition, recruitment by health care or pharmacy staff, who are often very busy, may not be workable. They may feel unable to put the time aside to discuss participation at busy times; they may feel uncomfortable approaching clients or may not remember to do so. If random or otherwise representative samples are required, researchers must be assured of the reliability of the recruitment procedures.

### Response Rates

High response rates greatly improve the value of any study, and every effort should be made to achieve the highest rate possible (see also Chapter 22). Unless a sufficiently high rate is achieved, the sample has to be viewed as self-selecting. Increasing the sample size does not compensate for bias introduced by a low response rate. A study protocol should include processes for maximizing response rates, as well as for collecting data on the number and, if possible, some characteristics of non-responders. In the analysis, if differences between responders and non-responders (or between responders and the wider population) can be identified, potential implications for the study findings can be assessed.

## OUTCOME MEASURES

### Primary and Secondary Outcome Measures

Assessments of efficacy and effectiveness aim to measure the extent to which specific objectives of a programme are met. In evaluating services, decisions must be made regarding the primary and secondary outcome measures. The features on which an existing or new service is to be evaluated will depend on the objectives of the service and the objectives of the evaluation. In an intervention study, the appropriate outcome measures will depend on the anticipated impact of the intervention. Endpoints may relate to specific biochemical or clinical measures, improved health status or broader aims regarding the delivery or quality of services. For an intervention study, one quantifiable measure will usually be designated as the primary outcome, as this will provide the basis for the sample size calculation.

Data will commonly be collected for secondary outcome measures as well. These may be alternative clinical measures, health status, psychometric measures such as quality of life or health beliefs, behavioural outcomes (e.g. adherence) or measures of satisfaction or perceived impact. The selection of these measures will depend on the wider anticipated impacts of the intervention. They can sometimes help provide context and explanation relevant to the primary outcome. If a significant impact on the primary outcome is not found, potential impacts on secondary outcomes are of particular interest.

Secondary outcomes may be included to assess factors that are important to different stakeholders. For instance, from the perspective of health policy makers, aside from technical standards of care, the costs of a programme may be of paramount importance. However, service users may be more concerned about the accessibility of a programme, the approachability of practitioners or the speed with which a service is delivered.

## Process Measures

The process evaluation will assess factors such as:

- Success of, and any difficulties in, the implementation and operation of the intervention
- Fidelity in delivery of the intervention (e.g. the extent to which the intervention was delivered as intended)
- Feasibility and acceptability:
  - Workability of the intervention from the perspectives of staff delivering the intervention and others who may be affected (e.g. by non-availability of colleagues)
  - From the perspective of participants (e.g. uptake, attrition [with possible reasons], timing, convenience and perceived value)

The process evaluation will provide insights into the extent to which and circumstances in which an intervention is deliverable in these settings. Failure of an intervention study to show an impact may be due to a lack of efficacy of the intervention, but difficulties in implementing the intervention can also be important contributory factors. Thus, in addition to assessing the extent to which specific objectives are met, the process evaluation may examine the extent to which an intervention is practicable in a pharmacy environment, acceptable to other health professionals and the public and appropriate to the needs and expectations of the consumers. The potential impacts of any intervention can be many, and unexpected.

From the perspective of community pharmacists, the acceptability of a service may depend on its practicability in a particular pharmacy. For example, a programme that requires the time of pharmacy staff may be difficult to accommodate at busy times, while some pharmacies may not have the space required to offer an extended service. Practitioners may be reluctant to promote a new service that they feel is inappropriate in a pharmacy environment, or when they do not believe that they possess the necessary skills. Factors such as these should be explored when evaluating the acceptability or feasibility of a service.

Consumers will also have views on the value of any intervention, its relevance and effectiveness in addressing their needs, the convenience of the timing, the suitability of the setting and in what ways it was or was not worthwhile.

## DATA COLLECTION

Data on the outcome measures must be accurate and the sources of information reliable. In some instances, these data may be available in routine information, but if not, or if this is not considered a dependable source, the data need to be collected by researchers specifically for the study. Data will, of course, have to be gathered in a similar way for the intervention and control groups. Common sources are patients' medical records, clinic notes or research interviews when these data are measured and obtained. Some measures are collected by questionnaire (e.g. health status measures and other psychometric measures). This could be by postal questionnaire or as part of a telephone or face-to-face research interview.

The reliability and validity of data are important considerations in all studies. The reliability of the data refers to the extent to which they are reproducible. For example, had the data been gathered by another researcher on a different occasion, would they be similar? During busy periods, could some information be missed? If data are being recorded retrospectively, might some cases be forgotten?

The validity of data refers to the extent to which they are a true reflection of events, activities or the views of individuals. For example, clients questioned about their views on a pharmacy service may be reluctant to express negative feelings. This may be particularly so if interviews are conducted in the pharmacy and the interviewee believes that pharmacy staff may overhear, or be privy to, the information they give. Interviews with clients should be conducted by independent researchers, preferably on neutral territory and with assurances of confidentiality. Questions should be carefully worded to be non-leading and provide equal opportunity for the expression of negative and positive viewpoints.

The presence of a researcher in a pharmacy and the knowledge that the study is taking place may influence the behaviours of those being observed. This is referred to as the Hawthorne effect, after the Hawthorne experiments which investigated the relationship between factory working conditions and productivity. In these studies, groups of workers were aware that they were being observed and modified their behaviour to the extent that changes as a result of the working environment were masked. In planning an observation study, researchers should endeavour to keep any effects of their presence to a minimum (e.g. causing minimal hindrance to normal pharmacy activities).

Reliance on pharmacy personnel, rather than on an independent researcher, to collect data can present difficulties in terms of both the reliability and validity of the data acquired. It has the advantage of enabling the involvement of a larger number of sites with limited resources, but, in depending on pharmacy staff to collect data, the researcher sacrifices control over the data-collection process. To promote fidelity to protocol and procedures, these should be as straightforward and undemanding as possible. Methods for the collection of data should be tested in preliminary fieldwork or a pilot study in order to check that they are acceptable to staff and workable in different types of pharmacy at busy and quieter times.

The researchers should also take steps to establish the extent to which the data obtained are an accurate reflection of events and experiences. Comparing data collected by a number of different methods (triangulation) is sometimes employed as a means of validation, especially if the evaluation includes data collected by a range of methods. For example, in a small number of sites, pharmacists' self-reports may be compared with data collected by an observer.

Validity and reliability are also important issues in the choice and development of instruments for an evaluation. The instruments are the questionnaires, interview schedules, data-collection forms for observation studies, report forms for data on non-responders, etc. Researchers must ensure that their instruments collect data on the relevant aspects of services (e.g. structures, processes and outcomes and pharmacist and client perspectives) according to the objectives of the intervention and the evaluation. They must be workable and reliable across different settings, environments and conditions and when used by different personnel.

## DATA ANALYSIS

Evaluation in terms of the primary outcome measure will follow a pre-determined analytical plan. This will ensure that a planned and robust assessment is made of the impact of the intervention. The usual practice is to conduct an 'intention-to-treat' analysis. This includes all participants recruited to the study, irrespective of whether or not they ultimately received the intervention as intended. This takes into account factors including implementation, delivery and uptake when assessing the impact of an intervention. These aspects which may be indicators of feasibility and acceptability to stakeholders will be important to an intervention's overall success. Sometimes, additional exploratory analyses are also planned (e.g. subgroup analyses). However, while these may provide some insights into the possible impacts of the intervention, caution should be exercised in their interpretation, as the study may not be adequately powered or designed for their robust evaluation.

Impacts on secondary outcome measures will also be assessed, in accordance with the analytical plan. These will provide additional information on the impacts of the intervention, independently of the primary outcome.

Data collected for the process evaluation may be collected by a variety of different methods – quantitative and qualitative – from a range of sources and in a variety of forms. Appropriate analytical procedures have to be followed for each data set (see Chapters 22 and 25).

## PROJECT MANAGEMENT

It is usual to have regular meetings with all members of a project team throughout the duration of the project. In addition, an advisory group is often convened with representatives of all stakeholders to meet periodically and advise on documentation and procedures and ensure that all perspectives are considered. This group can also be helpful in planning the dissemination of the findings.

## CONCLUSION

Given the current emphasis on service development and innovation in pharmacy services, evaluation of potential interventions is an important activity. This will provide an evidence base to inform future service development. Evaluations require scientific rigour combined with an element of pragmatism to ensure that findings are relevant to real life and diverse pharmacy settings.

## FURTHER READING

Bowling, A. 2014. *Research Methods in Health: Investigating Health and Health Services* (4th Edn.). Maidenhead: Open University Press.
Smith, F.J. 2010. *Conducting your Pharmacy Practice Research Project* (2nd Edn.). London: Pharmaceutical Press.

## REFERENCES

CONSORT 2010. Guidelines for Reporting of Randomised Controlled Trials. Available at: http://www.consort-statement.org.
Shaw, C. 1980. Aspects of Audit (1): The background. *Brit. Med. J.* 280: 1256–8.

# 28 Principles of Statistical Data Analysis

*Nick Barber*

## CONTENTS

---

### KEY POINTS

- Statistical tests are the part of the experimental process which aim to establish the truth of reality.
- Measurement can be divided into three levels: nominal, ordinal and interval rates/ratios.
- Statistical tests are used to determine whether a hypothesis is either true or false.
- Statistical tests may be used to determine the significance of any difference between two or more groups.
- Statistical testing leads to a probability value which is poorly understood and often misinterpreted.

---

## INTRODUCTION

Imagine a lecture theatre of 100 students. I give half of them tea to drink and the other half coffee; the 50 who receive coffee all die. Which statistical test should I use to determine whether the coffee was poisoned? The answer is 'none', as the answer is obvious. But what if I decided to try to improve my teaching, as 10% of students fall asleep in my statistics lectures? I revise my notes, slides, jokes, etc. and find that 6% fall asleep during my next lecture. Is my new lecture better? I don't think the answer to this question is obvious – the variation (a reduction from 10% to 6%) may be due to chance or it may be caused by the new teaching methods. We are uncertain – I say it's my brilliant new lecture, you say it's chance – how can we decide? It is here that statistical tests come to the rescue.

Statistical tests quantify uncertainty. They do not, contrary to popular belief, reveal what is true. Statistical tests are part of the experimental process; what is tested is an idea – a hypothesis – about reality. Statistics is part of the scientific process which tries to establish the truth about reality.

This chapter focuses on the choice and interpretation of statistical tests, rather than the details of how to execute them. The reason for this is that computers generally perform tests nowadays; the art is in the choice and interpretation of the findings.

Over the last half-century, around half of the papers in leading medical journals used the wrong statistical test. Most of these would have used the correct test if they had followed the simple principles outlined in this chapter. Most students who are taught statistics focus on calculations at the cost of the principles, but this is the wrong way round. There are many computer programmes that can do the calculation. The key to choosing a test is to understand the principles. We start by learning an enormously powerful principle that unlocks the choice of statistical tests – three simple levels of measurement.

## LEVELS OF MEASUREMENT

We are so used to measuring things that we forget that there are different 'strengths' of measurement. An understanding of these is the key to understanding the choice of statistical tests. Measurement can be divided into three levels: nominal (based on name), ordinal (based on order) and interval/ratio (based on a known interval between measurements). Interval/ratio is really two separate levels, but they can be treated in the same way for most statistical purposes.

### NOMINAL

Nominal measurement is the simplest, and is so much a part of life that we may not recognize it. It involves putting experimental findings into named categories (it is also called a 'categorical' level of measurement by some authors) – common examples are alive/dead, correct/incorrect, male/female, pass/fail and tablet/capsule/ injection. Each new measurement is allocated to its appropriate category; at the end of the study, the number in each category is counted. The data are therefore usually a form of frequency data. The categories must be mutually exclusive, and at this level of measurement it is assumed that all members of the same category are equal (e.g. no one patient is more dead than another). For each new reading, the decision to be made is whether it is equal or not equal to the other members in each category – if it is equal, count it as another member of that category (e.g. another male subject). No one category is higher or better than another.

## ORDINAL

Ordinal measurement is at a higher level as it allows categories to be put in some order. Examples are socio-economic group; pain scores on a scale of 1–5; palatability of formulations on a scale of +, ++ and +++ ; or measuring sedation as the distance from the right of a 100-mm visual analogue scale marked 'wide awake' at one end and 'nearly asleep' at the other. Not only can this information be categorized, as with the previous level of measurement, but the categories can now be related by putting them in order. This level of measurement is sometimes called a ranking scale. Although we can put the categories in order, we cannot precisely define the distance between them. For example, we cannot say that an increase in a pain score from 1 to 2 is the same 'aliquot of pain' as would raise the score from 4 to 5; nor can we say that someone with a score of 4 is in twice as much pain as someone with a score of 2. Any subjective measurement scale, where people rate themselves or others, must produce ordinal data. Expressed mathematically, in this scale the decisions made about a reading are whether it is equal, not equal, greater than or less than others.

## INTERVAL AND RATIO

Interval/ratio data are those upon which scientists are raised. The data are continuous (not in categories) and the intervals between reading are the same. Examples include height, weight, volume, temperature, concentration, pressure and time. Much more can be done with these data, as they have precise relationships. For example, 4 kg is exactly twice as heavy as 2 kg; two 1-kg weights added together weigh 2 kg. Mathematically, it cannot only describe whether readings are equal to or greater than each other, but also allows them to be added, subtracted, multiplied and divided.

# HYPOTHESIS TESTING

Science is based on people coming up with ideas (hypotheses) and then testing them by trying to prove them wrong (called falsification) – only the strong survive. We determine whether a hypothesis is true or false by experiment. First of all, two hypotheses need to be formulated. Then we conduct an experiment which forces us at the end to accept one or the other. It is a close parallel to a legal trial, in which evidence is collected and leads to a decision of either innocence or guilt.

Let us say, for example, that we have a hypothesis that community pharmacists can improve patient adherence by phoning up the patient one week after the patient receives the prescription and giving advice. We call this the alternative hypothesis ($H_1$). We must have a different hypotheses to test it against, and this is called the null hypothesis ($H_0$; null = zero). The null hypothesis is that the new service has no effect on adherence.

Our experiment would consist of taking a representative sample of pharmacies and randomly allocating the service to half of them. We would assess the adherence of patients perhaps two weeks after receiving their prescription. We would then choose an appropriate statistical test to test which of the hypotheses appear to be supported.

Note that technically we are interested in populations, yet we study samples. The uncertainty in statistical tests comes from this fact – if we measured whole populations, we would know if they were different. In the above example we would hypothesize that, if we introduced the new service into all pharmacies in Great Britain, adherence would increase. In real life this would be ridiculously expensive to study, so it is more cost-effective to take representative samples for the intervention and control group. Statistical tests then estimate, from the sample, the range of values that the population may have (it is a range as we cannot precisely predict a population from a sample). If both samples could have come from the same population, we accept $H_0$; otherwise, we accept $H_1$.

Statistical testing leads to a probability value, yet a dismally small proportion of researchers understand what this means. First, the basics – probability is denoted by the letter $p$, for example:

$p = 1$: certainty
$p = 0.5$: a 1 in 2 probability
$p = 0.05$: a 1 in 20 probability
$p = 0.01$: a 1 in 100 probability

When tossing a coin, the chance of it coming down 'heads' could be expressed as $p = 0.5$. A $p$ value is commonly quoted after testing an idea (hypothesis testing).

Many people misinterpret the $p$ value, so it is important to understand what it represents. When a hypothesis test has been applied (usually to determine whether two groups were different in an experiment) and a conclusion reached, the conclusion may be correct, or one of two types of mistakes could be made:

- It is decided that there is a real difference (choose $H_1$), when in reality there is not ($H_0$ is true).
- It is decided that there is no real difference (choose $H_0$), when in reality there is ($H_1$ is true).

The first of these (see Figure 28.1) is called a Type 1 error; the probability of it occurring is denoted by $\alpha$, and it is the probability value ($p$ value) usually quoted in experimental work. The experimenter should set a level for $\alpha$ (such as 0.05) before the study. The second type of error is rarely considered and yet is even more galling for the researcher – it occurs when $H_1$ is in fact true, but the results do not indicate that this is so. This is called a Type 2 error. The probability of it occurring is $\beta$. Although these are called errors it does not mean that we made a mistake in our experiment; it just reflects that our sample may not (by chance) be typical of its population.

A statement that one service is better than another ($p = 0.05$) means there is a 1 in 20 chance that the statement is wrong; in other words, that $H_0$ was true, there has been a Type 1 error and there was no real difference between the two groups. It is good practice when coming across a $p$ value in a research paper of, say, $x$ to say to yourself 'there is a one in y chance that this statement is untrue, where $y = 1/x$'. Considering the large number of published papers that make decisions at the $p < 0.05$

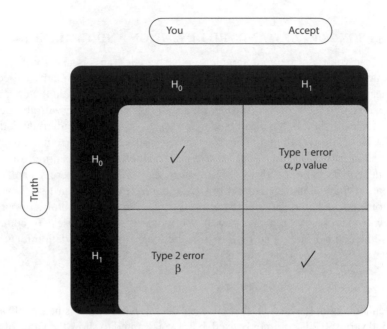

**FIGURE 28.1** Errors in statistical testing. In an experiment, you never know the truth (left side) of whether $H_0$ or $H_1$ is true. All you can do is accept one of these hypotheses (top) from your findings. If what you accept is true (✓), then you have accepted the truth. If you accept a hypothesis that is not true, you have made one of two types of error. The probability of making that error is $\alpha$ (Type 1) or $\beta$ (Type 2). $\alpha$ is the same as the $p$ value (often 0.05), which is taken as critical in statistical testing.

level, it is inevitable that quite a number (somewhere between 1 in 20 and 1 in 100, as $p < 0.01$ is the next level commonly reported) come to false conclusions. Remember that there is always some risk of a Type 1 error and rejecting $H_0$ when it is in fact true. A one in a million chance ($p = 0.000001$) will happen exactly one in a million times, even though you may be amazed that it has happened to you. This also illustrates that one experiment is never enough and can explain apparently contradictory findings in the literature.

How can these errors be reduced? The answer is to increase the sample size. Obviously, as our sample contains a greater proportion of the population we will be more certain of the population's characteristics. However, too large a sample is time consuming, expensive and often unethical. If it is too small, we are unlikely to discover a difference, even if it really exists.

There are several ways of calculating the correct sample size, but all depend on the same four factors:

$\alpha$
$\beta$
Expected difference between groups
Variance

**BOX 28.1   $N$, STANDARD DEVIATION AND VARIANCE**

How can you describe your sample to other people? This is usually done by giving the number ($n$) in your sample, a 'typical' result (technically called a measure of central tendency) and a measure of spread (how wide the data are spread around the typical result). For normally distributed interval/ratio data, the 'typical' result is the mean, and spread is given by the standard deviation (SD). Have you ever thought how you could measure deviation from the mean? The simplest way would be to measure the deviation of each reading from the mean and add them together. Unfortunately, they will add to zero, as half are negative. Statisticians get round this by squaring the deviations, so they all become positive, then adding them together. The size of this total will partly show the spread of the data, but will also increase as $n$ increases. To counter this, the number is divided by $n$ to give the mean squared deviation (or variance). If the square root of this is taken, we get the SD.

To calculate a sample size, you first choose $\alpha$ and $\beta$. Although $\alpha$ is nearly always set at 0.05, $\beta$ varies; 0.2 is commonly used, but if you wanted to show the value of a new pharmacy service, would you be happy that there was a 1 in 5 chance of missing it? A $\beta$ of 0.1 or even 0.05 may be more suitable, although this will markedly increase the sample size. We also need some idea about the expected size of the difference between the groups. If we expect them to be widely different we will need a smaller sample size to demonstrate it. If there is a small difference, a larger sample is needed. Finally, we need some idea of the variance within the sample (variance is a measure of spread – see Box 28.1). If the variance is large, we will need a large sample to reduce the confidence intervals and reveal a difference.

It can be seen that calculating a sample size is not easy. It requires judgement and prior knowledge about the distributions and effect size. The prior knowledge may come from previous research papers or, more often, has to be established by a pilot study.

## SIGNIFICANCE

There is a common and potentially misleading practice when describing results to refer to values of $p < 0.05$ as 'significant' and those of $p < 0.01$ as 'highly significant'. It is important to separate the $p$ value – the objective probability of a Type 1 error – from the subjective decision that the results have significance. To illustrate the difference, suppose I asked you to play a game of squash with me, but told you that there was a 1 in 20 chance ($p = 0.05$) of you being knocked by my racket. Most people consider this probability insignificant. However, if you were a haemophiliac, you would consider the same probability highly significant. The probability is the same, but the significance different.

There are two other consequences of linking significance and $p$ values. The first is that the opposite of 'significant' is 'insignificant', so experimenters who find a

$p$ value of greater than 0.05 tend to think of the experiment as a failure and the results as uninteresting. This is clearly wrong for two reasons. First, it is as important to know that a hypothesis is likely to be untrue as to know that it likely to be true; however, there is a publication bias in the literature that leads to under-reporting of 'negative' findings. To illustrate the problem with an extreme example, if 20 experimenters conducted the same experiment for which $H_0$ was true, by chance we would expect one may get a result of $p < 0.05$; this chance finding may be published and the others' papers may well be rejected or not submitted for publication. This also has implications for meta-analysis – the process by which studies which meet minimum design criteria are pooled and re-analysed to increase sample size and power. The second reason the $p = 0.05$ watershed is inappropriate is that it focuses on one value, so that a result of $p = 0.049$ is treated differently to one of $p = 0.051$, yet the difference is only 2 in 1,000.

The convention of using $p < 0.05$ as a level at which to reject $H_0$ grew from early workers who were trying to balance the high costs of pursuing too many false hypotheses (which would happen if $p$ was set at a higher level, such as 0.3) with the costs of conducting the large experiments needed in order to have a high level of certainty when rejecting $H_0$ and accepting $H_1$. However, there is no statistical reason why $p = 0.05$ was chosen – early authors said it was 'convenient', and it stuck. Probabilities should be interpreted intelligently, according to the study.

Some statisticians think that there is an excessive use of hypothesis testing, as it is beset by the problems discussed above and because the acceptance or rejection of a hypothesis tells us nothing about the size of any difference; instead they prefer the use of confidence intervals, described below.

## CONFIDENCE INTERVALS

A parametric distribution is defined by its mean and standard deviation (SD). From this we can calculate the standard error of the mean (SEM): $SEM = SD/\sqrt{n}$. We know that for a normally distributed sample, 95% of the results are within $\pm 1.96 \times SD$ of the mean. Using SEM, we can go further and extrapolate from the sample to the population. The population mean is 95% certain to be $\pm 1.96 \times SEM$ from the sample mean (i.e. there is a 1 in 20 chance, or $p = 0.05$, that the population mean is not in that range). As we are 95% confident, the mean $\pm 1.96 \times SEM$ is known as the 95% confidence interval (CI). The importance of this is easy to see when you remember that hypothesis testing is based on testing whether or not groups come from the same population. If two groups' 95% CIs overlap, then they could share the same population mean (i.e. come from the same population, supporting $H_0$); if they do not overlap, $H_1$ is supported at a level of certainty equivalent to $p < 0.05$.

To use an example, say two groups are treated with a potential anti-hypertensive or placebo. If the resulting diastolic pressures, shown as mmHg ($\pm 95\%$ CI) were 95(3) and 91(2), we would accept $H_0$ as their CIs overlap (92–98 and 89–93), so both could have come from the same population. Had the figures been 98(3) and 91(2), we would accept $H_1$, as the CIs do not overlap (95–101 and 89–93), so we are 95% certain that they do not come from the same population.

CIs can also be used for other types of data, such as proportions. If we introduced a new ward drug distribution system to reduce medication administration errors and the incidence of errors fell from 6% ± 1% (mean ± 95% CI) to 3% ± 1%, then as the CIs do not overlap, we would accept $H_1$, that there was a significant reduction in error rate.

Many medical journals prefer mean ± CI rather than hypothesis testing alone, because it is thought that it stops readers focusing on statistically significant differences, when a closer look would show the difference between the two groups to be clinically irrelevant. The use of CI ensures both the difference between groups and hypothesis testing are presented together.

## TESTS COMPARING GROUPS

Most pharmacists who ask about statistics are only interested in one thing – which test should they use for their data? This decision is relatively easy for most experiments as it depends on only three things:

- The level of measurement
- The number of groups being tested
- Whether the same subjects undergo each test condition

Once these three things are known, they lead to an appropriate test. All tests are based on assumptions and the data should be checked to see whether they have been met. Sometimes this is difficult to judge, and statisticians may disagree over which test is correct. Note that proportions and percentages should be reduced to the original data or have special tests applied. Incidentally, a common mistake is to start thinking about choice of test once you have the data. Beware: you may find no suitable test. Always choose the test when designing your study.

Of the three factors that determine the choice of test, the level of measurement has been dealt with above. The number of groups being tested is important because tests designed for two groups should only be applied to two groups. If three or more groups are being studied (e.g. A, B and C), it is wrong to compare A with B, B with C and A with C using tests for two groups. If more than two groups are tested, a form of analysis of variance (ANOVA) must be applied. The problem is that multiple testing of pairs of groups leads to 'false positives'. $p$ values are then misleading, as the true probability of a Type 1 error is much higher. The only exception to this is if the Bonferroni correction is applied. Sometimes only one group is tested (e.g. against population data).

The third factor in choosing a test – that 'paired' studies, in which subjects undergo all experimental conditions (e.g. each of two treatments), should be treated differently to 'unpaired' studies, in which a different group undergoes each treatment is unfortunately sometimes ignored. It is to the experimenter's advantage to use the correct tests. Experiments on the same subjects (e.g. in crossover studies) have less variation; so more powerful tests can be applied to them.

Once these three elements can be distinguished, it is easy to use a flow chart (Figure 28.2) to guide you to a suitable test. Other tests may also be suitable, and

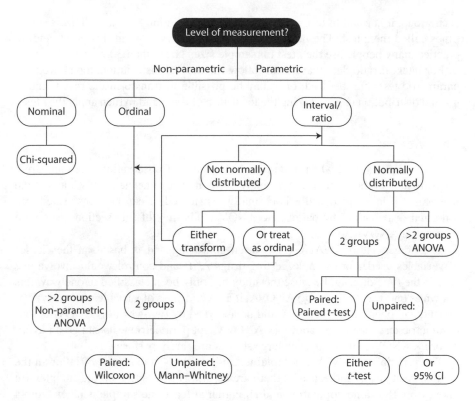

**FIGURE 28.2**   Flow chart for finding a suitable statistical test. Terms are described in the text.

may be alternatives if your data do not meet the assumptions of the test shown. Some more detail about the tests is given below, together with alternative tests.

For all tests of nominal data, the chi squared $(\chi^2)$ test can be used, independent of the number of groups. It can even be used to test against an expected frequency distribution (e.g. that the number of prescribing errors is independent of the day of the week [i.e. do a seventh of all errors appear each day?]). If the data form a $2 \times 2$ table (e.g. two treatments and two outcomes) then the $\chi^2$ test should have Yates' correction applied. If the assumptions are not met for larger tables, it may be necessary to merge categories until they are met. An alternative $2 \times 2$ test, which may be used on small numbers if the conditions for $\chi^2$ are not met, is Fisher's exact test.

Ordinal data from two groups can be compared using the Mann–Whitney test for independent samples and the Wilcoxon test for samples undergoing all conditions. In the Mann–Whitney test the results are pooled and put in rank order; special procedures should be followed if results in a group tie. An alternative to the Wilcoxon test is the sign test. These tests are powerful and easy to calculate.

The $t$ test (its full name is Student's $t$ test) is applied to two groups of small samples ($n < 30$) of data at the interval/ratio level that is normally distributed. If the samples are independent, then the 'unpaired' $t$ test is used; if the samples undergo all conditions, then the 'paired' $t$ test is used. If there are more than about 30 samples in each group, it is usual to test using the normal distribution $z$ statistic. This is sometimes called the $z$ test. The $t$ and $z$ values become very close at this point, and, in practice many people use the $t$ test for sample sizes larger than 30.

For interval/ratio data that do not follow the normal distribution, the above non-parametric tests can be used, or it may be possible to transform the results into a normal distribution (e.g. by taking the logarithm of them and to then apply the $t$ test).

## ANOVA

This technique is used when more than two groups of observations are compared. Measurement at the ordinal level is analysed by non-parametric ANOVA and at the interval/ratio level (provided it is normally distributed or can be transformed into a normal distribution) by parametric ANOVA. The rest of this section deals with parametric ANOVA.

The nomenclature in ANOVA is often confusing and is based on the classes of variables used. For example, testing drugs A, B and control would involve one class – the type of drug. Because the study has only been classified in one way, it is known as one-way (written 1×) ANOVA; if a second class of variable, such as type of patient, had been introduced, it would be analysed by two-way (2×) ANOVA. Non-parametric tests cannot go above 2× ANOVA, but parametric tests can go on to 3×, 4× or $n$× ANOVA, although such large studies are rarely performed.

The principle of ANOVA is explained in its name – it analyses variation in the results. As it is a hypothesis test, there are $H_0$ and $H_1$. $H_0$ is that all the samples are taken from the same population and $H_1$ is that at least one sample is taken from a different population. Taking 1× ANOVA as the simplest case, using the example above, the type of drug would either have no effect ($H_0$) on the patient or would have an effect ($H_1$). First of all, the variation *within* each group is calculated. Then the variation *between* each group is calculated. A measurement called the mean square is used to give the extent of deviation – remember that mean squared deviations were used in calculating variance and SD. If all samples have been taken from the same population, the two mean squares will be similar. This is calculated by the $F$ test.

$$F = \frac{\text{Mean square between groups}}{\text{Mean square within groups}}$$

The greater the value of $F$ (i.e. the variance *between* groups is greater than that *within* groups), the less likely it is that $H_0$ is true. Using tables of $F$ produces a $p$ value to support the alternative hypothesis. If there were only two groups, the $p$ value would be the same as if the $t$ test had been performed. Note that this test does not tell us where any differences lie, merely that all samples were not taken from the same population. Further testing is needed to find out where the differences lie (i.e. which groups are different from the control). Examples are the Scheffé test, the $t$ test with Bonferroni correction, Duncan's multiple range test and the Newman–Keuls method. The chances of finding a real effect are increased if there has been a good experimental design, which specifies a limited number of comparisons, rather than comparing everything with everything else in the hope of a significant result. Note that the results are only valid if the $F$ test has first been shown to be significant – it is incorrect, and may lead to false conclusions, to perform the other tests without a prior $F$ test.

Other assumptions important to ANOVA are that the sample size is the same in each group, as is the SD. If these assumptions are not met, then the data or calculations may have to be manipulated. In practice, equal sample sizes do not seem to be needed for $1\times$ ANOVA, although they should not be too unequal. It is important for $2\times$ ANOVA and above.

## REGRESSION

Regression describes the relationship between two or more sets of data. One of its key features is that it lets us predict one variable when we have the value of the other one. We usually want to make these predictions because we can measure the predictor variable more accurately or more easily than the thing we are trying to predict. Examples could be predicting the concentration of a drug at time $t_o$ from the concentrations at later times, or predicting, from Acute Physiology and Chronic Health Evaluation (APACHE) and other clinical scores, whether a patient on an intensive care unit is likely to live or die.

One of the hardest parts of regression is understanding the terminology:

The $x$-axis is called the predictor or independent variable.
The $y$-axis is called the outcome, response, yield or dependent variable.

The traditional names (independent and dependent) are being used less frequently in modern texts because they are not particularly informative. I shall use 'predictor' and 'outcome'.

We shall first deal with the simplest case – linear regression between two variables. We have measured $X$ and $Y$; in experimental settings, we have chosen the values for $X$ and measured $Y$ at each of them.

After plotting the points for our two variables, we want to fit a straight line. This is called a regression line and is calculated by a method called 'least squares'.

The straight line has the formula:

$$Y = a + bX$$

where $Y$ is the outcome variable and $X$ the predictor variable; $a$ is the intercept on the $y$-axis and $b$ the gradient of the line. What does this tell us?

$$Y = 0.13 + 0.82X$$

means that when $X$ increases by 1, $Y$ increases by 0.82, and that when $X$ is 0, $Y$ will be 0.13.

Although it is helpful to know the equation of the line, we want to know other things as well; for example:

- Does the intercept or slope differ significantly from zero?
- What is the CI of the line?
- What is the CI around $Y$ if I make a prediction for one patient from a value of $X$?

All of these are explained in more advanced statistics texts. There is another valuable calculation that can be made on regression lines, which is $100r^2$ (where $r$ is the correlation coefficient). This figure tells us the percentage of variation in $Y$ that can be explained by $X$. For example, if $r = 1$, $100r^2 = 100\%$; so for a given value of $X$ we could calculate $Y$ precisely. If $r = 0.7$, then $100r^2 = 49\%$, so approximately half of the variability of $Y$ can be accounted for by $X$, and our estimate of $Y$, given $X$, would be more uncertain.

In addition to simple linear regression there is multiple regression, in which there may be many predictor variables explaining the outcome variable. For example, the number of interventions made by hospital pharmacists to alter prescriptions on wards ($Y$) may be predicted by their grade ($X_1$), the type of beds they visit ($X_2$) and the time they spend on the ward ($X_3$). The technique is sometimes used the other way around to find out which of many variables predict an outcome; for example, 10 or 20 possible predictors may be fed into the regression model, and all the significant predictors will emerge, together with an $r^2$ value. This is often used in epidemiological studies: $Y$ may be a clinical condition such as blood cholesterol or having had a heart attack, and the $X$ values could be dietary and lifestyle factors. If the outcome can be only one of two possibilities (e.g. alive or dead), then a special technique called logistic regression is used.

## CONCLUSION

It has never been easier to perform statistical tests, and it has never been easier to misuse them. Statistical tests are there to test hypotheses. They depend on good experimental design and execution, careful exploration of the data, meeting the assumptions behind the test and intelligent interpretation of the findings. They do not reveal the truth, merely quantify uncertainty.

## FURTHER READING

These books are in increasing levels of advancement, and will provide more information on the concepts described here, on the tests themselves and on a variety of other tests.

Altman, D.G. 2011. *Practical Statistics for Medical Research* (2nd Edn.). London: Chapman & Hall/CRC.

Armitage, P., Berry, G. and Matthews J.N.S. 2002. *Statistical Methods in Medical Research* (4th Edn.). Oxford: Blackwell Science.

Bowers, D. 2014. *Medical Statistics from Scratch: An Introduction for Health Professionals* (3rd Edn.). Chichester: Wiley.

# Index